DR TIM PRIEST

Progress in Pain Research and Management
Volume 15

Psychological Mechanisms of Pain and Analgesia

Mission Statement of IASP Press®

The International Association for the Study of Pain (IASP) is a nonprofit, interdisciplinary organization devoted to understanding the mechanisms of pain and improving the care of patients with pain through research, education, and communication. The organization includes scientists and health care professionals dedicated to these goals. The IASP sponsors scientific meetings and publishes newsletters, technical bulletins, the journal *Pain*, and books.

The goal of IASP Press is to provide the IASP membership with timely, high-quality, attractive, low-cost publications relevant to the problem of pain. These publications are also intended to appeal to a wider audience of scientists and clinicians interested in the problem of pain.

We will achieve high-quality publications through careful selection of subjects and authors, well-focused editorial work at several levels of production, and a smooth flow of materials. In addition, we believe that we can restrain costs and prices by employing the administrative resources of the IASP central office and by obtaining grant support for selected publications.

Because we will keep the price of our books low and their value high, they will reach a wider audience than do similar books published by for-profit companies. Furthermore, our access to leaders in the field of pain research and treatment guarantees an outstanding selection of material and excellent editorial oversight.

Progress in Pain Research and Management
Volume 15

Psychological Mechanisms of Pain and Analgesia

Donald D. Price, PhD

*Departments of Oral and Maxillofacial
Surgery and Neuroscience, University of Florida,
Gainesville, Florida, USA*

IASP PRESS® • **SEATTLE**

Library of Congress Cataloging-in-Publication Data

Price, Donald D.
   Psychological mechanisms of pain and analgesia / Donald D. Price.
      p.   cm. — (Progress in pain research and management ; v. 15)
   Includes bibliographical references and index.
    ISBN 0-931092-29-9 (alk. paper)
    1. Pain. 2. Pain—Psychological aspects. I. Title. II. Series.
    [DNLM: 1. Pain—psychology. 2. Pain—physiopathology. 3. Pain—therapy. W1
    PR677BL v.15 1999]
    QP401. P75 1999
    616'.0472'019—dc21

                                                                99-039682

Published by:

IASP Press
International Association for the Study of Pain
909 NE 43rd St., Suite 306
Seattle, WA 98105 USA
Fax: 206-547-1703

Printed in the United States of America

Contents

Foreword

Every so often a book comes along that is truly inspired and unique. This is one of those books. Donald Price comes from a background in electrophysiology. Early in his scientific career he did some of the pioneering work on dorsal horn circuitry. While engaged in this sophisticated work, he expanded his focus to psychophysics and began to combine the tools of psychophysics and neurobiology. At this point, his work took on a more elegant and significant quality. Because of this psychophysical foundation, it was more obvious why certain experiments were done and what they meant. Although not alone in using this combination of techniques, Price realized that a focus on intensity, location, and time course of pain was unnecessarily limiting. He began to explore the dimensions of affect and meaning as well as the sources of variability in the pain experience. He clearly grasped that ignoring these critical factors would lead to incomplete, unsatisfying, and clinically irrelevant work.

In this age of explosive growth of the neurobiology of nociception, this book is a beacon of understanding. The attentive reader will be rewarded with a well-written guide to what is meaningful and significant in pain research. In fact, it is one of the few serious attempts to provide an all-encompassing description of the experience of pain. After all, as Price points out so clearly, pain is a subjective experience. To understand this experience is the task of psychophysics. Price concisely but rigorously reviews psychophysical methods as they have been applied in pain research. In the process, he sets a new standard for thinking about and measuring pain. In a brief but thorough review of anatomical, electrophysiological, and functional imaging data, he provides us with a significance map of the central nervous system from the unified perspective of psychophysics.

Donald Price is one of the most creative scientists in the field of pain research. While many are content with the certainty of a narrow focus, he demands significance and completeness. Instead of turning away from the difficult issues that surround subjective experience, he tackles them head on as valid targets of scientific inquiry. We benefit from his openness to the lessons about consciousness that the study of pain offers.

This book is a must for those interested in clinical research because it provides a breadth and level of understanding of pain measurement that are not available in any other single publication. For the same reason, it will also be helpful to those studying the neurobiology of pain in animals and in human subjects. From the beginner to the expert, anyone with a deep interest in the nature of pain will enjoy and be informed by this book.

HOWARD L. FIELDS, MD, PHD
Editor-in-Chief, IASP Press

Preface

The scientific study of pain has led to notable progress within the last 15 years in the areas of psychology, molecular neurobiology, neuropharmacology, and systems neuroscience. These advances continue to lead to new pharmacological strategies and principles for the treatment of pain. During the same time frame and particularly within the last 10 years, we have gained greater understanding of the psychological mechanisms of pain and pain modulation. We have achieved some degree of standardization and applicability across both clinical and experimental settings in the measurement and assessment of multiple dimensions of the human pain experience, overcoming the perplexing inconsistencies and paradoxes of the 1950s and 1960s. Improved methods of pain measurement and assessment, combined with technological advances such as neural imaging, have led to a scientific era in which questions that were considered unanswerable only 10 years ago are beginning to be addressed. For example, neurobiologists have begun to study placebo analgesia and hypnotic analgesia, and the distinctions between the multiple dimensions of pain experience are becoming increasingly clear from both a psychological and neurophysiological perspective.

Throughout the history of attempts to understand pain mechanisms, different emphases have been given to the multiple dimensions of pain experience. However, since the gate control theory of Melzack and Wall (1965) and its extension by Melzack and Casey (1968), it has become increasingly evident that pain is a multidimensional experience consisting of sensory, cognitive-evaluative, and affective-motivational dimensions. Pain is too complex to be explained purely in terms of neurophysiological, psychophysical, or psychological concepts; different approaches and disciplines are needed to promote more comprehensive understanding of this phenomenon. It is possible to combine and interrelate the advances within each scientific discipline so that discoveries in one field of science, such as psychophysics, can be directly applied to the body of existing knowledge in another field, such as neurophysiology.

Such an interdisciplinary approach has been especially successful in pain research and is leading to rapid advances in understanding the mechanisms of both normal and pathophysiological pain states.

With this interdisciplinary approach in mind, my purpose in writing this book was to synthesize and interpret existing scientific discoveries about the psychological mechanisms of pain and pain modulation. In choosing to revisit topics dealt with to some extent in previous works, notably *Psychological and Neural Mechanisms of Pain* (Price 1988), I have sought to examine them from the perspective of the new scientific knowledge of the past decade. This book is intended to provide explanations of psychological mechanisms that subserve the experience of pain and its modulation by psychological factors. In many instances, these explanations are further extended by consideration of general neurophysiological mechanisms that are associated with psychological mechanisms. Although the book contains discussions of neural mechanisms, their purpose is to amplify, extend, and further clarify psychological explanations of pain rather than to *reduce* psychological explanations to neurobiological or molecular constructs. Thus, the relationships between psychological and physiological concepts presented in this book are associative and not reductionistic. None of the explanations requires dualistic assumptions about two separate metaphysical substrates of pain, one belonging to the body and the other to the mind. Biological mechanisms are required for pain, yet pain is inherently an experience. Analogously, the hydrogen–oxygen bonds of water molecules make liquidity possible, yet liquidity is a physical property of water that is measurable and knowable without any reference to molecular bonds. In the same way, knowledge of psychological mechanisms of pain does not necessarily require knowledge of physiological mechanisms of pain processing. For both liquidity and pain, however, knowledge at the mechanistic level extends our understanding of these phenomena.

Chapter 1 defines pain, describes how pain is constituted in human experience prior to analysis or reflection, and discusses the biological roles of pain in relation to the experience of pain. This conceptual overview of the psychological and biological nature of pain is a starting point for explanations of the psychological mechanisms of pain and provides a basis for questions about the psychophysical attributes of pain and their relationship to the measurement and assessment of pain, which are elaborated in Chapter 2. Using the principles of psychophysics and pain measurement as a foundation, Chapter 3 explains the dimensions and stages of pain and the ways they can be measured in pain patients. Chapter 4 presents part of the neurophysiological basis for the psychophysical attributes of pain and discusses pain mechanisms at the level of primary afferent neurons and neurons of origin of major central somatosensory pathways. Chapter 5 discusses pain mechanisms at the level of the brainstem and cerebral cortex, explains how the central nervous system encodes information associated with pain, and provides neural representations of the different pain dimensions (i.e., sensory versus affective). Chapters 6–8 review the psychological modulation of pain: Chapter 6 deals with general mechanisms of pain inhibition and the general psychological factors that modulate pain, while the next two chapters focus on the specific psychological mechanisms by which placebo treatments (Chapter 7) and hypnotic suggestions (Chapter 8) modulate pain. Neurophysiological modulatory systems that are likely to be associated with these psychological mechanisms also are discussed. Finally, Chapter 9 summarizes the psychological and neurophysiological mechanisms of pain in relationship to the role of pain in culture and in human consciousness. In particular, pain is presented as a model for understanding interrelationships between perception, meaning, and emotions and thus for understanding the fundamental features of human consciousness.

DONALD D. PRICE

Acknowledgments

I am grateful to many colleagues who participated with me in studies described in this book and with whom I have had many discussions concerning the topics presented. They are listed in the references of several chapters. There are some individuals who have greatly influenced my thinking over the years about mechanisms of pain. Patrick Wall and Ronald Melzack gave me a testable theory with which to guide my graduate research on pain physiology and my graduate advisor, Irving Wagman, did his best to facilitate this research. David Mayer taught me how to construct heuristic models and to choose the best questions to guide research. Ronald Dubner and Rick Gracely broadened my thinking about the interface between psychophysics and neurophysiology of pain. Gary Bennett extended my understanding of pathophysiological pain states. Jim Barrell introduced me to phenomenology and to the idea of an experiential approach and method for studying pain. Howard Fields has continued to provoke and inspire me over the years and introduced me to new ways of thinking about pain modulation and placebo analgesia. Joe Barber has had a similar role in maintaining my enthusiasm for the topic of hypnotic analgesia.

I am grateful to members of IASP Press for their cooperation and assistance, particularly Elizabeth Endres who has done a superb job of editing. Finally, I wish to express deep appreciation to my wife Elizabeth for her encouragement and support.

DONALD D. PRICE

Psychological Mechanisms of Pain and Analgesia, Progress in Pain Research and Management, Vol. 15, by Donald D. Price, IASP Press, Seattle, © 1999.

1

The Phenomenon of Pain

A DEFINITION AND CHARACTERIZATION

According to the official definition of the International Association for the Study of Pain (IASP), pain is "an unpleasant sensory and emotional experience associated with actual or potential tissue damage, or described in terms of such damage" (Merskey and Bogduk 1994, p. 210). This definition is unique in that it was the first to recognize that the phenomenon of pain is an experience, yet one that comprises both sensory and affective dimensions (as proposed by Melzack and Casey 1968). Although I have supported the IASP definition in the past (Price 1988), I now think that it is confusing and that it is not experiential enough. The definition postulates an association between an experience of unpleasantness, sensation, and actual or potential tissue damage, but it is not at all clear from whose point of view such an association exists: is it based on the judgment of an outside observer or on the experience of the person in pain? Although this most likely was not the intention of its authors, the definition could be understood to imply that if an observer (e.g., a health care professional) cannot determine an association between the reported experience and actual or potential tissue damage, then the experience is not that of pain. A second and closely related problem with the definition is that an association between unpleasant sensation and tissue injury or even potential for tissue injury may be neither necessary nor sufficient for the experience of pain; it may not even be a common aspect of pain experience. Does someone with a stomachache associate the sensation with tissue damage or even the potential for tissue damage? Does someone who has tactile allodynia for several years associate the burning sensations with actual or potential tissue damage?

Given these ambiguities, I propose a new definition for pain that is more faithful to the actual experience of pain; I support it with a consideration of the phenomenology of pain experience and with the language that persons in pain use to describe their experience. The definition I propose is "a somatic perception containing (1) a bodily sensation with qualities like those reported during tissue-damaging stimulation, (2) an experienced threat associated with this sensation, and (3) a feeling of unpleasantness or other negative emotion based on this experienced threat." Notice that this new definition does not require anyone, including the person in pain, to "objectively" demonstrate actual or potential tissue damage, and it does not require that an association be made between sensation and tissue damage. This is helpful, because such a demonstration is often impossible.

Although the definition eliminates the unnecessary requirement that an observer establish an association between any of these components to tissue damage or potential tissue damage, it does not eliminate the putative relationship between pain and tissue damage. It simply indicates that an association with tissue damage is not a necessary component of pain experience. The definition would almost certainly be more appropriate for chronic pain patients, particularly those with neuropathic pain, because many such patients have long since disregarded the possibility of tissue damage.

However, two explanations are needed to support this new definition, the first for the assertion that pain is based on sensations like those that occur during tissue-damaging stimulation, and the second for the idea that threat and unpleasantness are associated with pain-like sensations. I will provide these explanations by considering the nature of sensory qualities of pain and the kind of meanings and unpleasant emotional feelings associated with these sensory qualities.

SENSORY QUALITIES OF PAIN

When body tissues are intensely stimulated, the resulting experience often includes unique somatosensory sensations that are not simply extensions of other sensory modalities but are like those objectively and subjectively associated with tissue damage. The uniqueness of such sensations can be illustrated by comparing what happens when a fold of skin is squeezed with increasing intensities with what happens when sound becomes increasingly loud. When the former occurs, sensations of touch or pressure are replaced with those described as "sharp," "stinging," or "aching." In contrast, when light becomes increasingly bright, it continues to be recognized as light and as remaining within the same sensory modality. Stimuli to body tissues at intensities that would produce damage either immediately or if they were maintained may be considered nociceptive stimuli (Sherrington 1906; Perl 1980). They often have qualities quite different from those resulting from less intense stimulation or from other types of somatosensory stimulation, such as vibration, cooling, or warmth. Nociceptive stimuli activate specialized types of primary afferent neurons, termed nociceptive afferents. Activation of such afferents, either by natural or artificial means, is usually closely associated with nociceptive sensations. The term "nociceptive sensations" describes qualities like those resulting from stimulation of nociceptive afferents. However, neither nociceptive sensations nor pain are inevitable consequences of such stimulation, and both can arise without such stimulation. Under certain circumstances, nociceptive afferent neurons are activated but central nervous system mechanisms of antinociception prevent pain. Alternatively, under pathophysiological circumstances, impulses in low-threshold mechanoreceptive afferent neurons can evoke burning sensations like those normally caused by impulses in nociceptive afferents and those that occur during tissue-damaging stimulation. It would be appropriate to term these sensations nociceptive because they are like those that normally result from stimulation of nociceptive afferent neurons. It would also be appropriate to term them painful if, in addition, they were unpleasant. Nociceptive stimulation, by definition, produces tissue damage either immediately or if maintained over time. Thus, the new definition of pain and the new term "nociceptive sensation" do not ignore the relationship between pain and tissue damage. They merely eliminate the requirement that the person experiencing or evaluating the pain associate a specific pain with tissue damage or describe it in such terms. In many cases, it is unlikely that the person in pain has any idea whether or not tissue damage has occurred or may ensue.

The sensory qualities of pain are diverse, and we perceive them in two distinct ways. One type of pain experience is to perceive pain as originating from an external source. Touching hot stoves or dry ice and unpleasant encounters with porcupines serve as examples. We say that the stove is hot or that the needle is very sharp, and readily notice that it is the stove or needle that presents the properties of "hotness" or "sharpness." We can confirm this by noticing that it is the exact point of contact between the object and the skin that feels painful, and that the pain lessens as contact ceases and can be repeated by touching the object again. By contrast, other types of pain do not refer us to an external source. They are simply there, inside us, with no reference to anything beyond themselves. Sensations arising from inflammation of deep tissues exemplify such types of pain.

A POTENTIAL LANGUAGE OF NOCICEPTIVE SENSATIONS

Perhaps the greatest contribution of Melzack and Torgerson in their efforts to devise a pain questionnaire has been the development of a language of pain that helps describe the qualities of nociceptive sensations and the sensory, evaluative, and affective qualities of pain. Fig. 1 lists words that patients use to describe sensory qualities and spatiotemporal features of their pain. Many appropriate words can describe the unique sensory aspects

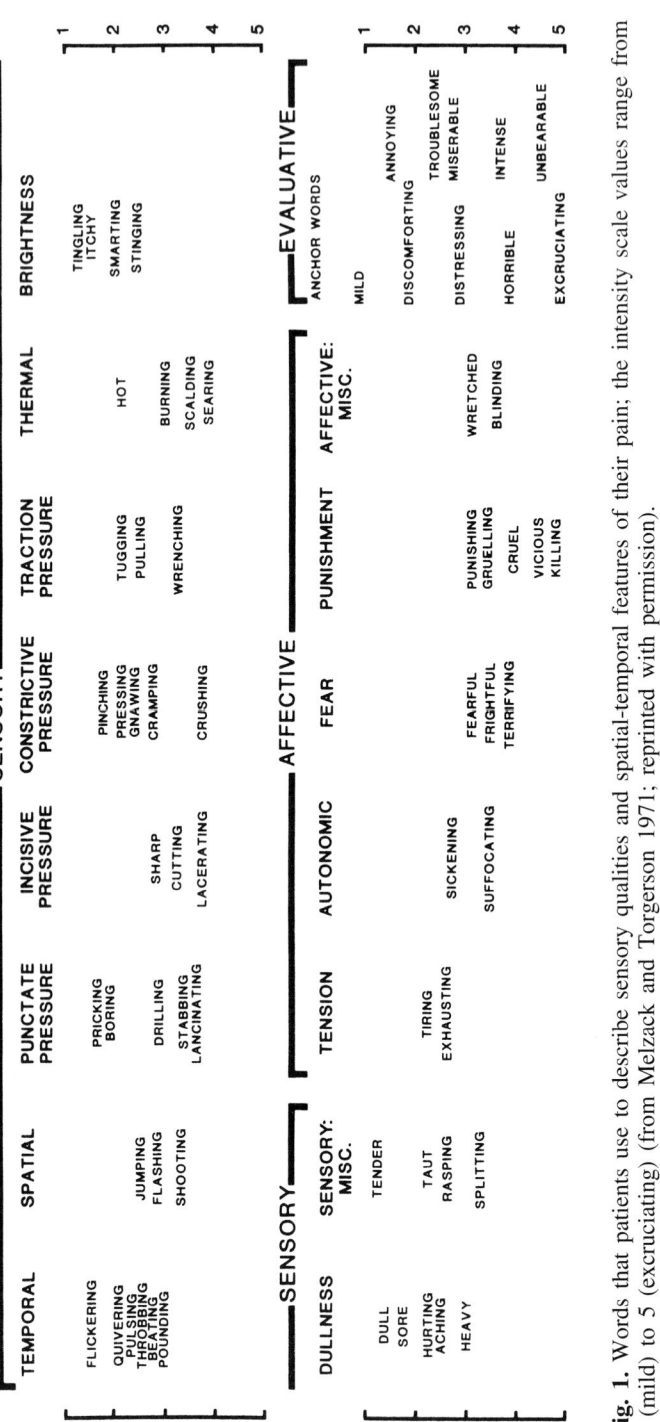

Fig. 1. Words that patients use to describe sensory qualities and spatial-temporal features of their pain; the intensity scale values range from 1 (mild) to 5 (excruciating) (from Melzack and Torgerson 1971; reprinted with permission).

of pain. Melzack and Torgerson (1971) collected such words and assigned them to categories that have formed the basis of the McGill Pain Questionnaire. An impetus was thus given to new approaches for describing and assessing pain. The sensations of pain are unique and have a tremendous variety of sensory-qualitative features. From an experiential perspective, these qualities often convey a sense of intrusion or assault upon the body, since painful sensations by their very nature dispose us to experience them as intrusive. The intrusiveness of pain is conveyed in various ways. Pain can be experienced as *constrictive pressure,* as implied by words such as "pinching," "pressing," "cramping," or "crushing." It can also be experienced as *punctate pressure,* as described by words such as "pricking," "boring," or "stabbing," or as *thermal sensation,* verbalized as "burning," "scalding," or "searing." Many of the words are metaphorical: patients may describe their pain *as if* their skin were being stabbed or burned. The intrusive qualities relate to the experience that the sensation is penetrating or invading the body in a way that could produce harm. This quality can be a sense of penetration (e.g., pricking, boring) and/or spatial spread (e.g., shooting, radiating, burning).

Thus, the sensory qualities of pain can often be dramatically distinguished from other somatic sensations that are perceived as being confined spatially and temporally. For example, a coin placed on the hand is perceived as being on the surface and as having clearly defined boundaries. The onset and removal of this stimulus also can be easily identified. In contrast, pain sensations are more often discerned as penetrating or spreading, and the onset and offset of the pain-evoking stimulus are not always easily identifiable. The sensory qualities that are unique to some types of pain, such as poorly defined boundaries, spatial radiation, and unclear onset and offset, relate to how pain is encoded within the peripheral and central nervous systems. As described in Chapters 4 and 5, these features are consistent with the neural mechanisms that code pain intensity and unpleasantness.

The penetrating qualities of some deep pains relate to the dimension of "phenomenal distality," as described by Bakan (1968). He used this term to describe the psychological distance between the experienced self and the object of consciousness. For example, a visual object is experienced as farther away from ourselves than a touch. On a 10-point scale of phenomenal distality, the visual object would appear close to 10, that is farthest away from us, and the touch of the body around 1, closest to us. Interestingly, pain would be at some negative number, since it appears to be *within* us (although separate from us). All of this suggests that although we have a body that is an extension of us, it is not our "home base," which remains interior to the body. The negative phenomenal distality of some types of deep pains is related to the sense of intrusion, which in turn is related to a perception of threat. These experiential dimensions are physically based meanings that contribute to the immediate unpleasantness of pain, which in turn provokes reflection and suffering.

It is extremely important to recognize that we can experience nociceptive sensations, described in terms of some of the qualities listed above, *without any experience of unpleasantness whatsoever.* This possibility has been verified several times in my own experience as well as that of my colleagues in pain research. We have all administered well-controlled nociceptive heat stimuli to our own skin to check the reliability of our thermal stimulators. Although the resulting sensations are intense and even have burning, throbbing, or stinging qualities, they serve merely to remind us that our thermal stimulators are working properly. The sensations that occur in this context *are not unpleasant.* Nociceptive sensation without unpleasantness has also been verified in hypnotic analgesia studies wherein several participants reported intense heat sensations with no unpleasantness (see Chapter 8). Thus, nociceptive sensation is not equivalent to pain, even though it may be strongly associated with pain and unpleasantness under most conditions.

THE IMMEDIATE UNPLEASANTNESS OF PAIN

Certainly, the sensory qualities associated with pain dispose us to experience them as unpleasant under all but the most unusual of circumstances (e.g., testing one's thermal stimulator). Thus, similar to nausea, intense thirst, or intense hunger, nociceptive sensations are usually closely linked to immediate unpleasantness. However, the immediate unpleasantness of pain often includes an additional component that is part of a more integrated perception. In order to illustrate this component, let us consider two hypothetical examples. Most of us have been stung by a bee. This unpleasant experience is accompanied by abrupt visual, auditory, and somatosensory attention to the bee. The stinging nociceptive sensation is only part of what is threatening. Seeing and hearing the bee at the same time makes the experience more threatening and frightening. The stinging sensation, the arousal, and the feelings of our own autonomic and somatomotor responses all culminate in an experience of sudden intense threat and consequent fear. Memories of past consequences of bee stings can also add to this perception; a bee sting would be even more unpleasant to someone who remembered a previous allergic reaction.

A second example illustrates that immediate unpleasantness can include an integrated perception that involves even more reflective evaluation. Suppose two patients have mild abdominal pain sensations, which both rate as 3 along a 10-point scale of pain sensation intensity. One patient has a history of indigestion and attributes her present abdominal sensation to just having eaten. She rates this experience as 2 along a 10-point scale of pain unpleasantness. The other patient has just been diagnosed as having cancer. He cannot help but consider the possible implications of this mildly intense abdominal sensation. Thoughts of these implications dominate his experience, and the sensation itself serves as a persistent reminder of them. He rates this experience as 8 along a 10-point scale of pain unpleasantness. Thus, both patients have similar intensities of sensation, but the cancer patient is responding to a radically different context than the woman who thinks she has indigestion.

Just as nociceptive sensation can exist without unpleasantness, unpleasantness can result from other types of somatosensory sensations, such as itching or dysesthesia from nerve injury. Thus, nociceptive sensation is neither necessary nor sufficient for unpleasantness. However, when nociceptive sensation and unpleasantness are associated, then the experience is that of pain; in other words, both dimensions are necessary to produce pain. Moreover, the unpleasantness of pain is unique in that it refers to a perceived physical threat to body tissues. Under most conditions, this meaning of threat is closely linked to the qualitative nature of the sensations (e.g., burning, stinging, crushing) and to the physical and social contextual aspects of the situation. It is important to recognize that this may or may not entail an experienced association between physical sensation and potential tissue damage. For example, such an association may not exist at all in the case of an ordinary stomachache, which nevertheless may be perceived as threatening. The definition of pain given earlier is consistent with these relationships between sensation, perceived threat, and unpleasantness.

As with human experience in general, an enormous variety of meanings can be associated with painful sensations and with the context in which they occur. The examples given above serve to illustrate that emotional feelings that contribute to pain experience are derived from meanings based not only on the physical sensations of pain but also on the context in which they occur. Part of the context may be the integration of different sense modalities, as in the case of the bee sting. Another aspect may be psychosocial and can lead to the association of pain sensations with dire or innocuous future consequences as a result of reflective evaluation. In either case, the affective dimension of pain is integrally related to the cognitive-evaluative dimension of pain. Cognitive evaluation is thus an integral component of the affective-motivational dimension of pain.

The experience of pain thus has three common elements that are each necessary and taken together sufficient for the phenomenon of pain: (1) bodily sensation(s) with qualities like those which occur during tissue damage or from stimulation that would cause tissue damage if maintained over time; (2) a meaning of threat to the body or self associated with this type of sensation; (3) unpleasantness and other negative emotional feelings associated with this perceived threat.

Dysesthesia from nerve injury, itching, and sensations from a spider crawling on one's leg may be threatening or unpleasant, but they are not examples of pain because the sensations do not have qualities like those associated with tissue damage. On the other hand, if sensations resulting from stimulation of oral nociceptors by capsaicin are like those that occur during tissue damage but are not unpleasant, then they would not be painful. Such nociceptive but nonpainful sensations might occur when enjoying tacos flavored with capsaicin from chili peppers.[1] The essential change in the new definition of pain outlined above is that the "association with tissue injury" is replaced by the concept that pain sensations have unique qualities that allow them to be identified as pain by those experiencing them. However, it eliminates the requirement that the person in pain or anyone else should make an explicit association between these sensations and tissue injury. Thus, the new definition is more closely aligned with the experience of pain. Moreover, it helps justify using the term "pain" for persons whose pain is *not* objectively or subjectively associated with tissue injury. Nevertheless, the definition retains the idea that painful sensations have at least a putative relationship to tissue injury because the sensations are *like* those that result from tissue injury.

THE EXPERIENCES, BEHAVIORS, AND BIOLOGICAL FUNCTIONS OF PAIN

PHENOMENOLOGY

The definition and characterization of pain given above are intended to be consistent with human experience; readers can judge for themselves

---

[1] To make tacos, grill filet mignon steaks and cut them into slices. Briefly fry corn tortillas using virgin olive oil to a point where they still can be folded. Fill the folded tortillas with steak slices, sharp cheddar cheese, cilantro, guacamole, and hot salsa (which includes capsaicin).

whether that is the case. However, direct reflection on what it is like to experience pain should include different types of pain, such as sudden acute pain and pain that has persisted over time. These two general types of pain have important similarities and differences, and each relates differently to biological roles of pain.

WHAT IS IT LIKE TO EXPERIENCE SUDDEN ACUTE PAIN?

The vast majority of us have experienced sudden acute pain from an injury. Upon reflection, we realize that this experience contains a rapid sequence of perceptions, evaluations, and emotions. Initially, there may be an intense, penetrating sensation accompanied by an alertness and orientation to the affected region. The sensation fills the space of our consciousness and comprises the immediate sense of our bodies to varying degrees. It is within us and will not be ignored. Our attention is commanded and directed toward the sensation and thoughts of concern: "Ouch!" "What has happened to me?" "Am I seriously hurt?" "This is really bad!" The questions contain physically based meanings of sudden intrusion and the possibility for harm. They implicitly relate to a desire for immediate termination of the sensation as well as an uncertainty about the possibility of avoiding harm or intrusion. The felt sense is usually that of fear, and this emotional feeling, like pain itself, is perceived as coming from the body. For example, one may feel one's heart racing or tension in the stomach area. The causes of pain-related fear are immediate and are embedded in the moment of such an experience. The intense sensation, the physically based meanings, and the fear exist nearly simultaneously and yet are causally interactive.

After a short time, thoughts of concern become more elaborate, reflective, and directed toward long-term consequences. Such thoughts also can be in the form of questions: "Have I broken my leg?" "Where can I get help?" "How long will it take to get better?" As with the immediate emotional reaction, the emotional dimension that is directed toward the ultimate consequences of the pain experience also has a felt sense. Anxiety, despair, frustration, or even anger are more likely to accompany this stage of pain. These feelings, like fear, also have referent sensations in the body. Both the immediate and more reflective stages of pain have two explicit or implicit dimensions of experience: a *desire* to avoid harm to some aspect of oneself and a less than certain *expectation* that such harm will be avoided. Pain always involves *some threat to the self,* a threat perceived as directed toward one's body, well-being, sense of psychological stability, or all of these aspects.

THE EMOTIONS OF LONG-TERM PAIN

When pain persists for even longer periods, such as several days, weeks, or months, reflection on both the long-term past and the future becomes even more elaborate. Whereas fear, anxiety, and anger may characterize the earlier phases of pain, despair, frustration, hopelessness, and depression develop during later phases. These differences relate to the likelihood that meanings of having pain for an extended period of time are somewhat different from those during sudden acute pain. A considerable number of meanings can be brought to bear on persistent pain and its context (Buytendyck 1961; Bakan 1968; Price 1988). These meanings are likely to be related to reflections on how the pain interferes with one's life, on how difficult it is to endure it over time, and on its ultimate consequences. These meanings, in turn, relate to desires to avoid or terminate the interference, the burden of enduring pain, and the ultimate negative consequences of having persistent pain, as well as expectations about whether these desires can be fulfilled (Price and Barrell 1980; Price et al. 1985a). High desires accompanied by very low expectations can accompany feelings of frustration or depression, whereas uncertain expectations can attend emotional feelings of anxiety. As will be discussed in Chapter 3, the factors of desire and expectation codetermine the intensity and nature of specific emotions that attend both acute and persistent pain.

THE EXPERIENCE OF PAIN IN RELATIONSHIP
TO BIOLOGICAL ROLES

The ways in which we experience different types of pain relate easily to the two major biological roles of pain, of which the first and most commonly experienced is that of a warning device to prevent or minimize tissue injury. The second is to promote recuperation and healing once tissue injury has occurred. Evidence for each of these roles is derived from different sources, and each role is associated with unique components of the pain experience.

Pain as a warning device

The most precise evidence that pain serves as a warning device comes from quantitative studies of heat-induced injury and pain (Hardy et al. 1952; Beecher 1959; Mountcastle 1974). Thresholds derived for both protective reflexes and pain occur at the same skin temperatures of 44.5°–45°C, regardless of rate of rise of skin temperature. Maintenance of skin temperatures at 45°C and above for extended periods of time (i.e., hours) will produce erythema, blister formation, and, finally, necrosis (Hardy et al. 1952).

Higher temperatures will produce the same responses at briefer durations. However, nociceptive responses generally occur *before* these changes take place. Moreover, as discussed in Chapter 2, there is an exquisitely precise relationship between intensity of pain and temperatures above 44°C, which, *if maintained,* will produce tissue damage."

Hardy et al. (1952) provided a simple and compelling case that pain and nociceptive responses, in general, are related to the rate rather than the amount of tissue damage or protein inactivation. Even though thermally induced pain and tissue damage have the same threshold temperature of approximately 45°C, these functions behave quite differently at temperatures above threshold. Pain intensity from heat stimulation increases as a direct function of skin temperature, but does not increase substantially with the duration that the skin is maintained at an elevated temperature. Thus, a second- or third-degree burn can be produced in response to a skin temperature of 45°C maintained for 5–6 hours. Conversely, a 49°C skin temperature can produce much more intense pain without perceptible tissue damage if the stimulus duration is only a few seconds. As shown in Fig. 2, the *rate* of tissue damage is a direct function of protein inactivation that, in turn, is a function of temperature. However, the *amount* of tissue damage is a function of both skin temperature and duration of stimulation (Hardy et al. 1952; Mountcastle 1974). Since heat-induced pain depends only on the temperature attained by cells of the skin and not on duration of stimulation, pain intensity follows the rate of tissue damage and not its total amount. One consequence of this phenomenon is that some extensive wounds may be less painful than slight wounds. Pain from tissues that have suddenly become inflamed, such as a toothache, is an example.

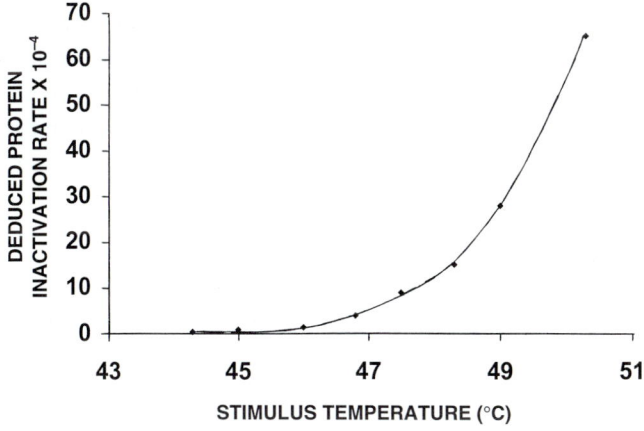

Fig. 2. The relationship between skin temperature and protein inactivation rate deduced by Hardy et al. (1952).

That some types of pain depend on the rate of tissue damage and on receptors that respond *before* actual injury takes place is strong evidence that both pain and nociceptive mechanisms serve the function of warning about potential injury. This function is not likely to be exclusively related to heat-induced pain because several types of nociceptors, including those responsive to mechanical and cold nociceptive stimuli, appear to have similar relationships to rate of tissue injury and have thresholds below those that would produce immediate injury.

The function of pain as a warning device also is supported by an abundance of common experience. Nearly all of us have touched an intensely hot object, only to pull our hand away and say "ouch." This rapid withdrawal is often accompanied by sudden pain. There is little doubt that far greater injury would occur in the absence of such responses.

Pain as a recuperative healing mechanism

When injury occurs in tissue, a sequence of changes occurs in nociceptive terminals and in our experience and behavior. Following injury, nociceptive afferent terminals undergo changes such as sensitization and, over time, peripheral and central sprouting (Wall 1979). These changes accompany the well-known inflammatory response and periods of primary and secondary hyperalgesia. Wall (1979) proposed that peripheral and central physiological changes accompany and support persistent pain states. He specified a sequence of behavioral changes that accompany the biological events that occur in relationship to injury and subsequent recuperation and healing. He proposed that three phases of behavior follow tissue injury in animals, including humans. The *immediate* phase is the period of time in which nociceptive afferent neurons are first activated. This is normally (but not inevitably) accompanied by pain-related behavior, autonomic responses related to fight or flight, and emotions of fear or anger. As described in Chapters 4 and 5, unique neurophysiological mechanisms are activated during this phase of pain behavior.

Pain behavior may be inhibited or suppressed in this immediate phase, particularly if other activities such as fighting, escaping, or obtaining safety take precedence. The extent to which pain experience is also inhibited under these conditions is not known with any clear degree of certainty, and it is very possible that under certain circumstances pain behavior may be suppressed while pain experience is not. The early studies of Beecher (1959) indicate that 40–50% of very different types of sudden injuries are not accompanied by pain behavior. Most of the time, however, sudden injury is accompanied by sudden pain.

Once the subject escapes the immediate danger of the situation, the immediate phase is replaced by the *acute* phase, in which behavior associated with recovery begins. During this phase, pain prompts the subject to cope with the perceived cause of injury, seek treatment, and prepare for recovery. This phase is likely to be accompanied by anxiety and behaviors indicative of distress, such as calls for help. These behaviors are directed toward seeking safety from the original threat and ameliorating the possible damage.

Finally, the *chronic* phase of pain consists of quiet inactivity and behavior related to rest, recuperation, and healing. This phase of relative immobility can be observed in many species of animals, including humans, days after injury. Extended periods of inactivity are accompanied by disturbances of eating, sleeping, grooming, and social interactions. Individuals may appear depressed during this phase. Wall claims that this phase may persist far beyond the necessary period for recovery and thereby may constitute part of the basis of chronic pain syndrome in humans. He further suggests that the chronic phase is analogous to a need state such as thirst or hunger. Just as hunger is associated with the search for food, Wall contends that pain can be associated with the search for treatment or optimal conditions for recovery. As in earlier phases of pain, neurophysiological mechanisms support the chronic phase of pain (see Chapters 4 and 5).

The concepts that pain has a warning function and a recuperative healing role are not at all mutually exclusive, but rather reflect different phases of protecting organisms from harm to body tissues. Persons born without the ability to feel pain provide dramatic testimony that pain serves both as a warning function and as a mechanism for protecting and healing injured tissue (Melzack and Wall 1983; Fields 1987). Such persons may sustain extensive bruises, burns, and lacerations during childhood and learn only with considerable difficulty to avoid inflicting severe wounds on themselves. The subtle but crucial role of pain as a warning device is further illustrated by the fact that persons with congenital insensitivity to pain often develop severe orthopedic problems. This results from failure to shift their weight when standing for long periods, to turn over during sleep, or to avoid postures that normally prevent inflammation of joints and soft tissues. Mild perceptions of pain normally serve to prevent excessive stress on joints or soft tissues, and thereby protect them from impending injury. Pain-insensitive individuals also provide evidence for the role of pain as a mechanism for recuperation and recovery because they often make little or no effort to protect injuries (Melzack and Wall 1983). As a consequence, healing does not take place and further complications develop, sometimes leading to death. For example, unprotected injured joints provide a source of dead or dying tissue in which bacteria and infection develop. Infection, accompanied by inflammation but not pain, can ultimately lead to death.

SUMMARY

The phenomenon of pain is clearly a sensory-emotional experience that is strongly linked to somatic sensations with somewhat unique qualities. The sensory qualities of pain are as diverse as the emotional feelings that are also an integral dimension of pain. The chapters that follow will explain how the dimensions and temporal stages of pain interact and how they can be modulated by psychological factors. Neurophysiological mechanisms of the various dimensions of pain will extend these explanations.

Psychological Mechanisms of Pain and Analgesia, Progress in Pain Research and Management, Vol. 15, by Donald D. Price, IASP Press, Seattle, © 1999.

2

Psychophysical Attributes of Pain and Their Relationship to Pain Measurement

Modern methods for measurement of pain have historical roots in psychophysics, the branch of psychology concerned with the relationships of physical stimulus properties to sensory experiences of humans and to behavioral responses of other animal species. Psychophysical studies are critically important for understanding both the psychological and neurophysiological mechanisms that underlie pain. Studies comparing psychophysical and neurophysiological data have characterized neurons and neural pathways that subserve pain by using quantitatively controlled stimuli in paradigms of threshold, discrimination, direct scaling, and detection (Price 1988; Price and Harkins 1992a; Gracely 1997). The psychophysics of pain also has led to critical improvements in pain measurement, particularly methods for measuring the different psychological dimensions of pain experience. Applications of psychophysics have great relevance for the treatment and management of acute and chronic pain. Psychophysical methods have provided crucial information about neural mechanisms of pain reduction and the relative efficacy of various pain-reducing treatments (Chapman et al. 1985; Price et al. 1985b, 1986b; Gracely 1997). This approach has raised the possibility of standardized, quantitative comparisons of different treatments for various types of clinical pain (Price and Harkins 1992a; Gracely 1997). In short, the psychophysics of pain has a pivotal role in understanding the neurophysiology of pain and for providing a scientific basis for modern methods of pain measurement and assessment.

This chapter has two interrelated objectives. The first is to briefly review modern approaches in pain measurement and to explain how psychophysical methods can be applied to assessment of both clinical and laboratory pain. The second objective is to review what is known about the basic psychophysical attributes of pain, including the neural, behavioral, and perceptual consequences of manipulating stimulus intensity, site, duration, and other spatial and temporal parameters. This review provides a framework for explaining how psychophysical studies of pain help us understand the psychological mechanisms of pain.

APPLICATION OF PSYCHOPHYSICAL METHODS
TO THE MEASUREMENT OF PAIN

Measurement of pain, like the optometrist's measurement of visual acuity, is directly dependent on the person who experiences the pain. Persons in pain are asked to match the perceived intensity of their pain to a scale. This can be done in various ways. For example, patients could match numbers or words to pain intensity, match an intensity of experimental pain to that of clinical pain, or use more than one of these procedures. In all such methods, the critical observer is the person in pain. The investigator or clinician also has a crucial role in providing the scaling procedures, recording the reported values, and using a measurement method known to be reliable and valid.

Persons in pain can be asked to notice and scale different dimensions of their experience. For example, they can observe and judge the relative intensity of the painful sensation, the degree of its immediate unpleasantness, and its spatial distribution and qualities. These separate judgments are by no means exclusive to pain and have a long history in the psychophysics of vision, audition, taste, smell, and somatosensory modalities. We can make separate and exquisitely precise judgments of intensity, pitch, timbre, volume, and density of the same sound stimuli as well as their pleasantness or unpleasantness.

All methods of pain assessment share the common goal of accurately representing the human pain experience. Pain threshold paradigms attempt to identify that point on a continuum of increasing stimulus intensity that distinguishes painful from nonpainful experience. Threshold and detection paradigms are useful in quickly ascertaining changes in pain sensitivity and are fairly reliable and generalizable measures (Chapman et al. 1985; Price 1988; Gracely 1994). Threshold measures of pain sensitivity are limited in that they do not assess changes in pain sensitivity that may occur over a wide range of nociceptive stimulus intensities. Partly due to these limitations, direct scaling methods were developed for pain measurement in both patients and normal volunteer subjects using two basic approaches (Guilford 1954; Gracely et al. 1978; Gracely 1994). In the first method, individuals rate pain intensity on scales with clearly defined numerical limits and intervals or on verbal rating scales whose words directly indicate a rank order. In the second method, direct ratings are made on continuous scales of sensation intensity or unpleasantness, without constraints of categories or whole numbers. Several investigators have used continuous scaling techniques to characterize psychophysical attributes of both normal and pathophysiological pain. This method involves direct scaling of both clinical and experimental pain; sometimes both types of pain are scaled within the same context.

CRITERIA FOR PAIN MEASUREMENT

Assessments of human pain have evolved from extensive reliance on threshold and tolerance measures to the use of a wide variety of psychological and physiological methods that recognize the multiple dimensions of pain experience and pain behavior. Despite their diversity of approach, all methods share a common goal of accurately representing the human pain experience, and there is general agreement on the principal requirements for an ideal pain measurement procedure. The following criteria include those originally suggested by Gracely and Dubner (1981) and others added by Price and Harkins (1992a). The ideal method would:

1) Have ratio scale properties.
2) Be relatively free of biases inherent in different psychophysical methods.
3) Provide immediate information about the accuracy and reliability of the subjects' performance of the scaling responses.
4) Be useful for both experimental and clinical pain and allow for reliable comparison between both types of pain.
5) Be reliable and generalizable.
6) Be sensitive to changes in pain intensity.
7) Be simple to use for pain patients and non-pain patients in both clinical and research settings.
8) Separately assess the sensory-intensive and affective dimensions of pain.

The goal of recent methods of human pain measurement has been to fulfill all or most of these criteria. Several general approaches to pain measurement are briefly described below in terms of their historical role in pain measurement as well as their capacity to fulfill the above criteria. Direct scaling methods are emphasized because they are likely to have the most direct and practical value in research and clinical pain assessment.

Attempts to quantify pain in volunteer participants or pain patients typically follow one or more of the following basic approaches (Chapman et al. 1985):

- Defining a threshold for pain and measuring changes in threshold.
- Defining tolerance for pain and measuring changes in tolerance.
- Assessing performance in laboratory tasks, usually to obtain measures of discrimination or detection.
- Rating pain intensity on numerical scales with clearly defined limits or verbal scales that indicate a rank order.
- Using magnitude scaling procedures to judge sensation intensity or unpleasantness by means of number assignment or cross-modality

matching techniques such as line production (drawing lines to represent perceived intensity) or handgrip force.

METHODS OF PAIN MEASUREMENT

PAIN THRESHOLD MEASUREMENTS

Guilford (1954) defined two general procedures for obtaining pain threshold. In the *method of limits,* stimulus intensity is gradually increased until the subject perceives the stimulus as painful, and is then gradually decreased to a point where it is no longer painful. The intensity midway between these two limits is considered the threshold. Multiple trials can improve the accuracy of this procedure. In the *method of constant stimuli,* stimulus intensity is increased in steps until the subject perceives one-half the stimuli as painful. Regardless of which procedure is employed, subjects are required to identify a point on the stimulus continuum that distinguishes painful from nonpainful experience.

Pain threshold measures are commonly used to infer a person's sensitivity to pain and changes in their sensitivity. Such measures can be useful in combination with other measures of pain, but they cannot provide direct information about pain intensity or ratios of pain intensity (criterion 1). Pain threshold can be strongly influenced by attentional, motivational, emotional, and sensory factors (e.g., touch) that are unrelated to pain. Threshold also can vary according to whether it is defined in sensory or affective terms (related to criterion 2). Pain threshold measurements require a stimulus continuum that is controllable by the tester, so they are more applicable to experimental pain than to clinical pain measurements. Nevertheless, clinical pain thresholds can sometimes be very important, as in the assessment of tender muscle points. Given adequate instructions, such thresholds can be reliable, generalizable across groups of people (criterion 5), and simple to obtain (criterion 7). However, under some experimental conditions, they are relatively insensitive to effects of clinically proven drugs (criterion 6), for reasons related to physiological mechanisms (Price 1996a). Stimuli used to test pain thresholds in humans and other animals are typically brief and have a rapid rate of increase in intensity. Rapid brief nociceptive stimuli produce neural responses mediated by peripheral Aδ nociceptive afferents. These responses are less sensitive to opioid analgesics than are slowly rising or sustained nociceptive stimuli that evoke tonic impulse discharge in C nociceptive afferents. Clearly, the latter are more likely to be relevant to most forms of persistent clinical pain states. Finally, depending on instructions that define the perceptual endpoint, pain thresholds can be obtained separately for sensory (e.g., pricking pain threshold) or affective (e.g., unpleasantness) dimensions of pain (criterion 8) (Blitz and Dinnerstein 1968; Price 1988).

ORDINAL RATING SCALE METHODS

Ordinal rating scales are relatively simple and are often used in clinical studies and even in many experimental studies of pain. Numbers on ordinal scales refer only to rank ordering and cannot be used to reflect ratios of magnitude (criterion 1). For example, if a person rates his or her pain as 4 but later changes the rating to 2, we can conclude that the pain has reduced in intensity but not that it has reduced by 50%. One type of ordinal rating scale has categories that clearly denote rank ordering; an example is the verbal scale designed by Melzack and Torgerson (1971) with five categories: mild, discomforting, distressing, horrible, and excruciating (see Fig. 2 of Chapter 1). Other ordinal scales are simple numerical scales (e.g., 1–5 or 1–10) that are anchored by descriptors of extremes, such as no pain and severe pain.

One major advantage of ordinal rating scales is that they can quickly determine whether pain intensity has changed (criterion 6), hence their relative simplicity (criterion 7). Clinicians commonly use ordinal scales to assess pain and the effects of treatment. Both health care professionals and patients can easily understand and respond to a 1–5-point scale, where 5 denotes severe pain. Ordinal scales can quickly assess both experimental and clinical pain (criterion 4), and they are reliable and generalizable (criterion 5). Similar to visual analogue scales, they can be adapted to assess both sensory-intensive and affective dimensions of pain (criterion 8) (Price et al. 1994b).

Unfortunately, ordinal scales have methodological problems and are widely misused and misinterpreted by both clinicians and researchers. One problem is that when pain intensity is classified into categories of scales, the category boundaries are not known; equal numerical intervals between the categories are often assumed without supportive evidence. For example, assigning numbers 1–5 to the categories devised by Melzack and Torgerson would not necessarily provide information about ratios or proportions of pain intensity. The numbers would only show rank order, and any data collected through the use of such scales should be analyzed with nonparametric statistics. This requirement is especially essential in view of Heft and Parker's (1984) demonstration that category boundaries of pain category scales are not equally spaced.

However, not all pain VAS are bias free or represent ratio scales. Comparisons of different types of VAS have shown that their sensitivity and reliability are influenced by the words used to anchor the endpoints, the length of the scale, and other factors (Scott and Huskisson 1976; Seymour et al. 1985). Scales that most clearly delineate extremes (e.g., "the worst pain," "the most intense pain sensation imaginable") and have sufficient length (≥10 cm) have the greatest sensitivity and are the least vulnerable to distortions. In contrast, a VAS anchored on the right with a weak superlative such as "intense pain" is likely to generate pain ratings that are concentrated toward the right end of the scale rather than being normally distributed.

EFFICACY OF PAIN MEASUREMENT TECHNIQUES

Reliability and generalizability (criterion 5)

When graded contact heat stimuli of varying intensity were randomly applied to the forearm, the stimulus-response functions obtained from VAS ratings and verbal descriptor scaling were power functions with exponents greater than 2.0, as shown in Fig. 2 (Price and Harkins 1987). These functions were very similar across different groups comprising pain-free participants and patients with low back pain or myofascial pain dysfunction. The same stimulus-response curve was generated within each group across different times, thereby demonstrating the reliability of the rating method for groups of participants. The test–retest reliability of the VAS was very high ($r = 0.9$) for participants in a study of pain evoked by electric shock (Kiernan 1995). Electrical stimulation is optimal for checking the reliability of a pain scale because it produces a highly reliable stimulus. The test–retest reliabilities of various types of VAS were also high ($r = 0.7$–0.9) for clinical pain patients tested over weeks without an intervening treatment (Wade et al. 1990). Taken together, these remarkably similar power functions and high test–retest reliabilities fulfill criterion 5 (reliability and generalizability).

Internally consistent measures of experimental pain and clinical pain sensation intensity (criteria 3 and 4)

Patients use verbal descriptor scales (Heft et al. 1980) and VAS very consistently to rate quite different types of pain, including low back myofascial pain, jaw muscle pain, and even experimental pain (Price et al. 1983, 1994a; Price and Harkins 1987). A specific psychophysical procedure was developed to determine whether patients use verbal descriptor scales or VAS as a common psychological scale to rate clinical and experimental pain (Heft et al. 1980; Gracely and Dubner 1981; Price et al. 1983, 1996). Known as the triangulation procedure, it tests the internal consistency of three response tasks, as shown in Fig. 3. First, patients make verbal descriptor or VAS ratings of various intensities of painful experimental stimuli, for which a regression line is plotted. Second, patients directly match experimental pain stimulus intensity to that of their clinical pain. Third and finally, they make direct verbal descriptor or VAS ratings of their clinical pain. If these three tasks are performed in an internally consistent manner, the direct stimulus match to clinical pain on the *x*-axis and the direct rating of clinical pain on the *y*-axis should intersect very close to the regression line of the stimulus intensity-response function. Thus, the triangulation procedure has shown

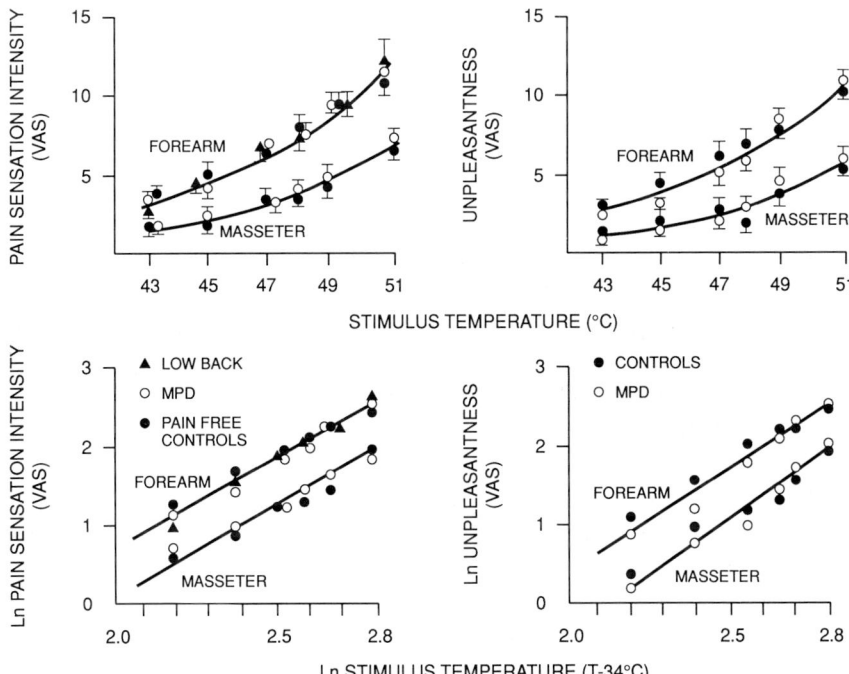

Fig. 2. VAS measurements of the relationship between temperature of the skin and the judgment of pain sensation intensity and its unpleasantness. The data were obtained from patients with low back pain and myofascial pain dysfunction (MPD) and pain-free control subjects, and are plotted in linear coordinates in the upper pair of graphs and in double-logarithmic coordinates in the lower pair. Data points represent the group average for a given temperature, and vertical lines represent standard errors of the mean (these conventions are followed in subsequent figures). Despite the substantial difference between the ratings of the intensity of the facial (area over the masseter muscle) and forearm stimuli on the pair of graphs to the left, the exponents (slopes) of the functions were identical (2.1). A similar result was obtained for ratings of unpleasantness (right), with the slopes equal to 2.4 and 2.7, respectively. Adapted from Price and Harkins (1987), with permission.

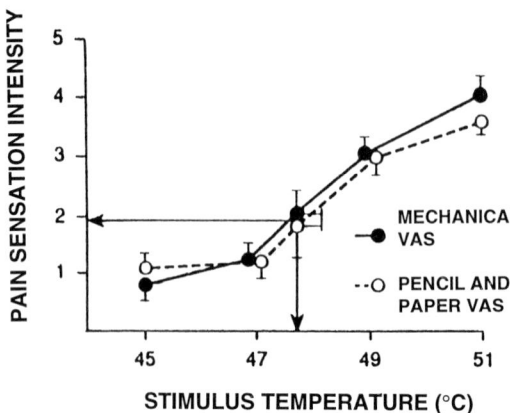

Fig. 3. Results of the triangulation procedure in 10 chronic pain patients. The intersection (i.e., the "match point") of the mean temperature match (vertical arrow) and mean VAS rating of clinical pain (horizontal arrow) occurs on the temperature stimulus–pain VAS rating curve. The consistency of these three responses demonstrates that the VAS is an internally consistent measure of clinical and experimental pain. Reprinted from Price et al. (1994c), with permission.

that the VAS can compare intensities of very different types of pain, including experimental pain.

If patients with different types of pain use a particular rating scale in an internally consistent manner to rate clinical and experimental pain, and if pain patients and pain-free groups have the same nociceptive stimulus–pain intensity curve, the curve can serve as a reference standard. Pain intensities of very different types of clinical and experimental pain could then be compared on a common scale that approaches a ratio scale level of measurement. A common scale and standard of pain intensity would permit quantitative comparison of different types of pain and of various palliative treatments, both within and across studies. Such comparisons are often hampered because different investigators use radically different and usually quite simplistic pain measurement methods such as category scales or other simple ordinal scales.

Sensitivity to pain-reducing treatments (criterion 6)

Direct rating can be a sensitive way to measure the relative efficacies of different pain treatments if the scale provides for a broad range of possible pain intensities and is not constrained by a small number of possible responses. Some verbal descriptor scales and continuous scales such as VAS fulfill this criterion. However, the empirical demonstration of the sensitivity of VAS to pain-reducing treatments comes from studies that tested low to moderate doses of opioid analgesics. In one study, low doses (0.06–0.08 mg/kg) of intravenous morphine produced statistically reliable reductions in VAS ratings of 45°–51°C temperature stimuli (Price et al. 1985b). In a second, similarly designed study in patients with chronic low back pain, low (0.8 µg/kg) to moderate (1.1 µg/kg) doses of fentanyl produced significant reductions in both experimental and clinical pain (Price et al. 1986b). The sensory intensities of clinical pain and experimental pain were reduced by an internally consistent amount. Experimental demonstrations of opioid analgesia have now moved well beyond the mere establishment of analgesic effects and have shown dose-response relationships, effects of infusion rates, effects of real or simulated potentiation, influence of central mechanisms, and the relationship between subjective report and neurophysiological indices (see Gracely 1994 for an excellent review). Experimental models of pain-reducing treatments offer considerable promise for screening new analgesic drugs and procedures.

Separate and independent measurement of sensory-intensive and affective dimensions of pain (criterion 8)

Pain scales can be adapted to separately measure pain sensation intensity and unpleasantness or emotional disturbance related to pain (Price 1988; Gracely 1994). When subjects are properly instructed and when the two scales have verbal descriptors or verbal anchors that clearly distinguish these pain dimensions, reliably different nociceptive stimulus-response functions are obtained for sensation intensity and unpleasantness (Fig. 2). Sensory and affective VAS ratings of 43°–51°C skin temperature stimuli are both positively accelerating power functions with exponents of about 3.0–3.5 for sensation intensity and 4.0–5.0 for unpleasantness. The two types of scale differ only in the verbal anchor points, for example, "the most intense pain sensation imaginable" and "the most unpleasant imaginable" for sensory and affective dimensions, respectively. The generally higher and more variable exponent for pain affect as compared with sensation indicates two measurably separate dimensions of experimental pain. Importantly, both unpleasantness and sensation dimensions have precise psychophysical relationships to stimulus intensity, and both are highly sensitive to small changes in stimulus intensity. These facts suggest that central nervous system neurons and pathways involved in pain affect have nociceptive stimulus-response functions that are as precise and discriminative as those obtained for pain sensation.

PSYCHOPHYSICAL ATTRIBUTES OF NORMAL PAIN

Valid direct rating scales of different dimensions of pain, methods for reliable determination of pain threshold, and paradigms for determination of detection of differences in stimulus intensity have led to a considerable literature on the fundamental psychophysical attributes of pain. One of the first systematic efforts to characterize the psychophysical attributes of pain and develop a quantifiable model of pain measurement was made by Hardy and colleagues (1940, 1952). Since then, there has been a gradual development of psychophysical methods for quantifying pain. Advances have accelerated within the past 20 years, partly because of increased interest in the fundamental neural mechanisms underlying pain, and partly because of methodological and conceptual progress in the use of quantifiable and controllable noxious stimuli in studies of experimental pain. A major step in quantifying the relationships between noxious stimuli and behavioral responses has been to move away from global measures indirectly related to the affective dimension of pain (such as pain tolerance), and toward direct magnitude scaling responses of suprathreshold components of pain. Furthermore, multiple scales have been developed for the sensory-discriminative and affective-motivational dimensions of pain. These advances have led to experimental paradigms that directly relate quantifiable suprathreshold stimuli to neural responses and quantifiable human judgments of different aspects of the pain experience.

The psychophysical attributes of pain have been characterized using several measurement methods, including thresholds for pain, adaptation, relationships between nociceptive stimulus intensity and pain intensity, discriminability, and temporal and spatial characteristics of suprathreshold pain.

HEAT-INDUCED THRESHOLDS FOR PAIN AND WITHDRAWAL REFLEXES

Hardy and colleagues (1940, 1952) were the first investigators to quantify stimulus parameters for pain and discover some of its psychophysical attributes. Using controlled radiant heat stimuli, they determined that the minimal skin temperature at which pain is perceived ranges from 42.7° to 45.7°C, with an average of 44.5°C. This threshold is remarkably similar to that for withdrawal reflexes (Hardy et al. 1952). Radiant heat pain thresholds are extremely reliable for any given body area but vary somewhat among different areas. For example, the thresholds are lowest for the thigh and lower back, averaging 42.6°C and 42.2°C, and highest for the finger pads and heel, averaging 47.1°C and 53.7°C, respectively.

Several types of withdrawal reflexes and escape behaviors are initiated in various mammalian species at a skin temperature close to 45°C, the pain threshold determined in man by Hardy et al. (1952). Furthermore, magnitudes of nonverbal pain-related behaviors and pain intensity increase monotonically as temperature is progressively raised above 45°C. Neural substrates for the various components of pain and pain-related behaviors may thus be common to all mammals. This assumption forms the basis for animal tests designed to evaluate the efficacy of analgesic drugs (Mountcastle 1974). Previous difficulties in demonstrating the effects of clinically accepted analgesic drugs on experimental pain in humans could have resulted from the inadequacy of using only threshold measures of pricking pain (Beecher 1956, 1959), which yield only one response measure per subject. Pain thresholds vary extensively among subjects, so large samples would be needed. Furthermore, models that rely on threshold stimuli do not evaluate how pain is perceived over a wide range of intensities. These considerations have led to the use of direct scaling of suprathreshold pain produced by multiple stimulus intensities.

ADAPTATION TO MAINTAINED STIMULATION

Adaptation, the diminution of perceived sensation with constant stimulus intensity, is believed to be a characteristic of all sensory systems. However, pain produced by a maintained nociceptive stimulus normally persists for as long as one attends to it. Adaptation may thus play a minimal role in pain, although experimental pain researchers may not fully appreciate this possibility, partly because tissue damage results from maintaining a noxious stimulus on the same area of skin.

Greene and Hardy (1958) were the first to test the hypothesis that pain perception has minimal adaptation to long-term stimulation. Five trained observers were asked to manipulate an unseen dial to maintain a radiant heat stimulus that would just continue to evoke the sensation of pricking pain. Rather than increasing the stimulus intensity, as would be predicted if adaptation were taking place, the subjects gradually lowered the intensity required to maintain the pricking pain. Over 13 minutes, the average threshold temperature decreased from about 45° to 44°C. These results indicate that adaptation is not a salient characteristic of heat-induced pain, and that neural mechanisms (i.e., those subserving hyperalgesia) decrease pain threshold during prolonged nociceptive stimulation. However, given the problems inherent in using only threshold measures for studies of pain, experiments of this kind should be repeated using suprathreshold temperatures. However, the risk of tissue damage would pose a problem for such studies.

A more recent study examined the adaptation of suprathreshold pain intensity to prolonged repetitive noxious heat stimulation. Repeated immersion of a finger in a water bath at a constant temperature between 45° and 49°C showed slight adaptation within the first 2 minutes, but no appreciable adaptation during the following 18 minutes (Coghill et al. 1993a). Pain intensity and unpleasantness ratings were both at their maximum values during the first 2 minutes and then declined to a level that was maintained for the remainder of the 20 minutes (Fig. 4). This profile of peak response followed by maintained response may relate to the different experiential and behavioral phases of pain response (discussed in Chapter 1). Thus, an imme-

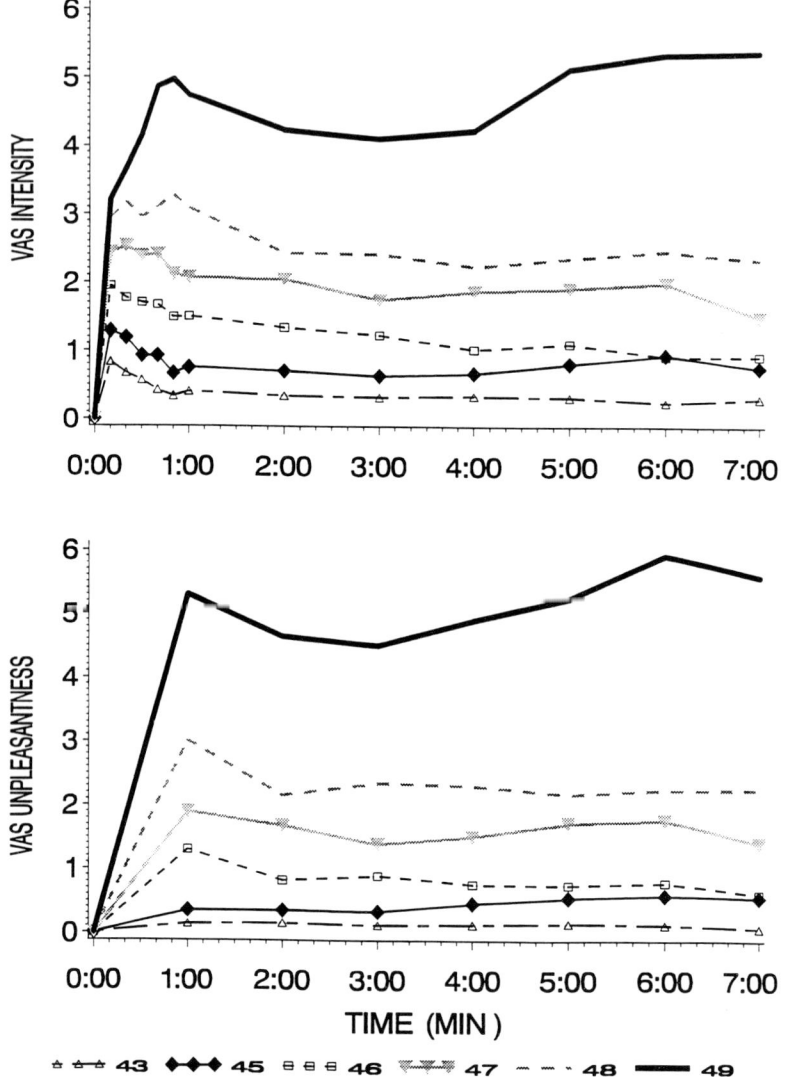

Fig. 4. Effects of prolonged stimulation (immersion of the finger in constant-temperature water bath) with nociceptive temperatures (45°–49°C) on VAS ratings. Ratings of both sensation intensity (top) and unpleasantness (bottom) displayed a rapid increase at the beginning of stimulation. After 1–2 minutes of stimulation, both intensity and unpleasantness ratings generally decreased slightly, but remained at stable levels thereafter. Reprinted from Coghill et al. (1993a), with permission.

diate phase of pain, accompanied by fear, flight or fight, and somatomotor and autonomic responses is followed by a second, acute phase during which pain-related behavioral responses are maintained at the same level. High peak responses followed by responses that remain stable over time have obvious adaptive significance, because the degradation of signals that lead to protective escape and avoidance behaviors in the presence of tissue-damaging stimuli would be maladaptive.

ENCODING OF PAIN INTENSITY

Contact heat-induced pain follows a positively accelerating power function (Price et al. 1983, 1987, 1994b, 1996; Price 1988; Duncan et al. 1989), as illustrated in Figs. 1 and 2. The exponent of the power function is consistently greater than 2.0, regardless of whether pain sensation intensity or unpleasantness is rated. Thus, for the data presented in Fig. 2, the exponent for unpleasantness is significantly higher than that for sensation intensity; both functions have exponents greater than 2.0 (Price et al. 1994b). The functions obtained using a VAS are very consistent across different groups of subjects, including both pain patients and pain-free volunteer groups (Fig. 2). The power function exponent is also independent of stimulus area. The stimulus-response functions of heat-induced pain differ markedly from those of warmth, for which the exponent ranges from 0.5 to 1.6, depending on the stimulus area (Marks 1974). However, the exponent for pain produced by radiant heat is close to 1.0 for different body sites (Adair et al. 1968; Price and Browe 1975).

A higher exponent for pain affect compared with pain sensation reflects the fact that unpleasantness ratings are systematically lower than sensory ratings when both are rated on VAS of the same length (Price et al. 1986a). This increases the slope when data are plotted in logarithmic coordinates. However, unpleasantness ratings are subject to a good deal of influence by psychological factors. The lower ratings in this case were due to assurances made to the participants that the stimuli would be brief, would not damage tissue, and would remain within tolerable limits. Very different ratings would most likely occur if subjects were to become anxious about the pain stimuli.

These data demonstrate that heat-induced pain is similar to other sensory modalities in that it follows a power function, which helps to characterize such pain as a somatosensory submodality. In addition to larger exponents for contact heat-induced pain (>2.0) than for contact-induced warmth (ca. 1.0), other major differences also exist between these sensory modalities. The perception of warmth intensity and the threshold for warmth depend on the rate of rise in skin temperature, whereas pain threshold and pain intensity are far less influenced by such factors (Hardy et al. 1952; Price and Browe 1975). Attributes of spatial summation (increased sensation as a function of increased stimulus area) also differ for pain and warmth. These clear differences in psychophysical attributes indicate that heat-induced pain cannot be construed as a simple extension of warmth and must be considered a separate sensory dimension. Considerable neurophysiological evidence also indicates that separate neuronal populations process warmth and nociception (Hellon and Mitchell 1975; Price and Browe 1975).

PAIN INTENSITY DISCRIMINABILITY

If we can detect the intensity of a noxious stimulus, we must also be able to detect differences in noxious intensities. The sensitivity of this capability is surprising. Both humans and monkeys can detect temperature shifts of 0.2°–0.3°C at nociceptive (≥47°C) intensity levels (LaMotte and Campbell 1978; Bushnell et al. 1983; Robinson et al. 1983), as shown in Fig. 5. This discriminative ability is even greater than that found for warmth. For example, temperature shifts of 0.3°–0.5°C from a baseline of 39°C are required for trained human observers to detect differences in warmth. The ability to detect very small differences of 0.2°–0.3°C within the nociceptive range (45°–51°C) is generally consistent with the 21 levels of just-noticeable differences obtained for radiant-heat-induced pain (Hardy et al. 1952). Contrary to the notion that discrimination of different magnitudes of pain is

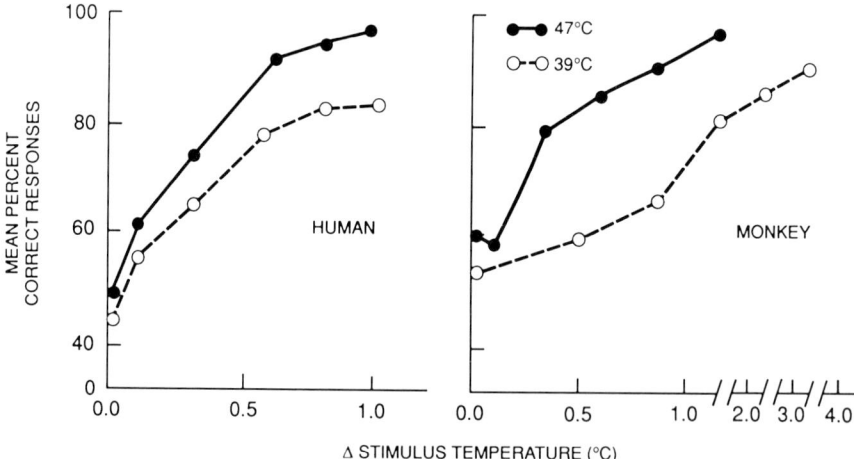

Fig. 5. Functions illustrating the capabilities of human subjects (left; $n = 3$) and a monkey (right) to discriminate small changes in temperature in the noxious (47°C, solid lines) and innocuous ranges (39°C, dashed lines). Each point represents the average of 100 trials. Note that small temperature shifts (0.2°–0.3°C) can be discriminated readily in both ranges. Adapted from Bushnell et al. (1983), with permission.

poor and unlike other sensory modalities, discrimination within the nociceptive stimulus intensity range is extremely refined. Both psychophysical studies and investigations of neurons at all levels within pain-related neural pathways consistently demonstrate the capacity of neurons, and of human observers, to discriminate 0.2°–0.3°C differences (Lamotte and Campbell 1978; Bushnell et al. 1983).

TEMPORAL CHANGES IN SECOND PAIN

A brief nociceptive stimulus, such as a 3-second heat pulse of 51°C or percutaneous electrical stimulation of A and C axons, can evoke two distinct pain sensations, called "first" and "second" pain (Price 1972; Price et al. 1977; Vierck et al. 1997). First pain is usually a well-localized, sharp, pricking sensation, whereas second pain occurs about a second later and is a dull, throbbing, or burning sensation. Second pain is often more spatially diffuse and less well localized than first pain and often lingers well beyond the brief nociceptive stimulus that evokes it. Cross-modality matching and VAS methods have been used to analyze the curious property of temporal suppression found in first pain and the temporal summation (increased sensation as a function of stimulus repetition) in second pain (Price et al. 1977; Vierck et al. 1997). The intensities of first and second pain respectively decrease and increase throughout a train of nociceptive heat pulses (i.e., 2.8 seconds at 51°C; Fig. 6). First pain, which is related to impulse input from Aδ myelinated axons, decreases in intensity whenever the interstimulus interval is 80 seconds or less, but only if the same spot on the skin is stimulated repeatedly. Second pain, related to impulse input from C unmyelinated axons, increases in intensity whenever the interstimulus interval is 3 seconds or less, but not when the interstimulus interval is 5 seconds or more. This slow temporal summation occurs even when the stimulus moves from spot to spot during the train of heat pulses, and even after total blockade of the peripheral impulses in the A axons necessary for first pain (Price 1972; Price et al. 1977). Thus, separate mechanisms subserve first pain suppression and second pain summation. Temporal summation of second pain usually results after several stimuli in a burning pain that often continues for several seconds after termination of the stimuli. This aftersensation has long been noted to be a common feature of pain evoked by stimulation of C nociceptive afferent neurons. As discussed in Chapters 4 and 5, temporal summation of second pain reflects mechanisms of pain that are related to central sensitization, secondary hyperalgesia, and persistent pain states. These phenomena may be related to the mechanisms that support the low rates of adaptation that occur during nociceptive stimulation of constant intensity.

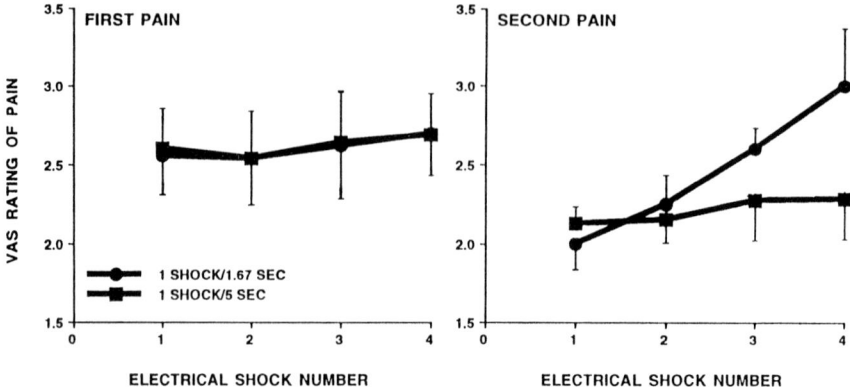

Fig. 6. Effects of repetitive heat pulses on first and second pain. Repeating a 51°C heat pulse produced a progressive decrement in the judged intensity of first pain (left). However, the same conditions produced very different results for second pain (right). In this case, judgments of second pain sensation intensity increased with each successive heat pulse only if the interpulse interval was 3 seconds or less. Apparently, a CNS mechanism exists for amplifying second pain with repetitive noxious stimuli. Reprinted from Price et al. (1994a), with permission.

These characteristics of temporal summation of second pain have been observed in several laboratories using different methods. Temporal summation of second pain occurs in response to repeated cutaneous electric shocks before and after blockade of myelinated axons (Price 1972). It also occurs in response to repeated brief heat pulses of 51°C (Harkins et al. 1996; Price et al. 1977, 1989b, 1994a; Fillingim et al. 1998; Maixner et al. 1998) or repeated 53°C heat taps to the skin (Vierck et al. 1997). Moreover, it occurs in response to direct electrical stimulation of C axons of a peripheral cutaneous nerve under conditions wherein the amplitude of the C compound action potential remains constant during repeated stimuli (Collins et al. 1960). Evidence indicates that slow temporal summation may occur with repetitive stimulation of muscle and visceral nociceptive afferents (Arendt-Nielsen et al. 1997). Temporal summation of second pain is enhanced and occurs at a lower frequency (i.e., 5 seconds) in patients with fibromyalgia (C.J. Vierck et al., unpublished manuscript) and in temporomandibular joint disease (Maixner et al. 1998). Because temporal summation of second pain reflects mechanisms that support central hyperalgesia and persistent pain states, it serves as a psychophysical model with which to study both pharmacological and nonpharmacological treatments for pain diseases (Arendt-Nielsen et al. 1997). Finally, sex and age differences affect the magnitude of temporal summation of second pain. Fillingim et al. (1998) found that women have greater temporal summation of second pain than do men, and Harkins et al.

(1996) showed that elderly persons (>65 years old) have less temporal summation of second pain than do younger individuals.

SPATIAL SUMMATION

Warmth shows considerable spatial summation at the threshold for warmth sensation, but pain exhibits much less spatial summation as its threshold (Hardy et al. 1940, 1952; Murgatroyd 1964; Stevens and Marks 1971; Marks 1974). Summation of warmth takes place generously over large areas of the body surface, and as stimulus area increases, so does the overall perceived intensity of warmth. However, the slope of the stimulus-response function obtained when relating stimulus temperature to perceived warmth (in double-logarithmic coordinates) decreases in magnitude with increasing stimulus area. Therefore, the same change in temperature over a small area has a proportionately greater effect than does the same change spread over a larger area. Furthermore, the perceived warmth intensity functions converge at a common point near the pain threshold (Marks 1974).

Psychophysical studies have only recently concluded that spatial summation exists for pain (Price et al. 1989a; Douglass et al. 1992; Coghill et al. 1993a); earlier studies had found equivocal evidence (Hardy et al. 1940, 1952; Melzack et al. 1962; Kenshalo et al. 1967). Given the potentially critical role of this property in understanding the neural mechanisms of pain and the obvious medical implications, it is astonishing that direct scaling analyses have been applied to testing spatial summation of pain only within the last 10 years.

In the five separate studies using direct scaling methods, human observers made direct ratings of pain sensation intensity and/or pain unpleasantness in response to contact heat (Price et al. 1989a; Douglass et al. 1992; Coghill et al. 1993a; Defrin and Urca 1996; Nielsen and Arendt-Nielsen 1997) or cold (Douglass et al. 1992). As shown in Fig. 7, considerable spatial summation occurred in both the intensity and unpleasantness dimensions of pain. Although spatial summation was evident throughout a wide range of temperatures, in all five studies it was far greater at temperatures that were suprathreshold for pain (47°–51°C) than at those near the pain threshold (43°–46°C). In contrast to spatial summation of warmth, that of heat-induced pain *increases* with increasing stimulus temperature (Fig. 7). Thus, for intensely painful stimuli, stimulus area is a particularly critical factor in determining pain level. The pattern of spatial summation of pain (Fig. 7) occurs for small areas of skin (Price et al. 1989a; Douglass et al. 1992; Defrin and Urca 1996), as well as much larger areas that extend across several dermatomes (Coghill et al. 1993a; Nielson and Arendt-Nielsen 1997),

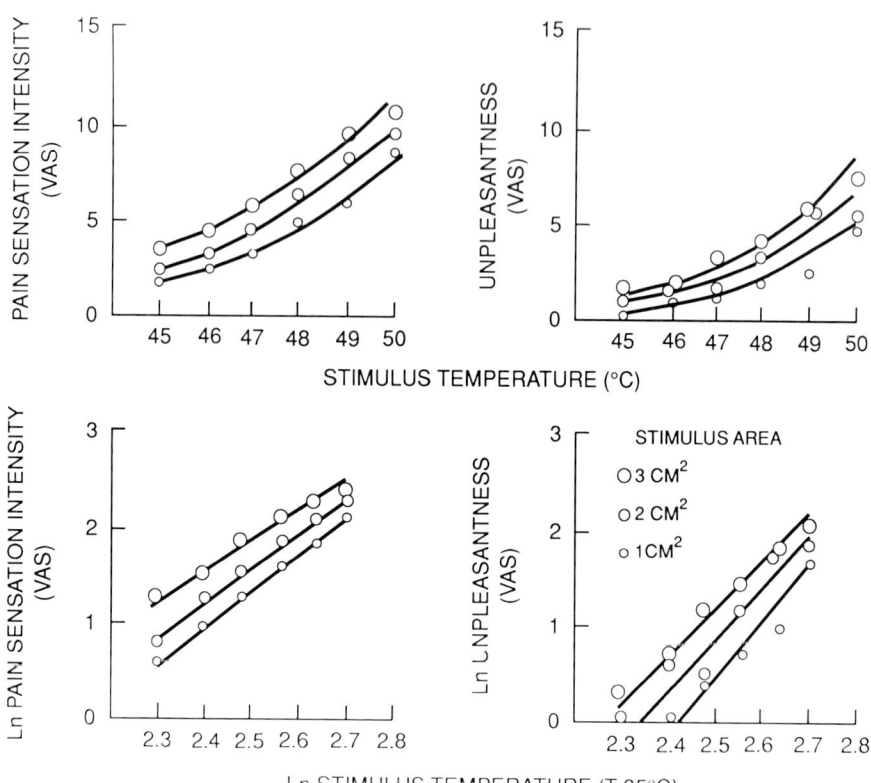

Fig. 7. Spatial summation of pain, showing sensory (left) and affective (right) VAS ratings of nociceptive temperatures; functions are plotted in linear (top) and double-logarithmic (bottom) coordinates. The magnitude of the stimuli (heat probes) is indicated by the size of the open circles. The functions are clearly positively accelerating in linear coordinates, and are linear in double-logarithmic coordinates, which demonstrates that spatial summation makes a greater contribution to subjective awareness as the stimulus size increases. Reprinted from Price et al. (1989a), with permission.

and even for multiple stimuli separated by as much as 20 cm (Price et al. 1989a). The fact that extent of spatial summation of pain is a function of both area and nociceptive stimulus intensity also has adaptive significance because these features are consistent with a mechanism that is sensitive to the total amount of biological threat to the integrity of body tissues. As discussed in Chapters 4 and 5, the psychophysical features of spatial summation are consistent with a pain-encoding mechanism that is heavily dependent on central neuronal recruitment.

The spatial summation of heat-induced pain is characterized by upward parallel displacement of the stimulus-response function in double-logarithmic coordinates (Fig. 7). A similar parallel displacement in double-logarithmic coordinates is evident, regardless of whether the various sized stimulus areas are small, large and extending across several dermatomes, or spatially separated. It also indicates that the power function exponent (the slope of the curve in double-logarithmic coordinates) is stable across different areas and various spatial patterns of stimulation. This consistent power function exponent differs markedly from that of warmth, whose slope and power function exponent decrease with increasing area.

Minimal spatial summation near the pain threshold is consistent with conclusions of previous studies (see Mountcastle 1974 for review), and helps to explain why the property of spatial summation of pain has long eluded investigators. This property of pain is very different from that of warmth, for which spatial summation occurs maximally near threshold. This difference, in turn, may be related to the fact that the steepest portion of the stimulus-response curve for warmth is near the warmth threshold, whereas that for heat-induced pain is well above the pain threshold. Central neural integrative mechanisms may also be quite different for pain and warmth.

Spatial summation is undoubtedly a clinically important attribute of pain. For example, evidence indicates that burn patients find larger areas of affected skin to be more painful than smaller areas. Atchison et al. (1991) determined a correlation coefficient of $r = 0.54$ ($P < 0.001$) between area of third-degree burn and patients' sensory ratings of pain. This association is strong, considering the additional multiple factors that contribute to pain intensity among burn patients. Spatial summation is not confined to cutaneous pain, but also occurs to a considerable extent in visceral and muscular pain (Arendt-Nielsen et al. 1997). Stohler and Kowalski (1999) demonstrated spatial summation for pain resulting from algesic chemicals injected into the masseter muscle. Clinical pain involving the same orofacial region also demonstrated spatial summation that extended over larger body areas for the affective than the sensory dimension and was enhanced if the pain was persistent rather than brief.

RADIATION

Another feature of heat-induced pain that is closely related to spatial summation, and may share common neural mechanisms with it, is the perceived spread or "radiation" of pain from the stimulus site. Thus, at or near pain threshold, the perceived area of the painful stimulus is confined to the actual area and location of the stimulus itself. However, as the stimulus intensity extends above pain threshold, the perceived area of painful sensation extends well beyond the boundaries of the actual stimulus. This property was demonstrated in a human psychophysical experiment (Price et al. 1978; Fig. 8). Five-second stimuli of randomly varied intensities were applied to the ventral forearm. The incidence of perceived spread of painful sensations increased from 0% near pain threshold (45°C) to 90% at 51°C. The spread of sensation did not result from conduction of heat on the skin, since at the highest temperatures used, skin temperatures 2–3 mm from the edge of the thermode remained unchanged.

Radiation also is a very common feature of many types of clinical pains, including myofascial pain and neuropathological pains such as postherpetic neuralgia, trigeminal neuralgia, and complex regional pain syndrome, type II (causalgia) (Noordenbos 1959; Travell and Simmons 1983; Price et al. 1994b). The extent of radiation often covaries with the intensity of the pain, remaining confined to a dermatome at low intensities and extending across dermatomes rostral and caudal to the stimulus site at high intensities.

PSYCHOPHYSICAL ATTRIBUTES OF PATHOPHYSIOLOGICAL PAIN

The psychophysical attributes of pain discussed thus far pertain to those evoked by brief stimuli that are not necessarily damaging. However, pain associated with tissue injury is often characterized by additional attributes, including spontaneous pain, hyperalgesia, and allodynia. Hyperalgesia is pain that is abnormally intense, such as severe pain evoked by mild- to moderate-intensity nociceptive stimulation. Allodynia is pain evoked by a

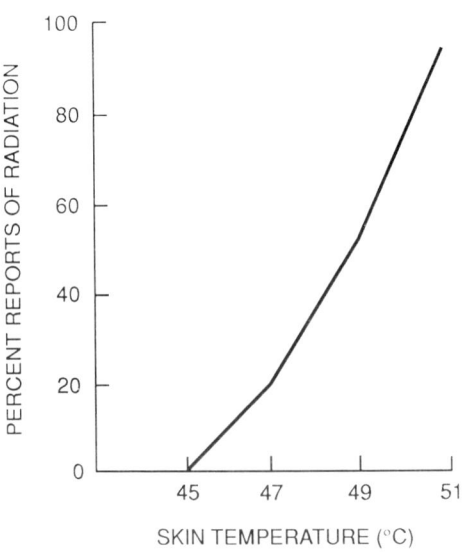

Fig. 8. Radiation of pain as a function of skin temperature. As skin temperature increases, the likelihood of reporting radiation of painful sensations increases. After Price et al. (1978).

normally innocuous (nonpainful) stimulus, such as light touch, cooling, or warmth. Both hyperalgesia and allodynia can be thermal or mechanical. It has been known for over 20 years that injury-induced sensitization of primary nociceptive afferent neurons accompanies and is the peripheral cause of hyperalgesia and allodynia (Campbell et al. 1988). More recent evidence showed that tissue injury is normally followed by increased responsiveness of nociceptive neurons of the spinal cord and of other regions of the central nervous system (Dubner 1991). Even more recent studies indicate that some types of pathophysiological pains caused by nerve injury represent exaggerated or abnormally triggered expressions of the same neural mechanisms that are evoked by tissue injury in general (Price et al. 1994b; Arendt-Nielsen 1997). The psychophysical attributes of pains related to inflamed injured tissues and neuropathic pains are critical in understanding the underlying neural mechanisms and consequently in providing appropriate treatments.

HYPERALGESIA AND ALLODYNIA

Examples of heat-induced hyperalgesia are shown in Fig. 9, which presents data from two patients with complex regional pain syndrome, type I (CRPS-I) (Price et al. 1992a). For both patients, exaggerated perceptions of pain occurred throughout a wide range of stimulus intensities (43°–49°C). However, the differences between the patients' abnormal responses to stimuli delivered to pathological zones, and normal responses to the same stimuli delivered to contralateral nonpathological zones, were greatest toward the lower end of the stimulus range, 43°–45°C (Fig. 9). This pattern of increased responsiveness is remarkably similar to that obtained for C-polymodal nociceptive afferents and for human ratings of pain after heat-induced injury of the skin (Meyer and Campbell 1981; Campbell et al. 1988). In both heat-induced injury and CRPS-I, hyperalgesia is likely to be dynamically maintained by tonic input from sensitized primary nociceptive afferents, particularly C-polymodal afferents (Gracely et al. 1992). The sensitization of such afferents in CRPS-I, however, appears to lack its usual association with injured skin. Based on the curves presented in Fig. 9, it is also likely that the thermal thresholds for pain were lowered in these patients, so that heat allodynia was probably also present. Cold allodynia also is a common characteristic of CRPS-I patients (Campbell et al. 1988).

Studies of neuropathic pain patients have shown pathophysiological conditions characterized by zones of skin in which heat hyperalgesia is present in some patients and larger zones in which mechanical hyperalgesia and/or allodynia exist in all or most patients (Gracely et al. 1992; Price et al. 1989b,

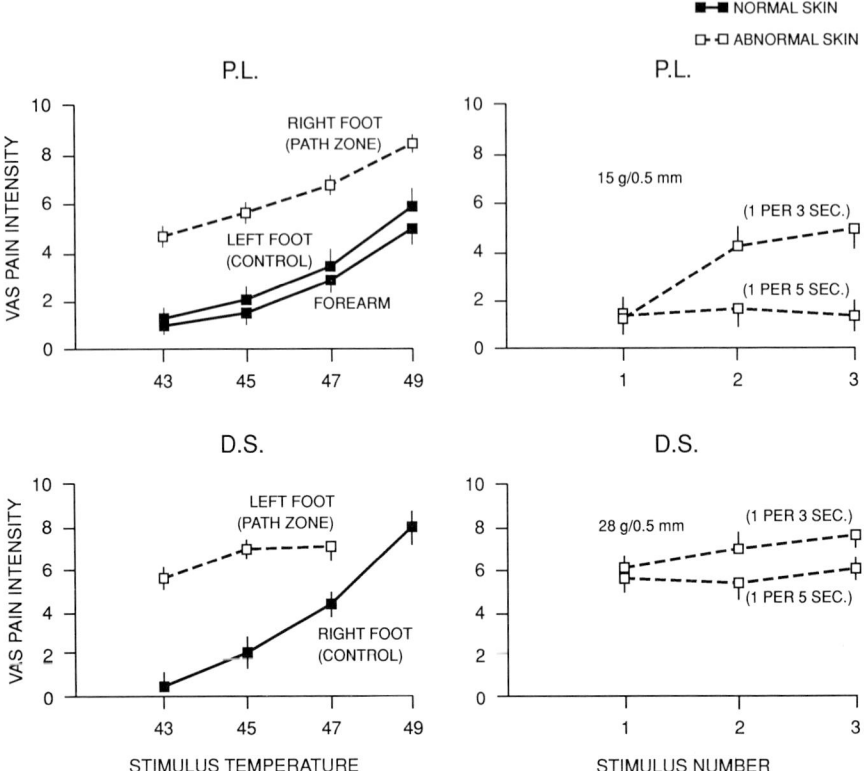

Fig. 9. Pain intensity VAS ratings of two patients (P.L. and D.S.) who both had heat-induced hyperalgesia (left graphs) and temporal summation of mechanical allodynia (right graphs) to repeated von Frey filament stimulation. Note that temporal summation occurred with stimuli delivered for 1/3 second but not 1/5 second (right graphs). From Price et al. (1992a), with permission.

1992a). Two distinct types of mechanical allodynia have been characterized in such patients. The first, low-threshold Aβ allodynia (Price et al. 1989b, 1992a), occurs in response to electrical stimulation of the lowest-threshold axons in nerves supplying the pathological zone and to very gentle mechanical stimuli. It is abolished by blockade of the largest, fastest-conducting axons within nerves and has a reaction time consistent with conduction in myelinated afferents (Gracely et al. 1992). It is also commonly characterized by the fact that moving or intermittent stimuli are more painful than static stimuli (Price et al. 1989b, 1992a). The second type of mechanical allodynia is characterized by evidence that Aβ afferents do *not* seem to be involved and that more intense but normally painless stimuli are required to evoke pain. For example, 15–600-g von Frey filament stimuli, which are well above threshold for Aβ primary mechanoreceptive afferents but are rarely painful under normal circumstances, evoke pain when applied to the pathological zones of these patients. Such "high-threshold" mechanical allodynia may well be mediated by nociceptive afferents that have thresholds below the normal pain threshold.

PATHOPHYSIOLOGICAL MECHANISMS OF SLOW TEMPORAL SUMMATION

Regardless of whether the mechanical allodynia is Aβ or high threshold, it is often similar to normal pain evoked by unmyelinated C nociceptive afferents (Price et al. 1994b). For some CRPS-I patients, slow temporal summation of burning pain occurs when gentle mechanical stimuli or electrical stimulation of Aβ afferents are applied at rates of once per 3 seconds (Fig. 10). For other patients, slow temporal summation occurs only with more intense but normally nonpainful mechanical stimuli. Still others do not exhibit slow temporal summation with these types of repetitive stimuli. Both mechanical allodynia and slow temporal summation of allodynia were almost completely reversed by anesthetic blockade of sympathetic ganglia, which indicates that these sensory abnormalities are dynamically maintained by sympathetic efferent activity, which presumably induces continuous input over nociceptive afferents. Slow temporal summation of mechanical allodynia, particularly that induced by stimulation of Aβ afferents, is abnormal, given that such types of stimuli do not evoke pain in pain-free subjects

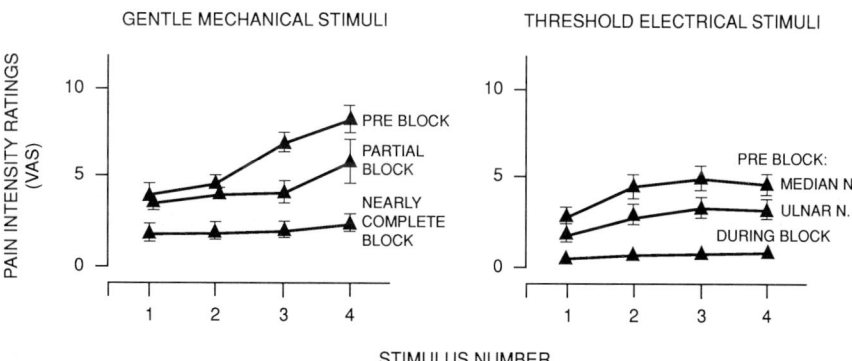

Fig. 10. Slow temporal summation of Aβ allodynia in a CRPS-I patient. The patient made pain intensity VAS ratings in response to trains of stimuli likely to activate Aβ afferents; ratings were made before and during successful sympathetic blocks. At left is shown the slow temporal summation of burning pain in response to trains of very gentle mechanical stimuli and its attenuation by sympathetic block. At right is shown the slow temporal summation of pain in response to transcutaneous electrical stimulation of Aβ afferents and its attenuation by sympathetic block. Adapted from Price et al. (1989b), with permission.

nor in pain patients when such stimuli are delivered to homologous contralateral pain-free zones. In fact, Aβ-afferent stimulation, even at extremely
high frequencies, does not evoke pain in normal human subjects (Collins et
al. 1962). Therefore, Aβ mechanical allodynia and abnormal slow temporal
summation of mechanical allodynia may represent an exaggeration or abnormal triggering of physiological mechanisms that already exist in pain-
free individuals. Such mechanisms can be demonstrated in the latter by
temporal summation of experimentally induced second pain, as described
earlier. Thus, under some pathological conditions after nerve injury, Aβ
input may somehow gain access to and trigger the same temporal summation
mechanisms normally activated by C-afferent stimulation. In other pathological conditions, sensitized nociceptors themselves are likely to be the
direct proximal cause of the slow temporal summation of mechanical
allodynia. Regardless of the exact mechanisms by which temporal summation of allodynia is generated, the phenomenon is likely to contribute to
ongoing "spontaneous" pain in CRPS-I patients. Patients who exhibit temporal summation of mechanical allodynia have higher magnitudes of ongoing pain than those who do not (Price et al. 1992a).

SUMMARY AND CONCLUSIONS

Different dimensions and mechanisms of pain can be measured in experimental paradigms that use controlled intensities of nociceptive stimuli.
These include combined studies of experimental and clinical pain. Psychophysical studies have demonstrated that the fundamental psychophysical
attributes of pain include highly reliable pain thresholds, minimal adaptation of pain intensity in the presence of maintained nociceptive stimulation,
slow temporal summation of pain mediated by C, but not A afferents, spatial
summation, and radiation of perceived area of pain sensation at suprathreshold levels of nociceptive stimulation. Pathophysiological mechanisms
of pain often represent exaggerations or abnormal triggering of the same
mechanisms observed for normal pain processing. Such expressions of pain
mechanisms can be identified in individual patients through the use of standardized sensory tests; they have important implications for treating various
types of pathophysiological pain.

The psychophysical analysis of pain has also created a scientific basis
for measurement and assessment of both experimental and clinical pain.
Different measurement approaches, including pain threshold measurement,
ordinal scales, and VAS, can be compared for their ability to satisfy several
criteria of ideal pain measurement. Both verbal descriptor scales and VAS

are likely to have ratio scale characteristics, and they are reliable and simple to use. They can be adapted to separately measure sensory and affective dimensions of pain experience. The following chapter will explore more refined assessment of the various stages and dimensions of pain processing.

Psychological Mechanisms of Pain and
Analgesia, Progress in Pain Research
and Management, Vol. 15, by Donald D.
Price, IASP Press, Seattle, © 1999.

3

The Dimensions of Pain Experience

Pain is associated not only with sensory-discriminative components such as intensity, duration, location, and quality, but also with emotional feelings such as anxiety, fear, annoyance, despair, and depression. Although both dimensions of pain have long been explicitly acknowledged, research studies of pain mechanisms and clinical studies of treatments for pain have placed greater emphasis on the sensory-discriminative than on the affective dimension. Considerable efforts have been directed toward understanding the sensory features of pain, such as discriminability and intensity coding. In contrast, fundamental questions about the nature and mechanisms of pain-related affect have received far less emphasis. Questions such as whether the two dimensions of pain are processed in parallel or in series, how they interact and differ under various psychological conditions, and the extent to which either dimension can be selectively modulated by psychological or pharmacological interventions have recently been given greater consideration. This chapter explains the affective dimension of pain as the end product of multiple contributing processes, including the pain sensation itself, arousal, autonomic and somatomotor activation, and finally and most critically, cognitive appraisal. Two quite different stages of the affective dimension of pain are described. The first stage is related to the *immediate* appraisal and emotional feelings associated with the sensory features of the pain and with the immediate context. The second stage is related to the *longer-term* implications of having pain. Fig. 1 is a diagram of this sequential model of pain processing. To support this multistage model of pain processing, I will consider the psychological nature of pain affect and review psychological studies of experimental and clinical pain conducted over the last 20 years. Finally, I will discuss the implications of this model for clinical pain assessment. Neurophysiological studies supporting this model will be the topic of Chapters 5 and 6.

THE PSYCHOLOGICAL NATURE OF AFFECT

A brief consideration of the psychological nature of emotions will help to explain how pain-related affect fits into the larger schema of pain experi-

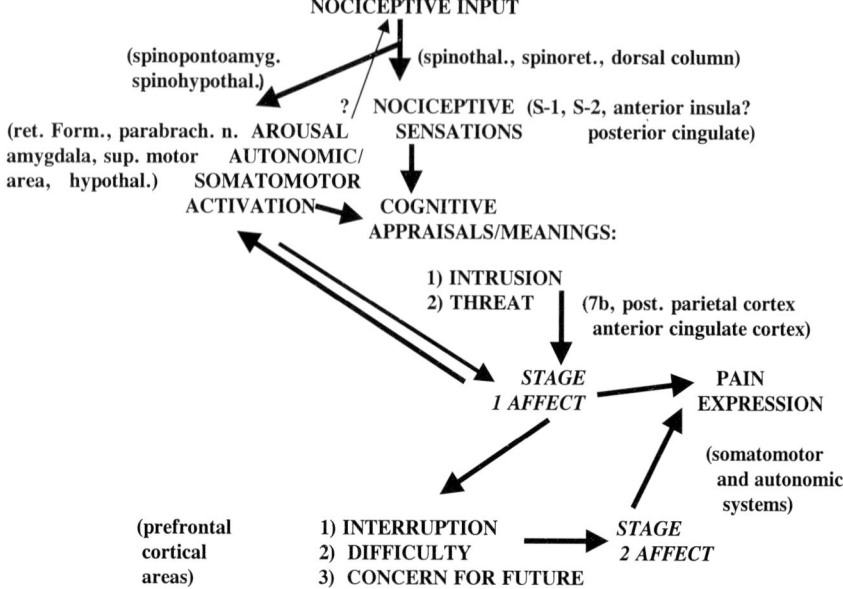

Fig. 1. A schematic used to illustrate interactions between different dimensions and stages of pain. Neural structures considered to have a role in these dimensions are shown in parentheses.

ence. As Buytendyck (1961) has pointed out, an adequate theory of pain requires an adequate theory of emotions in general. Therefore, this section will briefly review classical and current theories of emotions and the roles of arousal, bodily responses, and cognitive evaluation in human emotions. The following sections will discuss how pain-related emotional feelings can be explained in terms of general mechanisms of emotions.

ALTERNATIVE VIEWS OF EMOTION MECHANISMS

The James-Lange theory of emotions, first formulated in 1884, proposed that emotional reactions follow body responses (James 1950). Cannon (1927) attacked this theory by providing experimental evidence that the same physiological responses occur under quite diverse emotional states, thus making it difficult to understand how different emotional feelings can be experientially distinguished on the basis of physiological responses. To some extent, Schacter and Singer (1962) resolved these disparate views by performing experiments to determine how cognitive factors and physiological responses interact to produce emotional states. In general, they proposed that some minimal level of arousal and physiological activation is required for a variety of emotions. However, according to this view, a specific emotional state depends on the significance that one attributes to the situation—that is, the emotion experienced is largely dependent on cognitive processes. Although this theory probably overstates the similarity of physiological patterns of responses across different emotions, it is generally agreed that human emotions require an integration of such patterns with experienced meanings and intentions.

Damasio (1994) provides a modern view of emotional feelings that extends these classical theories by more precise explanation of the interrelationships between cognition and psychophysiological responses. According to his view, an emotional feeling requires that neural signals from viscera, muscles, joints, and neurotransmitter nuclei, all of which are activated during the process of an emotion, reach certain subcortical nuclei and the cerebral cortex. Endocrine and other chemical signals are introduced to the central nervous system via the bloodstream and other routes. Thus, the felt changes in the body produced by such inputs accompany specific thoughts or meanings. For Damasio, "the essence of feeling an emotion is the experience of such changes in juxtaposition to the mental images that initiated the cycle" (Damasio 1994, p. 145). I will return to this view of emotions in discussing the neural substrates of the affective-motivational dimension of pain (Chapter 5).

QUANTIFYING DIMENSIONS OF EMOTIONS

One major limitation of both classical and modern formulations of emotions is the lack of precise quantification of cognitive factors that underlie emotional feelings. Efforts to provide such a contribution come from an earlier theoretical formulation of Barrell and Neimeyer (1975) and from studies using psychophysical methods to study emotions in their natural context. Price and Barrell (1984) and Price et al. (1985a) could explain the intensities of at least some common types of emotional feelings on the basis of two major factors. The first is how much we *desire* something to happen or not happen, and the second is our level of *expectation* that something will happen or has happened. Neither of these two factors is specifically emotional, yet both factors are integral components of many ordinary emotions. Qualitative and quantitative evidence supports this two-factor model.

We used psychophysical methods to assess the influence of both desirability of an outcome and expectation of its occurrence on the magnitudes of emotional feelings. Prior to analysis, we developed ratio scales for each factor. Experiments using both VAS and line-production scaling procedures demonstrated that both factors interacted to influence both positive and negative emotional feelings. The magnitude of positive and negative feeling intensity was shown to be a multiplicative function of *both* desire for an outcome and its perceived likelihood (expectation) of occurrence. The nature of this interaction also was influenced by whether the goal was to avoid negative consequences (an *avoidance* goal) or to obtain pleasurable or satisfying consequences (an *approach* goal).

Over most of the range of expectation, emotional feelings are negative for avoidance goals and positive for approach goals (Fig. 2). We used these factors and their interrelationships to characterize human emotions such as depression, frustration, anxiety, excitement, and satisfaction (Price et al. 1985a). For example, anxiety was associated with avoidance goals and with mid-range expectation levels (Fig. 2), while frustration was associated with avoidance goals and low expectations. Depression was associated with very low expectation levels, and relief with avoidance goals and high expectations of avoidance. Excitement and satisfaction were associated with approach goals and high expectations.

These different emotions were also characterized in terms of specific types of intentions and the body feelings that reflected these intentions. As assessed by written reports, the feeling of frustration was characterized by a desire to move past an obstacle or through resistance. This intention was reflected in the person's thinking and in body feelings of tension, particularly in the neck and upper back, according to self-reports. On the other hand, anxiety was characterized by a more passive stance, wherein one either "waits out" the uncertain catastrophe or attempts to decide on the right

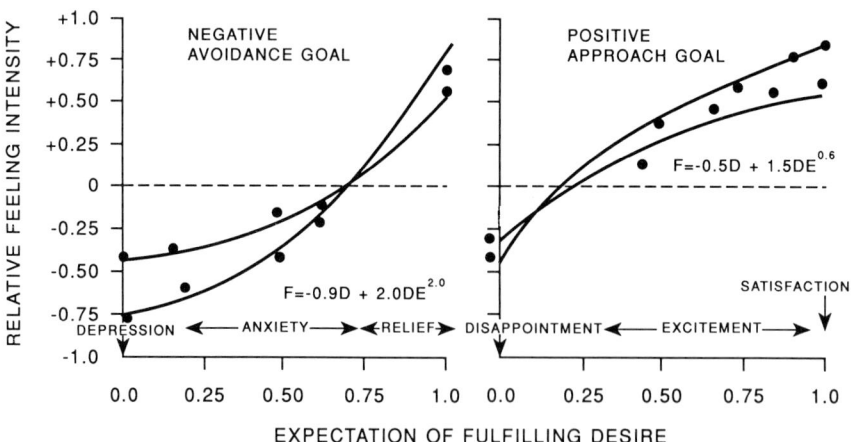

Fig. 2. Relationships of emotional feeling intensities to approach (left curves) and avoidance goals (right curves) and to different ranges of expectation. The expectation range of each emotion is shown by double-arrowed horizontal lines. F = magnitude of positive or negative emotional feeling; D = desire for goal; E = level of expectation of goal fulfillment. Reprinted from Price and Fields (1997), with permission.

course of action. The body tension in anxiety was directed inward and perceived as a more "visceral" sensation, as if to prepare for and absorb the shock of negative consequences. Both the thinking and the body preparation of excitement reflected a movement toward or an urge to move toward expected pleasure, whereas that of satisfaction was a whole-body feeling of being absorbed in the pleasure itself. Similarly, the whole-body feeling of weakness or heaviness in depression reflected the felt absence of goal fulfillment and the felt hopelessness of acting in the future.

In addition to characterizing common emotions, the model of emotions presented in Fig. 2 serves to explain how expectation, desire, and type of goal (approach or avoidance) interact to change emotional experiences. The focus on negative consequences during an avoidance goal has the effect that, unless one is close to certainty of avoiding these negative consequences, one will feel emotionally negative and often either anxious, frustrated, or depressed (Fig. 2). This aspect of emotional experience is captured by the positively accelerating curves in Fig. 2, which demonstrate that feelings are negative throughout most of the range of expectation. For example, if a person begins to undergo what he or she considers to be a moderately painful medical procedure with the goal of avoiding pain and a moderate level of uncertainty of avoiding it (50% chance), that person will have negative feelings. If expectation of avoiding pain increases to near certainty, he or she will feel some relief but not intense positive feelings. In fact, the best one can feel during a goal of avoiding negative consequences is relief. On the other hand, the focus on positive or pleasurable consequences with nothing or little to lose maintains emotional feelings at positive levels over most of the range of expectation (top curves, Fig. 2). Quantitative changes in desire and expectation can lead to qualitative changes in the type of emotion experienced. For example, as expectation of avoiding negative consequences diminishes, a shift is likely to occur in a person's relationship to his or her goal and intentions to take or avoid taking action. As expectation diminishes, the focus on uncertain negative consequences during anxiety may be replaced by a focus on obstacles to preventing catastrophe, and hence frustration. Likewise, frustration may be replaced by the felt hopelessness of depression as expectation lowers toward impossibility. A shift in goal orientation also can change the emotion experienced as well as the quantitative influence of expectation. For example, in receiving medical treatment for a persistent myofascial pain, a patient could focus for a time on the consequences of a more healthy condition of reduced pain and a moment later be thinking about avoiding the devastating consequences of a chronic pain condition. Even when expectations of these two possibilities remain uncertain, the shift from an approach goal (greater health) to an

avoidance goal (avoiding devastating consequences) would change a positive feeling to a negative feeling of anxiety (upper curve at expectation
[E] = 0.5 to lower curve at E = 0.5).

A CONCEPT AND DEFINITION OF EMOTIONS

Emotions require both cognitive appraisal and physiological activation
in an interdependent manner. Cognitive appraisals, in turn, often comprise
two general dimensions—significance or desire and expectation or level of
perceived fulfillment. As Arnold (1970) has pointed out, emotionally related
significance or desire is often in relationship to "something good for me" or
"bad for me"—that is, as something to be approached or avoided. The bodily
reactions during emotions reflect these factors. As discussed previously, the
feeling of unlikely fulfillment of a desire may be accompanied by felt body
tension if one focuses on the intention to remove the obstacle to fulfillment.
Similarly, feelings of weakness or heaviness accompany the meaning of
hopelessness of acting on one's desires during episodes of depression. The
extent of physiological arousal will generally increase with significance or
desire. The *pattern* of physiological response is co-determined by the nature
of one's intentions, attitudes, and expectations of fulfillment. For example,
intense frustration may arise when a chronic pain patient experiences a low
expectation of being able to carry out an important physical task. The felt
sense of this frustration is one of bodily tension accompanied by an urge to
remove the source of the interruption. The patterns of physiological arousal,
including both autonomic and somatomotor activation, help to provide the
felt sense of the emotion (Price et al. 1985a; Price 1988; Damasio 1994). The
felt sense of an emotional feeling comes from the body. Thus, an emotional
feeling is *the felt sense of a cognitive appraisal that occurs in relation to
something of personal significance, often in relation to desire and expectation.* Similar to previous theories of emotion, the quantitative-cognitive theory
recognizes the interaction between cognitions and physiological activation
patterns. It differs from previous theories in providing a means of quantifying emotional feelings along two scaleable parameters, desire and expectation, and in specifying how patterns of physiological response relate to
meanings and intentions. This is very different from the view that physiological activation patterns are similar across a variety of emotions.

THE IMMEDIATE AFFECTIVE DIMENSION OF PAIN

Emotional feelings, including feelings of unpleasantness, are integral
components of pain for several reasons. Painful sensations are somewhat

unique in that they dispose us to perceive them as unpleasant. Also, pain often occurs within a context that is threatening for reasons other than the pain sensation itself. For example, pain that is associated with disease or trauma may connote future negative consequences. The factors described above for emotional feelings in general apply to those that are a part of pain experience because unpleasant qualities of sensation and implications of negative consequences are almost inevitably accompanied by *desires* to terminate, reduce, or escape pain as well as related *expectations*. Pains have many unpleasant qualities and occur in a large variety of psychological contexts. Thus, many types of unpleasant emotional feelings are integral components of pain experience. The *immediate affective* dimension of pain comprises the moment-by-moment unpleasantness of pain as well as other emotional feelings that pertain to the present or short-term future, such as distress, annoyance, or fear. The immediate affective stage of pain often is closely linked with the intensity of the painful sensation and the associated arousal. The causal interactions between pain sensation and pain unpleasantness can be both immediate and cumulative. Thus, enduring a pain for a few moments may be unpleasant because of the qualities of the sensation and the experience of one's own somatomotor (e.g., startle, withdrawal) and autonomic responses associated with acute pain. However, the pain may be even more unpleasant if one must endure it for several hours.

Aside from the qualities of painful sensation, other psychological and physiological components may contribute to pain unpleasantness. These include coping with or attempting to reduce, escape, or deny the pain. Several additional components can also be a part of immediate pain affect. These include *arousal*, an immediate shift of *attention* to the bodily area of concern, *motor orientation* to this area, and *autonomic responses*. These *interoceptive* processes may be integral to an individual's affective reactions during pain. Indeed, just as multiple exteroceptive stimuli (e.g., sight and sound) can be integrated into the overall perception of bodily threat, interoceptive inputs related to autonomic and somatomotor responses also can influence this perception. For example, Barrell and Price (1975) found that the unpleasantness of painful electrical shock depended not only on the intensity of the evoked sensation but also on the unpleasantness of experiencing one's own startle response. The magnitude of both the startle response and the unpleasantness were, in turn, largely determined by the mind-set at the time of stimulus presentation. The point here is that even the *immediate* affective dimension of pain may be synthesized from nociceptive and other exteroceptive and interoceptive sensory processes. Pain sensation may be a salient but not the sole determinant of the affective state during pain. Thus, consistent with modern views of mechanisms of emotional feelings formulated by Damasio (1994), Arnold (1970), and Price et al. (1985a), the emotional state that accompanies the immediate unpleasantness of pain represents a synthesis from several psychophysiological sources. These include pain sensation, arousal, and autonomic, neuroendocrine, and somatomotor responses, all in relationship to meanings of the pain and to the context in which it occurs.

THE CONTRIBUTION OF NOCICEPTIVE SENSATIONS TO PAIN UNPLEASANTNESS

Pain-related sensations may not only be intense and persistent, but can be perceived as spreading, penetrating, and sometimes summating. They are experienced as an invasion of both the body and consciousness because their intensity and qualities are perceived as intense and penetrating (Buytendyck 1961; Bakan 1968). Therefore, a frequent meaning given to painful sensations is that of *intrusion*, a meaning that requires little reflection and occurs somewhat (although not entirely) automatically. It is the meaning conveyed by someone who says "It bothers me because it hurts!" Similar to states of nausea, dizziness, intense thirst, and intense hunger, part of the affective dimension of pain is closely linked to the nature of the sensations themselves. This being the case, both neural and psychological processes associated with pain-related sensation can be conceived as important causal links in the production of pain-related emotional disturbance. The qualities and intensities of pain sensations dispose us to perceive them as immediately unpleasant under most conditions. The painful sensation of a bee sting, for example, is unpleasant partly because it is experienced as an intense, sharply penetrating, and spatially spreading sensation. Its persistence and increasing intensity over time enhance unpleasantness. Thus, sensations evoked by nociceptive stimuli are one of the immediate causes of pain-related emotional feeling in the same way that sensations of dizziness or nausea are direct causes of unpleasant affective states. The close link between acute forms of pain-related sensation and immediate pain unpleasantness has been a source of confusion among psychologists, some of whom have questioned whether the dimensions of pain experience can be measured separately (Fernandez and Turk 1992). Psychophysical studies have clearly demonstrated that pain-related sensation and immediate pain-related unpleasantness or disturbance represent two separate dimensions of pain that demonstrate reliably different relationships to nociceptive stimulus intensity and can be separately influenced by various psychological factors (Price 1988; Price et al. 1992b; Rainville et al. 1992, 1997, 1999b). Human subjects rate intensities of experimental pain differently, depending on whether the VAS or verbal descriptor scales denote sensation or affect

(Gracely et al. 1976; Gracely 1979, 1994; Gracely and Dubner 1981; Price et al. 1983, 1987; Price and Harkins 1987, 1992a). For both VAS and verbal scales, the experimental pain stimulus-response functions are reliably different for pain affect compared to pain sensation intensity. In the case of sensory and affective VAS of identical lengths that differed only in the words used to anchor them, unpleasantness ratings were systematically *lower* than sensory ratings for all intensities of nociceptive temperature stimuli (Price et al. 1987). As discussed in Chapter 2, the lower ratings in this case were probably the result of assurances made to participants that the stimuli were to be brief, would not damage tissue, and would remain within tolerable limits. Very different ratings would probably have occurred if these assurances had not been made or if the stimuli had not been so brief. In support of this possibility, Rainville et al. (1992) showed that ratios of affective to sensory ratings of brief experimental pain stimuli (electric shock or 5-second heat pulses) were systematically less than 1.0, whereas those of long-duration pain stimuli (ischemia, cold pressor) were 1.0 or greater. Thus, systematic differences in ratios of affective to sensory ratings of nociceptive stimulus intensity occur as a predicted consequence of simple factors, such as stimulus duration and presence or absence of assurances. These differences constitute one line of evidence for measurably separate dimensions of pain sensation and pain affect.

Rainville and colleagues (1999b) helped to further establish the direction of causation between pain sensation intensity and immediate pain unpleasantness with a hypnotic analgesia study in which subjects immersed their left hands in a water bath heated to a moderately painful 47°C. Two experiments were compared, in which hypnotic suggestions were targeted specifically toward enhancing or decreasing either (1) pain unpleasantness or (2) pain sensation intensity. Ratings of pain unpleasantness, but not of pain sensation intensity, decreased in the first experiment, but *both* pain sensation intensity and pain unpleasantness ratings changed in parallel in the second experiment, despite the fact that the suggestions did not mention pain unpleasantness. The combination of these two sets of results helps to establish the direction of causation—pain sensation is one of the immediate causes of pain unpleasantness, but not vice versa. Pain really *is* unpleasant because it hurts!

THE CONTRIBUTION OF COGNITIVE EVALUATION TO IMMEDIATE PAIN UNPLEASANTNESS

Part of the confusion about the two separate sensory and affective dimensions of pain may stem from the fact that pain-related sensation intensity and pain unpleasantness are often closely linked under controlled labo-

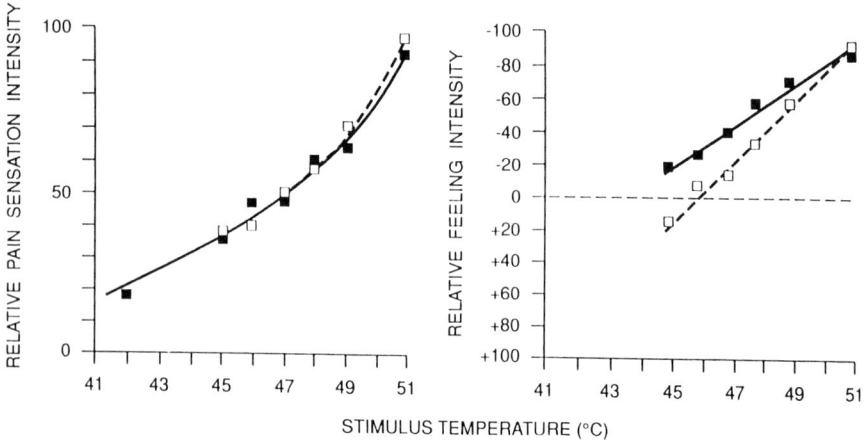

STIMULUS TEMPERATURE (°C)

Fig. 3. Selective effect of warning subjects that the stimulus will be intense on affective ratings of heat-induced pain. The painful sensation intensities (left) are unaffected by the warning signal, whereas unpleasantness ratings of the lower-intensity nociceptive temperatures are reduced. Adapted from Price et al. (1980), with permission.

tal pain, either by an anti-anxiety drug or placebo saline. Gracely and colleagues (1976) demonstrated that 5 mg diazepam (i.v.), a common tranquilizer, significantly reduced affective but not sensory descriptor responses to painful electrocutaneous shock (Fig. 4). Reductions were greatest for low-intensity noxious stimuli. In another study, Gracely (1979) found a very similar pattern for intravenous saline placebo injection. The results of these studies can be interpreted as a selective lowering of pain unpleasantness by a reduction in the anxiety associated with anticipating and receiving a noxious stimulus. As explained above and illustrated in Fig. 2, anxiety represents a state of wanting to avoid negative consequences, combined with an experienced uncertainty of avoiding them (Barrell et al. 1985; Price et al. 1985a). Regardless of whether anxiety is reduced by a drug or a cognitive manipulation that modifies expectation, the result is selective reduction of pain unpleasantness, with the greatest effects occurring for mildly painful intensities.

Expectations about the qualitative nature of pain sensations also selectively influence pain affect. Johnson (1973) found that subjects who had received a description of the painful sensations produced by ischemia of the forearm had lowered levels of distress when subjected to ischemia than did subjects who had only received a description of the procedure. As in the study by Price et al. (1980), pain sensation intensities were unaffected by this difference in description. Different kinds of expectations, either about the time of occurrence of pain or the types of sensations that will occur, can thus alter experienced unpleasantness without changing the intensity of experimentally induced painful sensation.

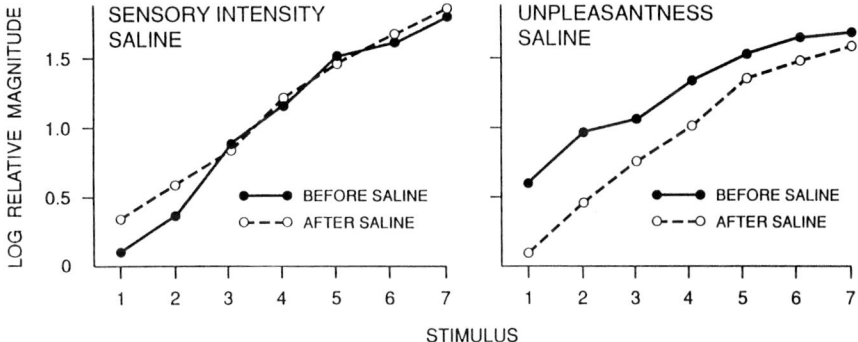

Fig. 4. Sensory intensity (left) and unpleasantness (right) descriptor scales of electrical tooth-pulp stimuli before and after the intravenous administration of saline placebo. Note that only the unpleasantness ratings were affected and that the greatest effect was at the lower end of the stimulus range, similar to the effect shown in Fig. 3. Modified with permission from Gracely, R.H. Psychophysical assessment of human pain. In: *Advances in Pain Research and Therapy,* Vol. 3, edited by J.J. Bonica, J.C. Liebeskind, and D.G. Albe-Fessard, Raven Press, New York, 1979.

The role of expectancy in experimental pain also has been examined within the context of social learning theory. Baker and Kirsch (1991) used various cognitive manipulations for coping with experimental pain to examine perceived self-efficacy and pain expectancy as potential mediators of pain perception and tolerance. They demonstrated that pain tolerance is predicted by perceived self-efficacy, which is in turn predicted by pain expectancy and the provision of incentives. Pain perception was strongly influenced by expectancy, but was unrelated to self-efficacy. Ohlwein et al. (1996), using a similar experimental paradigm, likewise found that response expectancy had a stronger relationship to pain responses than did self-efficacy. However, they did not replicate the finding that self-efficacy mediated the effects of response expectancy on pain tolerance. Although the mediating effect of self-efficacy remains to be clarified, a consistent finding across both studies is that expectations about pain intensity are somewhat predictive of perceived pain intensity itself. A limitation common to both studies is that sensory and affective dimensions of pain were not separately evaluated. Therefore, the question needs to be re-examined for both pain dimensions.

Studies that attempt to modify either experimental or clinical pain intensity by manipulations designed to change expectancy show either weak or negligible effects, as indicated in a meta-analysis by Fernandez and Turk (1989). An interesting finding was that 10 of 12 studies showed that, compared to other psychological strategies, expectancy manipulations were least effective in reducing pain. A distinct limitation of nearly all of these studies, however, is that the independent variable was a manipulation or instruction designed to persuade participants to develop a positive expectation rather than a measure of expectation itself. Therefore, whereas these studies emphasize weak or negligible effects of expectancy manipulations on pain intensity, it is not at all clear that direct effects of actual expectations have such weak effects. In fact, data published after Fernandez and Turk's analysis indicate that experiential manipulations of expectancy, such as repeated exposure to a pain-reducing agent, have stronger effects than do verbal manipulations of expectancy (Voudouris et al. 1990; Montgomery and Kirsch 1997a).

In summary, based on studies of experimental pain, it is apparent that expectations about different aspects of pain and about the contextual conditions surrounding pain influence pain differently. Expectations about when the pain will occur and what it means once it does occur may have relatively selective effects on the unpleasantness or immediate emotional disturbance associated with pain. Expectations about pain sensation intensity itself appear to have a modest influence on perceived pain intensity. Finally, manipulations designed to produce a positive expectation appear to have the weakest effect on pain intensity, although it is difficult to reach a definitive conclusion about this possibility because of the questionable pain measures used in most available studies.

The influence of expectancy on the immediate unpleasantness of clinical pain

In general, the factors of desire for relief and expectation appear to have a greater influence on pain-related affect in the case of clinical pain, where the implications are likely to be perceived as more open-ended and threatening than in experimental pain. Unfortunately, few studies have directly assessed the role of expectancy in clinical pain. Nevertheless, such a role is strongly supported by at least indirect evidence largely consistent with the idea that anxiety is a significant component of clinical pain affect. Price et al. (1987) hypothesized that affective ratings of clinical pain would be higher in patients whose pain is likely to be associated with a serious threat to health or life than in those whose pain is less threatening. Cancer pain and labor pain patients were chosen as representative of the former and latter, respectively. As a corollary to this hypothesis, we proposed that women in labor who focus mainly on the birth of their child would have lower ratings of pain unpleasantness than those who focus mainly on pain or on avoiding pain. We compared sensory and unpleasantness ratings of experimental pain to those of various types of clinical pain.

Different kinds of pain patients, including labor pain and cancer pain patients, used separate VAS to rate pain sensation intensity and degree of unpleasantness that occurred at different times during their condition, as shown in Figs. 5 and 6. In cancer pain patients, unpleasantness ratings were higher than sensory ratings (Fig. 5), whereas the reverse was true for labor pain patients (Fig. 6). Furthermore, we observed significant differences in pain affect ratings among labor pain patients as a function of whether the patient focused primarily on pain or avoiding pain or on having the baby. Patients who focused primarily on having the baby, an approach goal, rated the unpleasantness of their pain as approximately one-half that of patients who focused primarily on pain or on avoiding pain (Fig. 6, right panels). This difference occurred for each stage of labor. In contrast, no significant differences in pain sensation intensity ratings occurred between patients with these two orientations at any stage of labor (Fig. 6, left panel).

All these results combined indirectly indicate that a person's goals, desires, and expectations about outcomes strongly influence emotional feelings associated with different clinical pain conditions. The influence of these factors is most apparent when divergent psychological orientations exist *within* a clinical pain condition. Thus, the unpleasantness brought about by the immediate implications of cancer pain, including the reminder that pain sensation is a signal for the presence of a progressive disease, appears to add to the unpleasantness directly related to the pain sensations. One of the implications of having labor pain, on the other hand, is that birth of a baby is imminent. The positive emotional consequences appear to offset to some degree the unpleasantness of labor pain. This interpretation is supported by the different results for women who focused on avoiding pain rather than on the birth of the baby. Part of what constitutes pain unpleasantness is the *immediate* implication of the pain condition. The implication, in turn, is related to a goal and a desire and expectation associated with that goal.

Results obtained in studies of experimental pain indicate that certain pharmacological and psychological manipulations can selectively, and sometimes powerfully, reduce the immediate unpleasantness of pain. Some can be quite simple, such as different stimulus duration or the presence or absence of a warning signal. Others, such as hypnotic suggestions, may be much more complex and relate to restructuring the meanings associated with pain. Manipulations can also enhance pain unpleasantness. The identification of experimental manipulations that can selectively modify affective components of pain is critical for developing experimental strategies to identify neurons, central pathways, and brain regions that are uniquely involved in the immediate affective dimension of pain.

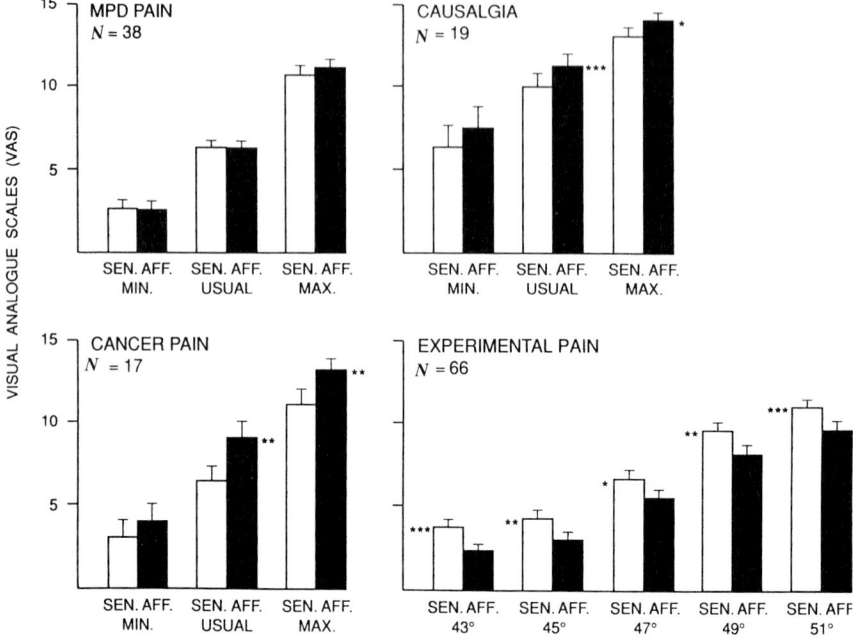

Fig. 5. Sensory (white bars) and affective (black bars) VAS ratings (mean + 1 SEM) for three types of clinical pain (MPD = myofascial pain dysfunction) and one type of experimental pain. VAS ratings of chronic pain patients were obtained at minimum, usual, and maximum levels experienced during the week prior to their clinical visit. Affective and sensory ratings were compared using paired t tests (*$P < 0.05$, **$P < 0.02$, ***$P < 0.001$). Asterisks to the right and left of the black bars indicate higher affective and sensory ratings, respectively. Adapted from Price et al. (1987, p. 302).

THE SECONDARY STAGE OF PAIN AFFECT

Similar to many types of biological threat, pain sometimes contains both immediate and long-term implications. Cognitive appraisals of these implications constitute the link between the sensory features of pain and emotional feelings and their expressions. Cognitive appraisals, in turn, often are associated with specific and complex desires and expectations and therefore complex emotional feelings. An understanding of these feelings must take into account the meanings that are common to the experience of pain and pain-related suffering.

Both empirical studies of experiential factors of pain and consideration of the experience of pain itself indicate that there are two stages of pain-related emotional feeling (Price 1988; Price and Harkins 1992b). A sequential processing model of pain proposes that the two stages are distinguished by the time frame over which cognitive appraisals are made. These stages

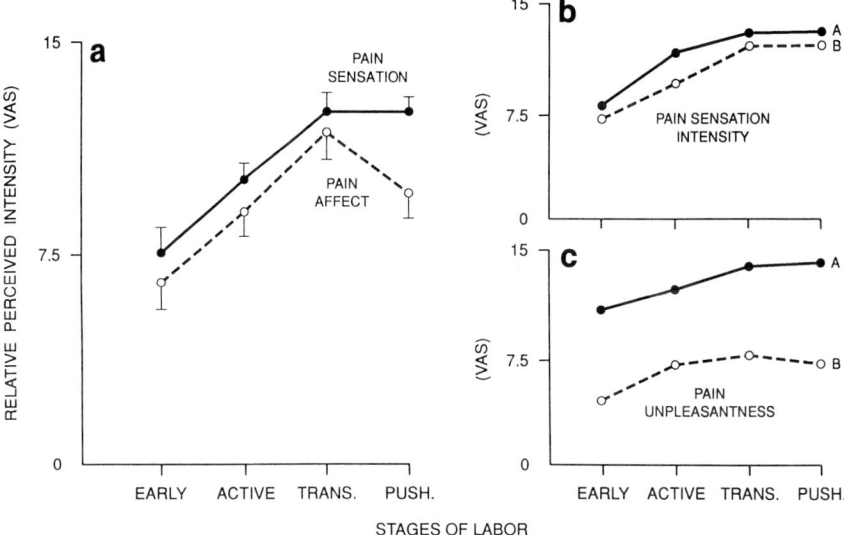

Fig. 6. (a) Mean sensory and affective VAS ratings of pain of 23 labor patients at various phases of labor (vertical lines are standard errors). (b) Sensory VAS ratings of women who focused mainly on pain or avoiding pain (Group A) compared to women who focused mainly on the impending birth (Group B). Note that both groups gave very similar sensory ratings. (c) Affective VAS ratings of groups A and B. Note that affective ratings of group B are approximately one-half those of group A. Adapted from Price et al. (1987, p. 303).

and their interrelationships with nociception, arousal, and cognitive appraisals are illustrated schematically in Fig. 1. The first, discussed previously, is the *immediate affective* stage comprising the moment-by-moment unpleasantness, distress, and possible annoyance that are often closely linked with the intensity of the painful sensation and the accompanying arousal. The *secondary* stage of pain-related affect is based on more elaborate reflection and relates to memories and imagination about the implications of having pain, such as the way pain may interfere with different aspects of one's life, the difficulty of enduring pain over time, and concern for the long-term consequences. Persistent pain can be experienced as a serious threat to one's freedom, to the significance of one's life, and ultimately to one's self-esteem (Buytendyck 1961; Bakan 1968; Barrell and Neimeyer 1975). Whereas the immediate affective stage is based on the present and short-term future, the secondary stage is based on the past and long-term future. A person may be fearful, anxious, or annoyed about the short-term implications of having pain or chronically anxious or depressed about the long-term implications. Pain is often experienced not only as an immediate threat to one's body, comfort, or activity, but also to one's well-being and life in general. Thus, the cognitions and accompanying negative emotions related to the meanings of how pain influences one's life activities and future constitute much of the second stage of pain-related affect, a stage that may be thought of as suffering.

A psychological distinction that helps further clarify the two stages of pain affect is that of *state* and *trait* manifestations of emotions, such as anxiety. *State anxiety* is the anxiety someone is feeling in the moment, whereas *trait anxiety* refers to a person's general disposition to feel anxious or to have anxious feelings about one's life in general. Similarly, whereas immediate pain unpleasantness contains negative affective feelings associated with pain in the present or immediate future, secondary pain-related affect contains feelings about pain as they relate to the long-term future or to one's life in general.

The sequential processing model of pain indicates that immediate pain unpleasantness is the proximate cause of the secondary stage of pain affect (Fig. 1). To use the spatial metaphors of vertical and horizontal causation described in Chapter 1, pain unpleasantness causes secondary pain affect in two ways. Over an extended period of time (days, weeks, months), pain unpleasantness provokes meanings related to suffering (horizontal causation). Conversely, most brief acute pains and almost all experimentally evoked pains contain only the sensory-discriminative and the immediate unpleasantness stages of pain, because time is required for the development of more complex meanings and future implications. However, pain unpleasantness also can serve as an immediate cue for the meanings related to the secondary stage of pain affect once these meanings have been established over time; that is, it can act "vertically" as well. A sudden exacerbation of low back pain can instantly remind the patient of how long he or she has had to endure the interruption of normal life activities and of the unlikely prospects of relief. The secondary stage of pain affect is often a component of pain itself. Thus, for our low back pain patient, the experience of the pain sensations, immediate unpleasantness, and meanings and emotions of suffering can exist simultaneously as a coherent, integrated structure.

The second stage of pain-related affect is based on three potential meanings (Buytendyck 1961; Price 1988). The first is that the painful condition will continue to *interrupt* one's ability to function or to live a meaningful life. The second is that the painful condition and its domination of one's consciousness are a *burden that one has endured for a long time*. Finally, the condition of persistent pain may mean that *something permanently harmful might happen or has happened*.

The meanings attached to intrusion during the first stage and to interruption, endurance, and concern for the future in the second stage of pain affect relate to the painful sensations, the context in which they occur, and their immediate and long-term implications. Each of these meanings, in turn, is easily related to a desire to avoid or remove the interruption, burden, or negative consequences. Numerous contextual factors regarding the nature of the painful condition and potential means of avoiding or reducing the pain and its negative consequences converge to determine one's level of expectation that pain and its consequences will or can be reduced. As such, emotional feelings associated with the first and second stages of pain-related affect may be determined to some extent by desires and expectations, factors that determine many common human emotions (Price and Barrell 1984; Price et al. 1985a). The following discussion provides empirical support for the construct of the secondary stage of pain affect and for the types of negative emotional feelings that constitute this stage of pain processing.

ASSESSMENT OF THE SECOND STAGE OF PAIN AFFECT

The number and types of cognitive appraisals during pain are a function of both the intensity of the painful sensation and several psychological contextual factors, so it is not surprising that the negative emotional feelings experienced during pain are also diverse. Thus, patients in pain may feel anxiety, frustration, depression, anger, or fear to different degrees depending on the nature of the appraisals and the time frame toward which they are directed. The prevalence and relative magnitudes of these feelings are illustrated for different types of pain patients in Fig. 7. Patients were instructed to rate these feelings as they specifically pertained to their chronic pain and not to other, unrelated problems. Moreover, except for labor pain patients, they were asked to rate how strong these feelings had been over the previous week (analogous to a "trait" assessment). Whereas chronic frustration was the most common emotional feeling of patients with musculoskeletal types of pain, depression and frustration were predominant in patients with CRPS-II (causalgia). Anxiety and fear were the most common negative feelings of patients with labor pain, and were more reflective of immediate pain affect because they pertained to how the patients were feeling at the time (i.e., a "state" assessment). Importantly, all five emotional feelings were present in different types of chronic pain patients to varying degrees.

The secondary stage of pain processing has been assessed by administering VAS for each of the five pain-related negative emotions shown in Fig. 7 and for cognitive factors that are likely to mediate these emotions (Harkins et al. 1989; Wade et al. 1990, 1992, 1996; Bush et al. 1993). The combined ratings of these emotions and ratings of interruption, difficulty of enduring the pain, and concern about the consequences represent a psychological stage that is unique and separate from that of immediate pain unpleasant-

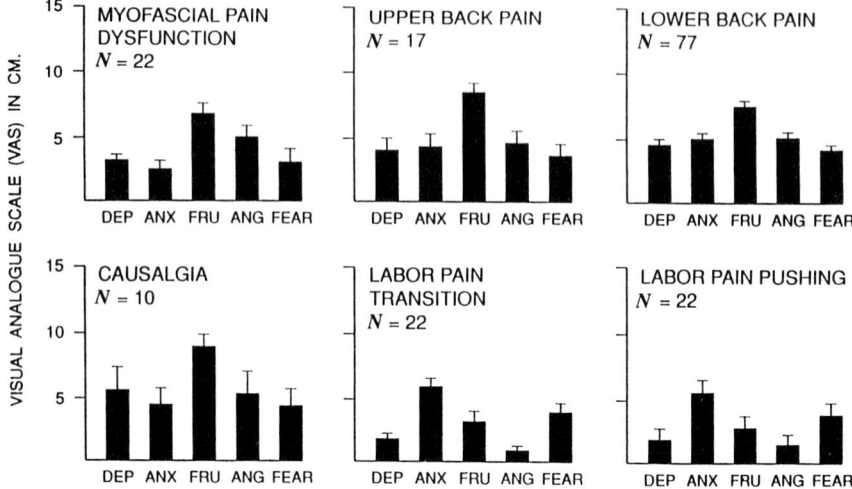

Fig. 7. Profiles of VAS ratings of five distinct types of emotional feelings (DEP = depression; ANX = anxiety; FRU = frustration; ANG = anger; and fear) during different types of clinical pain. Adapted from Price (1988, p. 59).

ness (Harkins et al. 1989; Wade et al. 1990, 1992, 1996). The evidence for this separately measurable stage comes from three types of studies. The first shows associations between VAS measures and other indices of emotional disturbance, such as the Beck Depression Inventory (Wade et al. 1990). The second shows selective effects of personality traits or demographic factors on VAS measures of secondary pain affect (Harkins et al. 1989; Wade et al. 1992). The third directly tests the sequential model shown in Fig. 1, using the method of linear structural equation modeling (LISREL) (Wade et al. 1996).

Effects of extraversion and neuroticism

Wade et al. (1990) used canonical correlation and multiple regression methods to demonstrate significant associations between the composite of VAS for the five negative emotions shown in Fig. 7 and other indices of depression (Beck Depression Inventory and Minnesota Multiphasic Personality Inventory depression scales). Each emotion scale was shown to assess a unique and separate emotional feeling. Importantly, the study determined that emotion VAS were not simply redundant measures of the *immediate* unpleasantness of pain as assessed by the unpleasantness VAS.

Two separate studies have shown that personality traits exert their largest effects on the secondary stage of pain affect. The differential influence of two personality traits, neuroticism and extraversion, on pain sensation intensity, on the immediate unpleasantness stage, and on the secondary stage of pain-related affect was assessed in a group of myofascial pain dysfunction (MPD) patients (Harkins et al. 1989). Eysenck's (1975) personality inventory was used to measure neuroticism and extraversion, and VAS methods were used to measure the various dimensions and stages of pain. Neuroticism is a personality trait characterized by Eysenck (1967) as high emotionality and arousability, as well as a predisposition to engage in maladaptive behaviors and negative emotions. First, neither the personality traits of extraversion nor neuroticism had any influence on VAS sensory ratings of experimental heat pain in these patients (Fig. 8A,C). Patients with high and low scores on these two personality dimensions had nearly identical sensory VAS curves for nociceptive temperature. Second, these high- and low-score groups did not significantly differ with respect to their sensory ratings of their clinical pain (Fig. 9A,B). Therefore, these two personality traits do not appear to influence the first stage of pain, i.e., sensory discrimination. Third, neuroticism but not extraversion was associated with a modest but statistically significant enhancement of VAS unpleasantness ratings of experimental heat pain (Fig. 8B,D) as well as their clinical pain (Fig. 9A,B). Thus, neuroticism appears to exert a small but reliable effect on the immediate stage of pain-related affect, in both experimental and clinical pain.

Finally, it was at the secondary stage of pain-related affect that the personality trait of neuroticism appeared to exert its largest influences (Fig. 10). As hypothesized, patients with high neurotic scores evidenced more intense emotions related to suffering (i.e., depression, frustration, anxiety, etc.) than did patients with low scores. Extraverts and introverts did not differ in their ratings of these emotions. Precisely the same overall pattern of results was replicated by Wade et al. (1992), who used canonical correlation analysis to assess the influence of neuroticism and extraversion on both stages of pain in 205 chronic pain patients. This study differed from that of Harkins et al. (1989) in using the NEO (neuroticism, extraversion, openness) Personality Inventory (Costa and McCrae 1985) to assess neuroticism and extraversion and in including patients with various types of chronic pain such as low back pain and CRPS-I. Despite these differences, the results again clearly demonstrated that neuroticism (and not extraversion) exerted its largest influences *not* on early stages of pain sensory processing and immediate unpleasantness, but on the secondary stage related to higher-order cognitive processes and suffering. Although several studies (Harkins et al. 1989; Wade et al. 1992; BenDebba et al. 1997) suggest that extraversion is also related to suffering, its relationship is weaker than that of

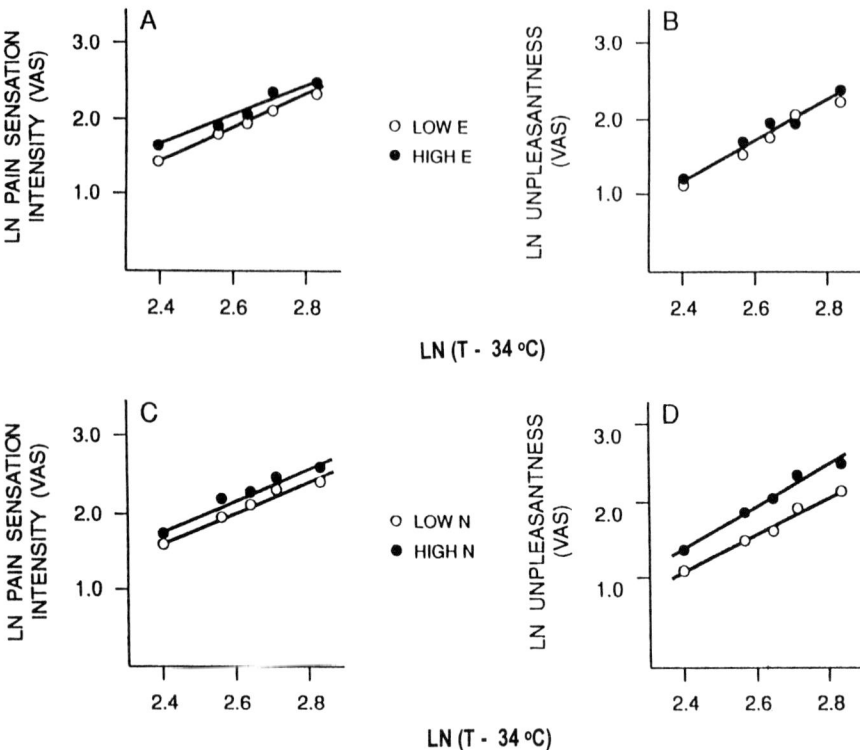

Fig. 8. VAS ratings of pain sensation intensity (left) and unpleasantness (right) of experimental noxious temperatures administered to patients with myofascial pain dysfunction, plotted in double-logarithmic coordinates. Patients with high neuroticism (N) scores (bottom panels) gave significantly ($P < 0.05$) higher unpleasantness ratings than did those with low N scores. Sensory VAS ratings were unaffected by neuroticism score. Both sensory and unpleasantness ratings were unaffected by extraversion score (E) (top panels). Adapted from Harkins et al. (1989), with permission.

neuroticism. In Wade et al.'s (1992) study, assertiveness, a component of extraversion, was the most important predictor of pain suffering. Assertiveness and activity level were the only subscale scores associated with illness behavior. The relationship between extraversion and behavior is complicated. Highly assertive subjects manifested more pain behavior at home and during clinical interviews when they were unobtrusively observed. In contrast, they also reported less lifestyle disruption (i.e., sickness impact) and fewer incidents of solicitous behavior (e.g., from family members) that could represent secondary gain. Several reports (Eysenck 1967; Gordon and Hitchcock 1983; Harkins et al. 1989) support the finding that extraverts express their suffering more frequently than do introverts.

Fig. 9. Affective VAS responses to clinical pain plotted as a function of sensory VAS responses to clinical pain for myofascial pain dysfunction patients with (A) high and low extraversion (E) scores and (B) for patients with high and low neuroticism (N) scores. Sensory-affective functions were similar for extraversion groups, while the affective ratings of high N patients were higher than those of low N patients for equivalent sensory intensity ratings. Adapted from Harkins et al. (1989), with permission.

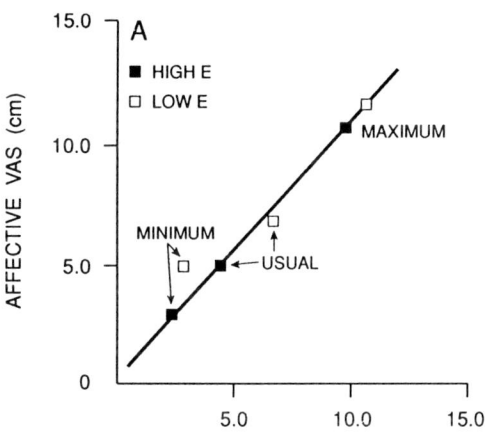

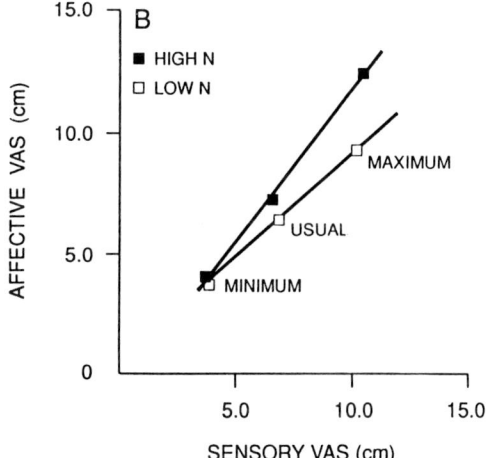

Effects of culture, gender, and age

Since the classical writings of Aurelius and Sophocles, investigators have considered the impact of demographic factors on pain processing. The literature addressing the association between ethnicity and pain has come to contradictory conclusions (see Wade and Price 1999 for review). A major problem with nearly all such studies is that each examines only one or two simple measures of pain or psychophysiological response. Thus, a literature review by Zatzick and Dimsdale (1990) concluded that little evidence supports cultural differences in responses to pain.

For the most part, pain and gender studies suggest that compared to men, women have a lower pain threshold (Leon 1974; Ellermeier and Westphal 1995) and lower pain tolerance (Woodrow et al. 1972; Dubreuil and Kohn

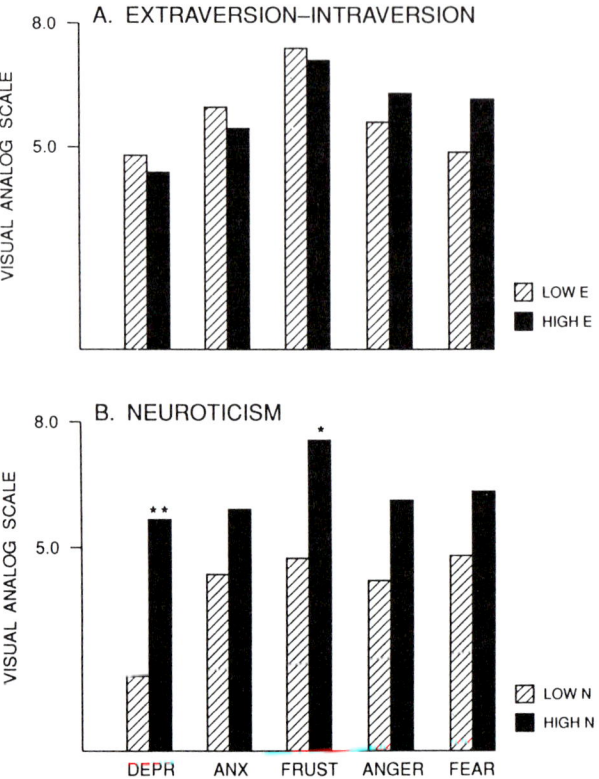

Fig. 10. Mean VAS ratings of the same patients as in Figs. 8 and 9 in response to judgments of magnitudes of depression (DEPR), anxiety (ANX), frustration (FRUST), anger, and fear. Patients with high neuroticism scores rated depression and frustration higher than did those with low scores (**$P < 0.01$; *$P < 0.05$). Adapted from Harkins et al. (1989), with permission.

1986). These studies used a variety of experimentally induced pain techniques such as heat, cold, pressure application, and electric shock. A meta-analysis conducted by Riley et al. (1998) concluded that women have slightly greater pain sensitivity than men; however, the effect sizes across studies were relatively small. Similar to the ethnicity and age literature, most of the gender and pain studies focus on the sensory-discriminative dimension and give little regard to other components of pain. One study included an assessment of immediate pain unpleasantness and the secondary stage of pain affect (Bush et al. 1993). This study detected no gender-related differences for pain sensation intensity or immediate pain unpleasantness associated with either experimental or clinical pain, and also found no such differences the secondary stage of pain affect.

Studies examining the relationship between age and pain are similar to the pain and ethnicity literature for two reasons. First, these studies have focused primarily on the first stage of pain processing–pain sensation intensity. Second, their findings are contradictory (Woodrow et al. 1972; Harkins et al. 1986; McMillan 1989; Sorkin et al. 1990). The earlier studies using a variety of experimental pain stimuli and threshold or tolerance measures point to an increase in pain threshold with advancing age (Chapman and Jones 1944; Sherman and Robillard 1964; Procacci et al. 1970; McMillan 1989). Other studies (e.g., Mumford 1965) have found no age effects for pain tolerance or threshold. More recent studies (Harkins et al. 1986) have used direct scaling techniques to evaluate threshold and suprathreshold levels of experimental pain sensitivity and demonstrate a much stronger similarity than variability across the lifespan.

Bearing in mind the limitations of most previous demographic studies of pain, Harkins and Price (1992) examined the extent to which age influenced the magnitude of the various stages of pain processing in chronic pain patients. As shown in Fig. 11, no effects of age were evident for pain sensation or immediate unpleasantness ratings, consistent with previous results obtained for experimental pain (Harkins et al. 1986). Thus, no age

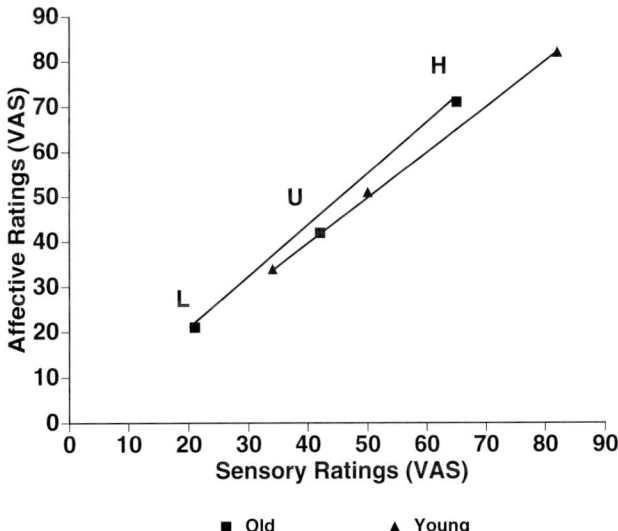

Fig. 11. Mean VAS ratings of pain sensation intensity and pain unpleasantness in elderly (mean age 69 years) and young (mean age 37 years) chronic pain patients. Sensory ratings are plotted on the *x*-axis against unpleasantness on the *y*-axis. Ratings are for chronic pain at its lowest (L), usual (U), and highest (H) levels over the past week. No significant group differences were observed. Based on Harkins and Price (unpublished data).

effects were observed for in the first two stages of pain processing. However, age had large (>1.5 VAS units) and selective effects on the secondary
stage of pain affect and illness behavior, with older adults (>65 years old)
manifesting lower mean ratings of negative emotional feelings as compared
to younger patients. Older pain patients had considerably lower ratings of
anxiety, frustration, anger, and fear (Fig. 12) and significantly lower composite ratings of the five pain-related emotional feelings. J. Riley et al. (unpublished manuscript, 1999) also observed a highly selective and relatively
potent effect of age on the secondary stage of pain affect in 1712 chronic
pain patients. This effect was perhaps related to lower lifestyle disruption
and less concern for future consequences in the elderly. For example, older
pain patients would be less likely to be dealing with concerns such as the
interaction of pain with their employment, their children's college tuition, or
other mid-life issues. Older adults may view pain as less of a long-term
threat, resulting in less suffering. Similar to the studies of personality factors on the stages of pain processing, this study further validates the sequential model of pain processing by showing a selective impact of a given
factor on the secondary stage of pain affect.

Personality factors and age (but not gender) have their greatest influence on later stages of pain processing—suffering and illness behavior. This
finding reinforces the uniqueness and separateness of these later stages of
pain. Although the literature cited above demonstrates an association

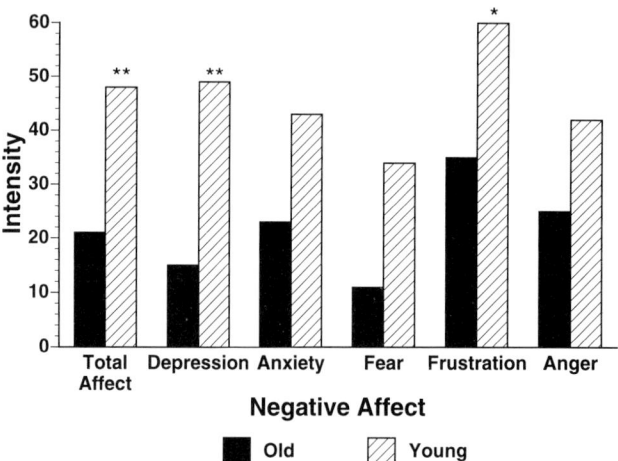

Fig. 12. Ratings of pain-related emotions in chronic pain patients. Old and young
patients (as in Fig. 11) rated levels of depression, anxiety, anger, and fear specifically
associated with their chronic pain. Elderly patients had reduced VAS ratings of pain-
related emotional feelings, but did not have reduced ratings of pain sensation or
unpleasantness (* $P < 0.05$; ** $P < 0.01$). Based on Harkins and Price (unpublished data).

between measures of normal personality (mainly neuroticism and extraversion) and pain-related suffering, it does not clearly assign a causal relationship between these variables. One possibility is that life-long depression and enduring anxiety contribute to a pattern of catastrophizing that exacerbates emotional disturbance in chronic pain patients. An alternative explanation is that increasing lifestyle disruption resulting from pain leads to an intensification of suffering. The latter hypothesis is a particularly plausible explanation for age effects on secondary pain affect. Thus, although pain sensation and immediate pain unpleasantness may be similar across age groups, less lifestyle disruption and consequently less suffering may occur in the elderly.

TESTING THE SEQUENTIAL MODEL WITH LINEAR STRUCTURAL EQUATION MODELING

A final line of evidence for the sequential model of pain processing comes from multivariate (LISREL) analysis (Wade et al. 1996). Path analysis with chronic pain patients demonstrated that VAS could be used to assess pain sensation intensity and pain-related unpleasantness and suffering (stage two affect). Structured interviews (Getto and Heaton 1985) and self-report inventories were shown to be adequate means of assessing pain-related behavior, which was conceptualized as a final stage of pain processing. This stage reflects the activities of daily living that are influenced by pain (e.g., number of hours spent in bed during the day). Exploratory analysis of data from 506 patients and confirmatory analysis of data from a second sample of 502 patients confirmed a high goodness of fit for the sequential model. Comparison of the model to alternative ones that contain parallel processing showed that the sequential model provided the best fit.

IMPLICATIONS OF THE SEQUENTIAL PROCESSING MODEL FOR PAIN MEASUREMENT AND ASSESSMENT

If pain comprises different dimensions and stages of processing, and if psychological, pharmacological, and physiological factors can selectively influence a given stage of processing or dimension, then measurement and assessment of pain ideally should address each of these dimensions and stages. For example, just as some personality traits and age strongly and selectively influence the secondary stage of pain affect, so might some psychological therapeutic interventions exert their greatest influence at this level. Multidimensional assessment appears most critical for chronic pain management. If chronic pain is multidimensional and multiple treatments are used in its management, then its assessment likewise needs separate measures of nociception, immediate pain-related affective disturbance, affective disturbance reflective of suffering, and overt pain behavior.

As discussed earlier, cancer pain patients give significantly higher VAS affective ratings of their pain as compared to sensory ratings, whereas the reverse is true for women in labor. Thus, simple antinociceptive treatments that are directed mechanistically toward reducing the sensation of pain may not offer adequate pain control for some cancer patients, for whom any amount of pain may carry a strongly negative implication. Thus, psychological therapies may be especially important in pain management in such patients. Similarly, personality traits such as neuroticism may enhance the overall sense of hopelessness and anxiety associated with living with chronic pain. In such cases, group therapies and support groups may allow us to become aware of the processes by which different patients develop meanings associated with the secondary stage of pain affect. Nevertheless, even when a strictly antinociceptive treatment is given for a chronic pain patient, its impact on the several stages of pain processing may vary as a function of several possible intervening psychological factors. Consequently, the assessment of various stages of pain is of paramount importance in chronic pain patients—even when the treatments given for such pain are directed only toward reducing nociceptive processing. Studies of the secondary stage of pain-related affect can only be carried out in chronic pain patients, since this stage involves more reflective cognitive processes that occur during suffering. The secondary stage of pain-related affect, based on cognitive processes directed toward long-term implications and more elaborate meanings, is of considerable importance for patients with cancer pain and for others with severe, debilitating chronic pain. Just as some pharmacological and psychological factors can reduce pain sensation intensity and immediate pain unpleasantness, others may selectively reduce the secondary stage of pain-related affect.

These considerations also have important implications for neurophysiological analysis of the affective-motivational dimension of pain. Even the identification of neurons, pathways, and central nervous system regions involved in pain-related affect depends on our capacity to relate their responses to measurable aspects of the affective dimension of pain, similar to the approach required for identification of neurons involved in the sensory-discriminative dimension of pain.

Psychological Mechanisms of Pain and Analgesia, Progress in Pain Research and Management, Vol. 15, by Donald D. Price, IASP Press, Seattle, © 1999.

4

Primary Afferent and Dorsal Horn Mechanisms of Pain

Previous chapters have emphasized that pain has unique sensory qualities, psychophysical attributes, and associations with several levels and types of emotions. This brings us to question which peripheral nociceptive and central neural mechanisms are related to these characteristics of pain and how these mechanisms can help to explain the qualities of pain. This chapter describes primary afferent and dorsal horn mechanisms that underlie the encoding and transmission of somatosensory signals related to pain. The following chapter will discuss brain mechanisms that further explain the encoding and transmission of these signals and how different components and dimensions of pain are represented within the central nervous system (CNS).

PRIMARY AFFERENT NOCICEPTIVE NEURONS

Throughout the body, certain receptors respond optimally to stimuli that would result in tissue damage if maintained over time. These receptors, termed nociceptors, are innervated by primary afferent neurons (Fig. 1), and the impulse activity they generate results in pain under most conditions. Although critical for pain, such receptors are not called pain receptors, because pain is not an inevitable consequence of activation of nociceptors. Pain can occur without activation of nociceptors, and nociception can occur without pain. The functions of primary nociceptive afferent neurons are to transduce chemical, thermal, or mechanical energy into action potentials and then to transmit information about the intensity of nociceptive stimuli. This information is coded by the frequency of action potentials in the population of nociceptive afferents. Transmission also involves the release of neurotransmitters by nociceptive afferent neurons onto second-order neurons of the dorsal horn of the spinal cord (Fig. 1). The latter, in turn, transmit nociceptive information over ascending pathways to the brain, where such information is further processed and is likely to result in the experience of pain. Nociceptive neurons also elicit a variety of responses at

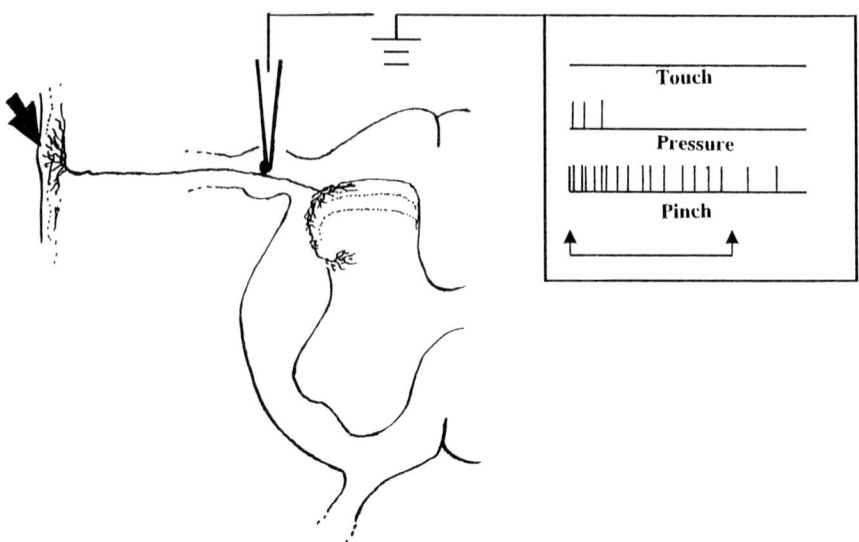

Fig. 1. Primary nociceptive afferent neuron and its synapse projected onto neurons of the dorsal horn of the spinal cord. Intracellular recording of the neuron allows a tracer (horseradish peroxidase) to be injected into the cell so that the neuron can be anatomically characterized. Recordings of action potentials from similar types of neurons allow their physiological characterization.

several levels of the CNS, including spinal cord withdrawal reflexes and autonomic and neuroendocrine responses, as well as the behavioral consequences of general alertness, arousal, and orientation.

EARLY DISCOVERIES LEADING TO FUNCTIONAL CLASSES
OF PRIMARY NOCICEPTIVE NEURONS

The general characteristics of nociceptive primary afferent neurons became known concurrently with studies of axons within peripheral nerves and studies of general functions of classes of axons. However, prior to the development of methods for physiological and anatomical characterization of axons within peripheral nerves, Henry Head concluded in 1893 that the skin was served by *epicritic* and *protopathic* afferent systems, each of which gave rise to its own particular types of sensations (Head 1920). Epicritic pain, for example, was considered to be accurately localized, to not outlast the stimulus, and to provide precise qualitative information about the nature of the stimulus. Thus, epicritic pain could be elicited by mild pricking of the skin with a needle (a test for which Head and other neurologists since his time have developed a strong penchant). In contrast, protopathic pain was described as less well localized, slow in onset, often outlasting the stimulus, and summating with repeated stimulus application. Protopathic pain was considered more difficult to endure and to contain special feelings of unpleasantness or "feeling tone." Head based these ideas largely on observations of his own experiences of pain after cutting his own cutaneous peripheral nerve and during the course of nerve regeneration.

With the advent of modern electrophysiological and neuroanatomical techniques, it became clear that pain depended on two types of peripheral nerve axons: thinly myelinated Aδ axons and unmyelinated C axons, whose conduction velocities range between 3 and 30 m/s and between 0.5 and 2.0 m/s, respectively. Based on their differences in conduction velocity and reminiscent of Head's functional dichotomy, Zotterman (1933) hypothesized that Aδ and C afferent axons could account for first and second pain that often occurs in response to a brief, intense stimulus to the hand or foot. Landau and Bishop (1953) explicitly related first pain to epicritic pain and second pain to protopathic pain. Interestingly, their approach was similar to that of Head. They carefully observed and recorded their own pain experiences in response to "experimental" pain stimuli before and after selective conduction block of Aδ or C axons of peripheral nerves. They used local injections of dilute solutions of procaine to selectively block C axons within small nerve branches in order to study pain from impulses in Aδ axons. They selectively blocked all myelinated axons in peripheral nerves of their lower arms by means of a 250 mm Hg pressure cuff to assess the types of pains evoked by impulses in C axons. They applied various types of painful stimuli to skin, fascia, and periosteal surfaces, including bee stings, turpentine injections, intramuscular potassiun chloride injections, and application of deep and sharp pressure with mechanical probes. When they blocked C axons with procaine, well-localized, stinging, sharp pains of brief duration, such as those elicited by pin pricks, were preserved, but prolonged, deep, and diffuse burning pains evoked by inflammatory stimuli, such as the delayed pain from a bee sting, could no longer be elicited. When they blocked all myelinated (A) axons by means of the blood pressure cuff, however, the latter types of pain were more intense than they were before blockade of myelinated axons. These general observations have since been corroborated in studies using individuals other than the investigators themselves as subjects (Collins et al. 1960; Price 1972). Collins et al. (1960) monitored compound action potentials by placing stimulating and recording electrodes under the sural nerve of cancer patients undergoing anterolateral cordotomy for relief of pain. Stimulation of Aδ axons produced sharp, painful sensations that were accurately localized. When Aδ axons were blocked by cold, stimulation of C axons at a rate of 3 impulses/second resulted in unbearable summating pain that was diffuse, burning, and less well localized.

Confirmation of *epicritic* and *protopathic* pain and their relation to Aδ and C axons does not require such elaborate extremes and need not place such burdens on experimental observers. Observations can be made while the ulnar nerve is partially blocked by pressure so that the lateral portion of the hand becomes very numb (i.e., "falls asleep"). Folds of skin can be briefly pinched as the hand becomes more numb (i.e., the block progresses). At about the time at which myelinated axons become blocked, quickly pinching a fold of numb skin evokes pain, but only after a delay of a second or more. Compared to painful sensation evoked by a similar pinch of normal skin, the pain is stronger, lasts much longer, and has more of a burning quality. This "experiment" demonstrates that even Aβ afferents contribute to the sensory qualities of both first and second pain. When the hand becomes numb to the point at which light touch is no longer perceived, the qualities of pinch-induced pain, including first and second pain, become less blunt, sharper, and longer lasting (Price 1972).

The association of first and second pain with impulses in Aδ and C axons and the relationship of these two types of pain to epicritic and protopathic pain have pivotal roles in the history of pain research. However, like all functional dichotomies, it is important not to overgeneralize their explanatory role, for example, to prematurely label different central pain-related pathways as "epicritic" or "protopathic." Head himself (1920) warned against this type of error when he concluded that epicritic and protopathic systems *recombine once they entered the dorsal horn.* Thus, although he found zones of relatively pure epicritic or protopathic sensibility after dorsal root or peripheral nerve lesions, he never observed such zones after lesions of the spinal cord or brain. More than 40 years before electrophysiological studies were conducted on dorsal horn nociceptive neurons, Head anticipated the synaptic convergence of two functional types of primary nociceptive afferents (known since as Aδ and C) onto neurons of the dorsal horn.

Aδ and C nociceptive afferents are rarely activated in isolation; most acute pains are likely to reflect a combination of input from both types of nociceptive afferents, and in some cases from non-nociceptive afferents as well. Indeed, the *composition* of input from different types of afferents undoubtedly contributes to the diverse qualities of both painful and nonpainful somatic sensation. However, many pains of long duration, especially those that are diffuse, inflammatory, and particularly unpleasant in their "feeling tone," may depend to a greater extent on tonic input from C than from Aδ nociceptive afferents. Initial pains from abrupt injuries (e.g., stepping on a tack) are likely to depend heavily on Aδ nociceptive afferents.

FUNCTIONAL CHARACTERIZATION OF PRIMARY NOCICEPTIVE AFFERENT NEURONS

With the advent of modern electrophysiological methods, Perl and his colleagues (Perl 1968; Burgess and Perl 1973) developed techniques for recording and physiologically characterizing distinct classes of primary afferent nociceptive neurons. Based on interrelated lines of evidence, several types of primary nociceptive afferents have been well characterized as having a critical role in nociception and hence pain.

The first stage in the characterization of primary nociceptive afferents is to establish that the type of neuron in question has both peripheral and central anatomical connections that are consistent with a role in nociception. For example, using intracellular microelectrode recording, electrophysiologists such as Light and Perl (1979) have recorded action potentials from a single dorsal root ganglion cell in response to nociceptive stimuli (e.g., mechanical pinch) applied to the receptive field of that neuron (Fig. 1). The receptive field is that region (or structure) which upon stimulation causes an increase in action potential frequency. Receptive field mapping established the peripheral anatomical connectivity of primary nociceptive afferent neurons. The central connectivities of such neurons were established by injecting a tracer, such as horseradish peroxidase, into them by means of the same microelectrode used for recording, and then anatomically examining their central terminals and synapses within the dorsal horn (Fig. 1). These elegant experiments demonstrated that some types of primary nociceptive neurons respond optimally to nociceptive stimulation and have peripheral and central anatomical connections consistent with a role in nociception and pain.

The second stage is to establish that the neuron in question responds to and can convey precise information about nociceptive stimulus intensity, consistent with human psychophysical ratings of similar stimuli, as described in Chapter 2. Thus, some $A\delta$ mechanothermal and C-polymodal nociceptive afferent neurons respond in a positively accelerating manner over the range of skin stimulus temperatures that would evoke increasing pain ratings in human observers (Fig. 1). Both the psychophysical ratings and neural responses are power functions with an exponent greater than 2. Moreover, some of these neurons, like psychophysical subjects, respond differentially to very small differences in nociceptive stimulus intensity, within the order of 0.2°–0.3°C. Taken together, these types of data establish that some types of primary nociceptive neurons can code precise information about nociceptive stimulus intensity and detect small differences in intensity.

A third and critical line of evidence for an important role in nociception and pain is that selective stimulation of a given type of primary nociceptive neuron gives rise to pain. For example, selective blocking of myelinated axons of a peripheral nerve provides the capacity to determine whether impulses in C nociceptive afferents are necessary or sufficient for pain. In primate cutaneous limb nerves, over 90% of C axons are from nociceptive neurons (Burgess and Perl 1973; Beitel and Dubner 1976a,b). Thus, nociceptive heat stimulation of skin that is functionally innervated only by C axons is likely to selectively activate C nociceptive neurons. Under conditions wherein A afferents of a nerve are blocked by asphyxia or pressure, a heat pulse of 51°C delivered to the skin results in a delayed burning pain, the "second pain" identified in experiments described earlier (Price et al. 1977). Similarly, both "first pain" and brief latency responses of Aδ heat-nociceptive afferents can be evoked by a heat pulse of 51°C, suggesting that input from this type of nociceptive afferent is sufficient for pain (Price et al. 1977). Microstimulation of different types of nociceptive afferents also gives rise to pain (Torebjork and Hallin 1974). Thus, selective stimulation of various types of primary nociceptive afferent neurons, including Aδ and C nociceptive afferent neurons, can elicit pain in human subjects.

Taken together, these lines of evidence have established the role of specific classes of primary nociceptive afferent neurons in nociception and pain. Several types of primary nociceptive afferent neurons have been characterized and implicated in pain over the last 35 years.

EVIDENCE FOR INVOLVEMENT OF CLASSES OF NEURONS IN NOCICEPTION AND PAIN

Cutaneous nociceptive afferents

Aδ nociceptive afferents. Three types of Aδ cutaneous nociceptive afferent neurons have been characterized (Treede et al. 1998). These include high-threshold mechanoreceptive (HTM) afferents and type I and II mechanothermal (MT) nociceptive afferents. HTM afferents respond exclusively to intense and potentially damaging mechanical stimulation of skin, whereas type I and II Aδ MT afferents respond to both intense mechanical and heat nociceptive stimuli. Important differences were found when type I and II MT were compared for responses to an intense heat stimulus (53°C, 30 seconds). Type I was characterized by a long latency (mean 5 seconds) and a late peak discharge (16 seconds), and type II by a short latency (mean 0.2 seconds) and an early peak discharge (0.5 seconds). Type I neurons exhibited faster conduction velocities (25 vs. 14 m/s) and higher heat thresholds than type II neurons (53° vs. 47°C, 1-second duration). Thus, type II MC neurons are most likely to provide the basis for the first pain sensation induced by a brief noxious heat stimulus. They are also likely to account for brief latency escape responses of primates and other mammals to rapid noxious heat stimuli. On the other hand, type I A-fiber nociceptors likely signal pain associated with long-duration heat stimuli and may contribute to first pain sensation evoked by mechanical stimuli.

C-polymodal nociceptive afferents. This is an extremely important group of nociceptive afferents because it comprises the vast majority of unmyelinated cutaneous afferents in primates (80–90% in monkeys and more than 90% in humans) (Burgess and Perl 1973; Price and Dubner 1977); unmyelinated afferents outnumber myelinated ones by three or four to one. They are optimally responsive to at least three distinct forms of nociceptive stimulation, including thermal, mechanical, and chemical stimuli (Burgess and Perl 1973). Hence, the term "polymodal nociceptor" has been used to designate this class of primary afferent neuron. Approximately one-third of C-polymodal nociceptive neurons also respond to noxious cold stimuli (<10°C) (Burgess and Perl 1973). Similar to Aδ mechanothermal neurons, their responses to graded intensities of nociceptive temperatures are monotonic, positively accelerating functions, with maximum sensitivity in the 45°–53°C range (Beitel and Dubner 1976a,b). These neurons can respond differentially to very small differences in intensity (0.2°–0.3°C) within this range (LaMotte and Campbell 1978). They may account for the ability to scale differences in slowly rising or long-duration heat pain, but cannot account for first pain or rapid escape responses to sudden noxious heat stimuli.

Both Aδ and C-polymodal nociceptive neurons can undergo sensitization. After damage to the skin or during inflammatory conditions, such neurons can become spontaneously active, have lowered thresholds to mechanical and thermal stimuli, and show enhanced responses to suprathreshold stimulation. Sensitization of primary nociceptive afferent neurons is the basis of primary hyperalgesia and represents a vast topic that is covered in detail by others (Meyer and Campbell 1981; LaMotte et al. 1982).

Muscle nociceptive afferent neurons

Several types of primary afferent neurons innervate muscle, including those classified as low-threshold mechanosensitive afferents and others that are nociceptive (Kumazawa and Mizumura 1976, 1977a). Similar to cutaneous nociceptive afferents, those innervating muscle include slow-conducting, unmyelinated (C) and possibly Aδ afferents. Presumably, muscle nociceptive afferents supply many free nerve endings found in connective tissue of the muscle, between muscle fibers, in blood vessel walls, or in tendons (Mense and Schmidt 1977; Willis 1985). Although the evidence for Aδ muscle nociceptive afferent neurons is equivocal, there is substantial support for the role of unmyelinated C muscle nociceptive afferent neurons in pain (Kumazawa and Mizumura 1976, 1977a). They are excited by algesic chemicals and are optimally responsive to strong, presumably nociceptive, mechanical stimuli. According to Kumazawa and Mizumura (1976), C muscle nociceptive afferents are similar to C-polymodal nociceptive afferents that innervate the skin; muscle C afferents that were excited by nociceptive heating were also excited by mechanical stimuli and by algesic chemicals. Mense and Stahnke (1983) found that many C muscle afferent neurons responded weakly or not at all to muscle contractions and yet responded quite vigorously to the same intensity of contractions during ischemia. They suggested that such afferents might contribute to ischemic muscle pain.

General evidence suggests that activation of Aδ and C muscle nociceptive afferent neurons results in excitation of dorsal horn sensory projection neurons (Mense and Schmidt 1977; Willis 1985). Since pain can be evoked in humans from the types of stimuli used to activate C muscle nociceptive afferents, their selective activation may well be sufficient for pain. Thus, available studies of C muscle nociceptive afferent neurons provide several lines of evidence for their involvement in pain.

Visceral nociceptive afferents

Visceral pain has several unique features that distinguish it from muscular and especially cutaneous pain. First of all, visceral pain often is not well localized or discriminated in terms of the type of stimulus evoking it (Gebhart 1995). Second, visceral pain is often referred to a cutaneous somatic region (Arendt-Nielson 1997), which can become tender. This tenderness is likely to be a form of secondary hyperalgesia or allodynia. Finally, at least in a general sense, visceral nociceptive afferent neurons evoke central effects generally similar to those evoked by cutaneous C-polymodal nociceptive neurons; visceral pain demonstrates considerable spatial and temporal summation and is often accompanied by long-duration autonomic and somatic reflexes (Gebhart 1995; Arendt-Nielson 1997).

The general characteristics of visceral primary nociceptive afferent neurons can be illustrated by the work of Kumazawa and Mizumura (1977b), who studied testicular nociceptive afferent responses to precisely quantified mechanical and thermal stimuli and algesic chemicals. Both Aδ and C afferents responded to mechanical pressure applied to dogs' testicles over a range of 30–2000 g. The lower end of this range would not be at all painful and the upper end would be distinctly painful when applied to dog or human testicles. Thus, the response range of these afferents is consistent with human experience. Mechanical pressure applied to the testicles can elicit both nonpainful and painful sensations, depending on stimulus intensity. The same afferents also responded to algesic chemicals and reacted in a graded fashion to increasing nociceptive temperatures, becoming sensitized when the latter stimuli were repeated. Therefore, these afferents have similar physiological characteristics to C-polymodal nociceptive afferents that innervate the skin. Monkey spinothalamic tract neurons of the dorsal horn of upper lumbar segments respond to similar stimuli applied to the testicles (Willis 1985). Thus, it is likely that Aδ and C testicular afferents of the type just described synaptically converge on and excite these central neurons. However, it is not known whether selective stimulation of either Aδ or C testicular afferents is sufficient to evoke testicular pain. Thus, available studies of testicular nociceptive afferent neurons provide moderately strong evidence for their involvement in pain.

Similar evidence demonstrates that both Aδ and C nociceptive afferents innervate the heart, gastrointestinal tract, bile duct, and urinary bladder (Gebhart 1995). Primary afferent neurons presumed to innervate structures near capillaries of the lung, called type J receptors (Willis 1985; Gebhart 1995), are activated by lung deflation and large lung inflations, as well as by stimuli that irritate lung tissue. Many of these are likely to have a nociceptive function and are unmyelinated.

Although much more research is needed to characterize primary nociceptive afferent neurons innervating noncutaneous structures, it is becoming evident that similar principles in nociceptor functioning extend across different tissues (Burgess and Perl 1973; Price 1988; Gebhart 1995; Arendt-Nielson 1997). First, for most innervated tissues, classes of primary nociceptive neurons can be distinguished from low-threshold mechanoreceptive and thermoreceptive neurons. Second, C-polymodal nociceptive afferent neurons similar to those innervating the skin comprise a large proportion of the nociceptive neurons innervating visceral organs. Similar to cutaneous C-polymodal nociceptive neurons, C nociceptive afferent neurons innervating viscera and muscle may well account for pains that are diffuse, poorly localized, and poorly discriminated in terms of sensory modality. These pains are especially prevalent in inflammation and in certain diseases. Third, at least for some visceral structures such as the testicles and gastrointestinal tract, many primary nociceptive afferent neurons respond over a broad stimulus range, extending from intensities that would not be at all painful to those which would be extremely painful (Gebhart 1995). Such a broad response range is consistent with human experience. We experience gastrointestinal sensations every day that range in intensity from barely detectable and not at all painful to distinctly painful.

DORSAL HORN MECHANISMS OF NOCICEPTION AND PAIN

NEURONS OF ORIGIN OF ASCENDING PATHWAYS FOR PAIN

All types of primary nociceptive afferent neurons described in the preceding section converge on and synaptically excite neurons of the dorsal
horn of the spinal cord and medulla (trigeminal dorsal horn) (Fig. 2). The
dorsal horn neurons that receive this input are of two general physiological
types and constitute the main origin of pain pathways that ascend from the
spinal cord or medulla oblongata to the brain (Willis 1985; Price 1988). The
first type, termed *nociceptive-specific* (NS) neurons, receive exclusive input
from primary nociceptive afferents (Fig. 2, top right). Consistent with this
restricted input from nociceptors, these second-order sensory neurons respond nearly exclusively to intense and often painful levels of somatic stimulation. The second type, termed *wide-dynamic-range* (WDR) neurons, receive synaptic contacts from low-threshold mechanoreceptive primary

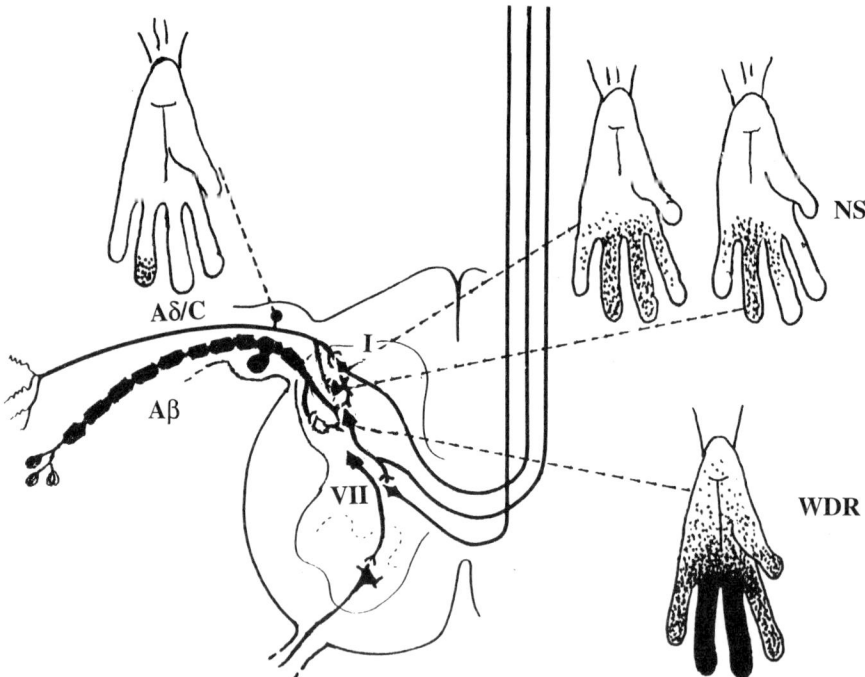

Fig. 2. Synaptic convergence of primary nociceptive afferent neurons onto nociceptive-specific (NS) and wide-dynamic-range (WDR) dorsal horn neurons. Similar to
primary nociceptive neurons, these second-order neurons have stimulus-response functions that are consistent with the types of primary afferent neurons that synapse onto
them. They project their axons into ascending spinal pathways for pain.

afferents (related to touch and other nonpainful types of mechanoreceptive sensibilities) as well as from primary nociceptive afferents (Fig. 2, bottom right). As a consequence of these multiple types of input, WDR dorsal horn neurons respond with increasing impulse frequencies over an extensive range of stimulus intensity, extending from very gentle touch to distinctly painful levels of stimulation.

Both WDR and NS neurons have axons that project to multiple levels of the brain and often have collateral axonal branches that project to several brainstem sites (Fig. 3). These central targets include reticular formation nuclei of the lower brainstem and midbrain, deep layers of the superior colliculus, the periaqueductal gray, parabrachial nuclei, hypothalamus, and various ventrolateral and medial thalamic nuclei. To some extent, these multiple projections reflect multiple functional consequences of nociceptive input and are likely to contribute to many components of pain behavior and experience (discussed in Chapter 5).

Consistent with the types of somatosensory information conveyed by neurons of origin of these ascending pathways, anterolateral quadrant lesions that interrupt axons of these major ascending pathways produce profound temporary analgesia and deficits in temperature and tactile sensations (White and Sweet 1969). On the other hand, electrical stimulation of the anterolateral quadrant produces pain, tactile sensations, or innocuous thermal sensations, depending on the frequency and intensity of stimulation (Mayer et al. 1975; Coghill et al. 1993b).

CONVERGENCE OF CUTANEOUS, MUSCULAR, AND VISCERAL PRIMARY AFFERENTS ONTO DORSAL HORN NOCICEPTIVE NEURONS

Primary afferent nociceptive neurons that innervate muscle, skin, and viscera have synaptic terminals on dorsal horn nociceptive neurons. These neurons, from diverse tissue sources, often converge on and synaptically activate the same dorsal horn neuron, thereby explaining in part how pain is referred from such tissues (Foreman 1977; Foreman et al. 1977; Willis 1985). A fascinating pattern of convergence occurs in these neurons: the location of cutaneous, visceral, and muscular "receptive fields" can be predicted on the basis of known patterns of referred pain. For example, stimulation of cardiac sympathetic nerve axons excites WDR and NS spinothalamic tract neurons that are located at upper thoracic segmental levels of monkeys' spinal cords (Foreman 1977). The cutaneous receptive field of these neurons often extends along the inner aspect of the forearm, the pattern of pain referral in angina pectoralis. Similarly, spinothalamic neurons of upper lumbar segments can be excited both by nociceptive stimulation of the testicle

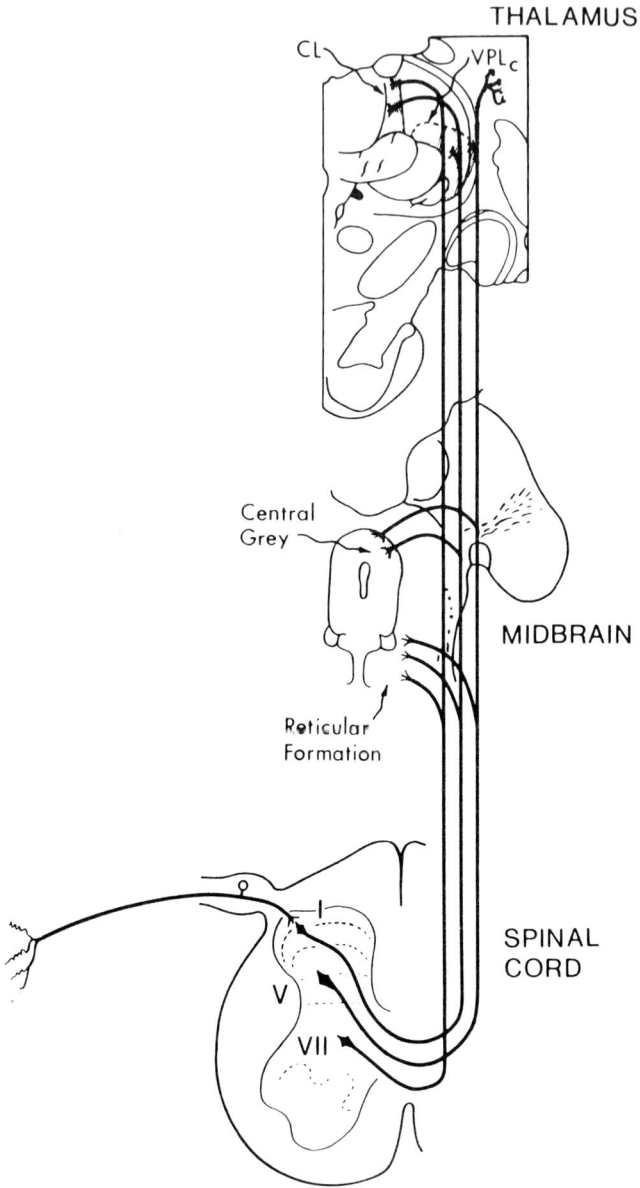

Fig. 3. Ascending brain projections of dorsal horn nociceptive neurons.

and by nociceptive and non-nociceptive stimulation of the upper flank and lower abdominal skin areas, areas of pain referral in testicular injury (Milne et al. 1981; Willis 1985). Some of these neurons also can be excited by overdistension of the urinary bladder.

The patterns of pain referral and tenderness in humans are strikingly similar to patterns of input from skin, viscera, and muscle nociceptive afferent neurons onto spinothalamic neurons of the dorsal horn of the spinal cord (see Willis 1985 for review). The parallel between patterns of pain referral in humans and patterns of physiological convergence observed in the monkey dorsal horn supports the convergence theory of referred pain. From psychological and physiological perspectives, this finding means that central pathways and central encoding mechanisms for visceral, muscular, and cutaneous pain are not likely to be radically different.

SPINAL CORD CODING MECHANISMS OF NOCICEPTION

Both NS and WDR dorsal horn neurons respond incrementally to increased nociceptive stimulus intensity. For example, both types of neurons follow positively accelerating power functions to increasing nociceptive temperatures, and these stimulus-response functions are very similar to those obtained in the psychophysical experiments described in Chapter 2. However, WDR neurons but not NS neurons have a very high discriminative capacity, as demonstrated in studies of WDR neurons recorded in awake monkeys trained in a discrimination task (Dubner et al. 1986; Maixner et al. 1986). Consistent with the monkeys' ability to detect very small shifts within the nociceptive temperature range, WDR neurons responded with distinctly higher impulse frequencies to shifts as small as 0.2°–0.4°C, as shown in Fig. 4. NS neurons were much less sensitive to these small differences. Therefore, dorsal horn WDR neurons represent a critical class of neuron necessary for the encoding of pain intensity. Their capacities to encode nociceptive stimulus intensity and small differences in the intensity of stimulation are like those of primary afferent neurons and are consistent with the discriminative capacity of human subjects in psychophysical experiments (see Chapter 2). Similar to other sensory modalities such as audition and vision, pain intensity is encoded partly by the frequency of action potentials.

These studies underscore the fact that pain is a highly discriminative sense as well as a powerful motivator of behavior. However, these two roles are interrelated. A monkey picking berries out of a thorny bush or an animal stalking prey across hot rocks pursues these tasks in order to eat. The animal must carefully weigh the painfulness of thorns or hot rocks against its need for food. In making such decisions, it must assess whether different objects in the environment or movements in different directions will result in *more* or *less* pain.

One apparent paradox that pertains to WDR neurons is that they respond to *both* gentle mechanical and nociceptive stimuli, yet are likely to be

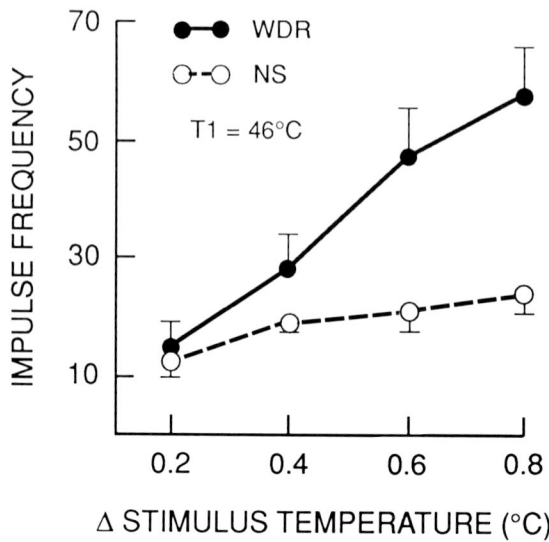

Fig. 4. Discriminative capacities of nociceptive-specific (NS) and wide-dynamic-range (WDR) neurons. Stimulus temperature was shifted in small increments (abscissa) from the baseline temperature of 46°C. WDR but not NS neurons significantly increased their impulse frequency (ordinate) in response to temperature shifts above 0.2°C. Reprinted from Maixner et al. (1986), with permission.

critical for conveying precise information about nociceptive stimulus intensity. As illustrated in Fig. 5, WDR neuron receptive fields have a relatively small area of skin within which increasing stimulus intensities ranging from extremely gentle to distinctly nociceptive produce graded differential responses (hence the term "wide dynamic range"). Surrounding this small zone is a much larger one in which only nociceptive stimuli evoke impulse discharge; they do so at a lower frequency than that evoked by touching the most sensitive zone. If gentle stimulation of the "sensitive" zone and nociceptive stimulation of the "surround" zone evoke the same frequency of action potentials, how can a single WDR neuron encode the distinction between a nociceptive and non-nociceptive stimulus?

The resolution of this paradox may emerge from the distinctive receptive field organization of WDR neurons, which may provide part of the basis for the neural encoding of pain at the spinal cord level (Price et al. 1976, 1978; Price 1988; Coghill et al. 1993b). Increases in receptive field size induced by peripheral and central sensitization mechanisms may partially account for allodynia and hyperalgesia found in neuropathic pain states and in other pain diseases (Dubner 1991; Price et al. 1994b). Given this common receptive field organization and a rostrocaudal somatotopic organization of WDR neurons within the dorsal horn along various spinal segments (e.g.,

Fig. 5. Receptive field organizations of two WDR neurons in anesthetized monkeys (designated A and B). The central portions (shown in black) of the receptive fields are areas wherein the neurons responded over a very wide range of stimulus intensities, as shown in both A and B. The surround areas (shown in stipple) were less sensitive, and only nociceptive stimuli were effective.

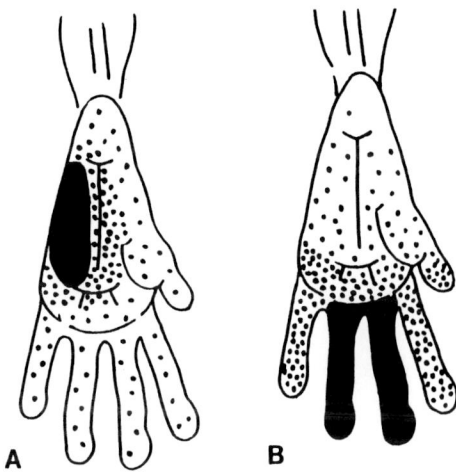

L2–S1), we would predict that a nociceptive stimulus would activate a much larger number of WDR neurons in comparison to a non-nociceptive stimulus. Furthermore, we would predict that progressively more intense nociceptive stimulation would recruit more and more spinal cord nociceptive central neurons along a greater number of spinal segments. For example, a gentle mechanical stimulus to the third or fourth toe would evoke a low-frequency impulse discharge in the WDR neuron whose receptive field is shown in Fig. 5 (right panel). It would not activate the neuron shown at the left in Fig. 5 because the toes are within the less sensitive zone of its receptive field. However, a strong nociceptive stimulus, such as pinch or 51°C to the third or fourth toe, would activate *both* WDR neurons because these sites are within the nociceptive zones of both neurons. The recruitment of both neurons as stimulus intensity progresses from gentle touch to painful levels could provide part of the basis for encoding the distinction between painful versus nonpainful somatosensory events as well as nociceptive stimulus intensity. Thus, although pain intensity is encoded by impulse frequency, it is the total impulse frequency in a large population of dorsal horn neurons that is critical.

Coghill et al. (1991, 1993a,b) used the ^{14}C-2-deoxyglucose (2-DG) method to further test the predictions of this concept of population coding based on WDR receptive field characteristics. The advantage of this technique is that it allows the simultaneous examination of responses of multiple CNS areas to a stimulus or behavioral condition. It does so by measuring local glucose utilization rates during a relatively long period (30–40 minutes). Thus, the technique is particularly suitable for mapping neural activity during prolonged noxious stimulation or ongoing nociception. The critical advantage of this technique is that it can provide a three-dimensional comparison of the spatial extents of dorsal horn neural activation resulting from different stimuli (Coghill et al. 1991; Porro 1991). Coghill's team compared responses to intense but innocuous stimulation, consisting of vigorous brushing of the rat's hindpaw, with nociceptive simulation from immersion of the same area of the hindpaw into a heated water bath. Mapping of spinal cord activity by the 2-DG method revealed that a nociceptive water temperature of 47°C activated extensive dorsal horn regions extending from L1 to L5 (Fig. 6). In contrast, vigorous but innocuous brushing evoked neural activity confined to the dorsal horn within L3. Thus, as predicted from previous studies of receptive field characteristics of WDR neurons, the distinction between non-nociceptive and nociceptive somatosensory events is at least partly reflected by differences in the spatial distribution, and hence, the relative numbers of spinal cord neurons activated by nociceptive and innocuous stimuli. This experimental approach also demonstrated that increasing levels of nociceptive heat stimuli resulted in progressively greater rostrocaudal activation within the deep layers of the dorsal horn, consistent with the hypothesis that intensity of nociceptive stimulation is partly represented by the number of neurons activated.

Pain intensity and the distinction between painful and nonpainful sensations evoked by electrical stimulation depend on both the intensity of electrical current (and hence number of axons activated) and the frequency of action potentials. In a series of studies of 21 patients undergoing percutaneous anterolateral cordotomy for relief of pain, an electrode was positioned within the anterolateral quadrant, that sector of spinal white matter that contains ascending spinothalamic and spinoreticular axons (Mayer et al. 1975; Coghill et al. 1993b). The patients were awake and were instructed to make judgments of pain threshold and pain intensity, which provided an unusual opportunity to determine the separate contributions of number of axons stimulated and frequency of action potentials to pain intensity. A precise trade-off was determined between these two factors, as is illustrated in Fig. 7. High frequencies of anterolateral quadrant stimulation (i.e., high action potential frequency) combined with low-stimulus currents (i.e., low number of axons activated) produced painful sensations such as burning or aching, as did low stimulus frequencies combined with higher stimulus currents. Furthermore, the intensity of pain increased when the investigators

---

Fig. 6. Spatial distribution of increased neural activity in response to immersion of the hindpaw in 35°C water (left), vigorous brushing of the hindlimb (BR; middle) or immersion of the same area of the hindpaw in a 47°C water bath (right). These maps are based on autoradiographs of metabolic rate increases as measured by the 2-DG method. Note the extensive rostrocaudal activation with 47°C stimulation in comparison to vigorous brushing. Reprinted from Coghill et al. (1993b), with permission.   ⟶

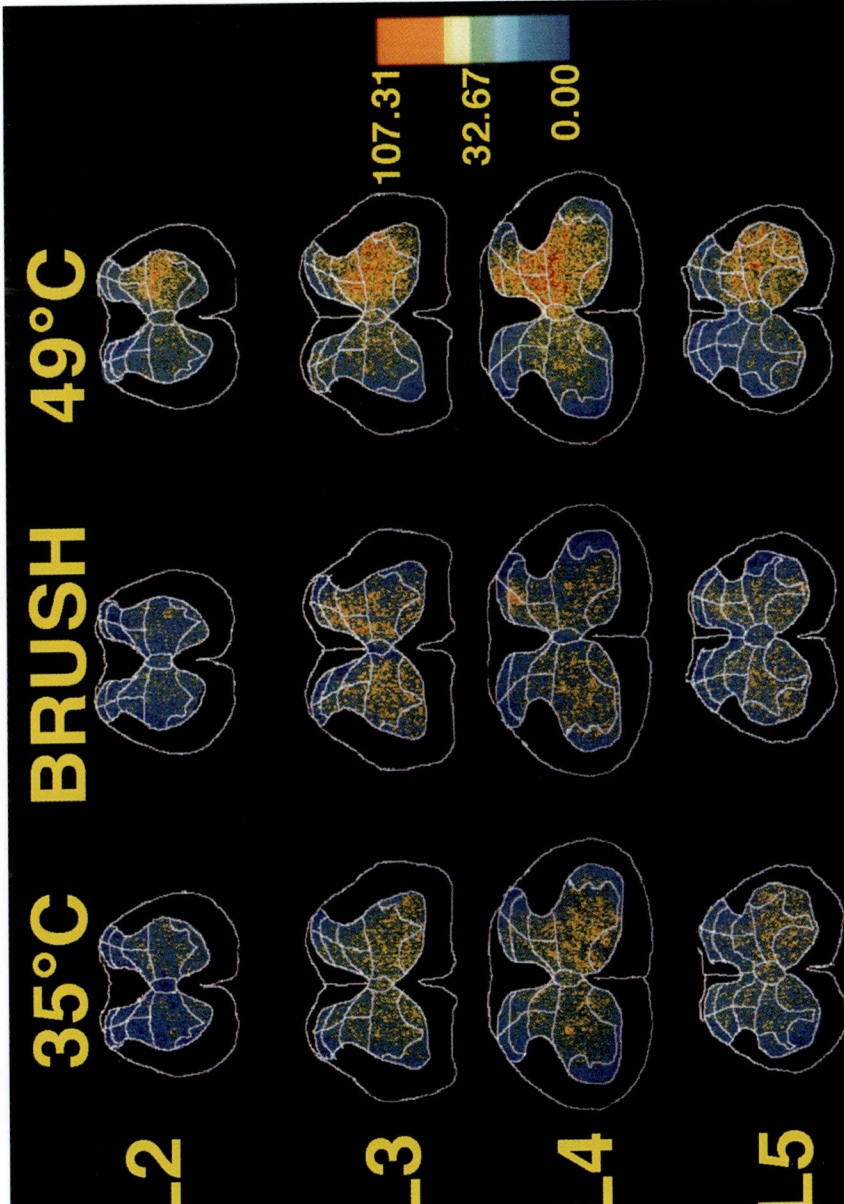

DONALD D. PRICE

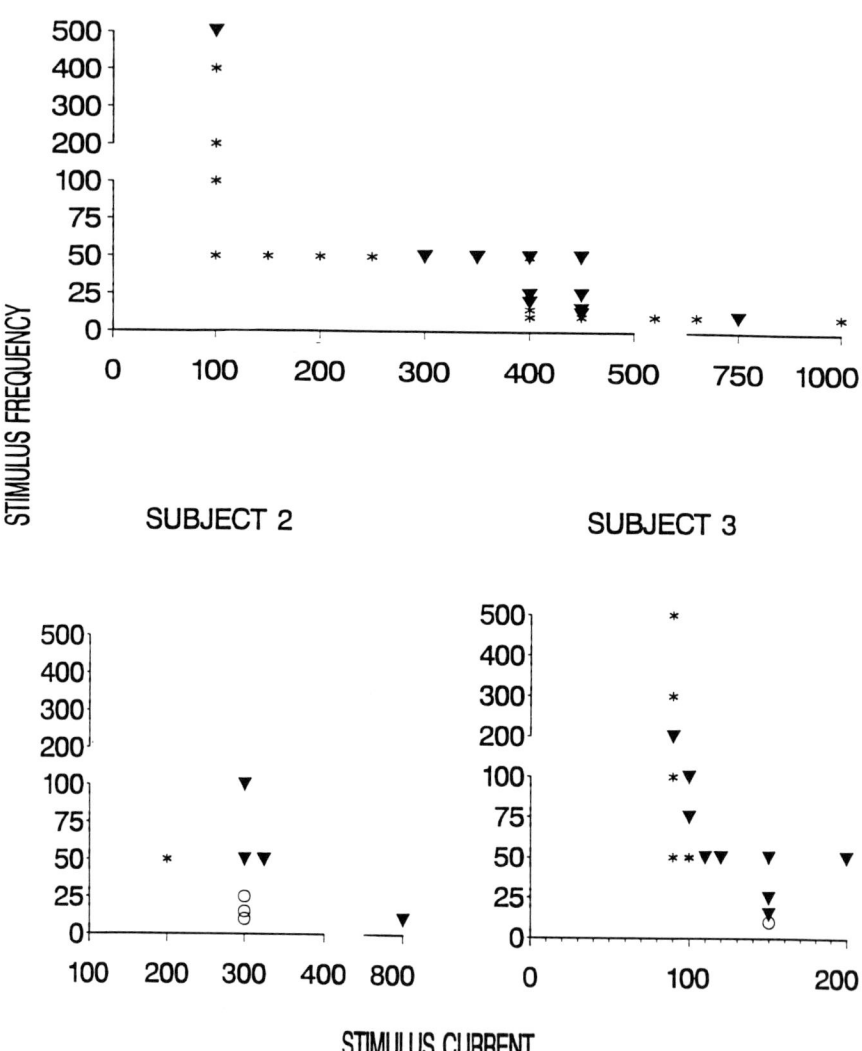

Fig. 7. An example of the relationship between stimulus frequency (Herz) and stimulus current (microamperes) with sensations elicited by anterolateral quadrant stimulation in awake patients. Different combinations of frequency and current (i.e., number of axons activated) produced no sensations (open circles), innocuous sensations (asterisks), or painful sensations (black triangles). From Coghill et al. (1993b), with permission.

raised the frequency of stimulation while holding stimulus intensity constant. It also increased when they raised the stimulus intensity (i.e., number of axons activated) while holding stimulus frequency constant. The trade-off between frequency and number of axons activated to evoke pain represents critical evidence that pain intensity is co-determined by action potential frequency and number of neurons recruited.

The results of these three separate types of studies—characterization of WDR neuron receptive field, 2-DG mapping, and anterolateral quadrant stimulation—converge to support an important hypothesis about pain-encoding mechanisms in the spinal cord. Both the frequency of action potentials and the total number of dorsal horn neurons activated contribute to the overall perceived intensity of pain and to the perceived distinction between painful and nonpainful somatic sensations. This hypothesis helps to explain two fundamental psychophysical properties of pain discussed in Chapter 2— spatial summation and radiation. Since increasing the area of nociceptive stimulation would activate more peripheral and central nociceptive neurons, spatial summation of pain would result from an increase in total number of neurons activated. However, simply increasing nociceptive stimulus intensity would also increase the total number of dorsal horn neurons activated along the rostrocaudal axis of the spinal cord, as demonstrated by the 2-DG experiments. This recruitment would include neurons of many spinal segments that represent multiple dermatomes, so the perceived area of pain should increase with increasing stimulus intensity. Hence, spatial radiation of pain would be expected to result from higher-intensity nociceptive stimuli, as described in Chapter 2. The proposed encoding mechanism also is consistent with results of psychophysical experiments that demonstrate spatial summation of pain even when the stimulus area extends across several dermatomes or across multiple stimulus sites that are separated by wide distances (see Chapter 2).

DORSAL HORN MODULATORY MECHANISMS

The dorsal horn is a critical integrative site of multiple inhibitory and facilitatory interactions, which take place both at a local level and with descending systems and determine the extent to which nociceptive information will be conveyed to higher levels of the CNS. Different functional types of primary afferent neurons make synaptic contact with nociceptive neurons of the dorsal horn (Fig. 2). Low-threshold mechanoreceptive primary afferent neurons also exert inhibitory effects on WDR neurons by means of inhibitory interneurons (Fig. 2). Both WDR and NS neurons are subject to descending inhibitory and facilitatory modulation from the brain. Thus, brief excitation followed by inhibition is evoked in WDR neurons by large, fast-conducting Aβ mechanoreceptive afferents. The Aβ-evoked inhibition has figured prominently in major theories of pain mechanisms, particularly the gate control theory (Melzack and Wall 1965). The local inhibitory effects of Aβ input on WDR neurons help to explain why pain can sometimes be reduced by repetitive stimulation of large-diameter axons, either by transcutaneous electrical nerve (TENS) or dorsal column stimulators (Dubner and Bennett 1983; Willis 1985). According to the gate control theory, this form of inhibition represents a means of "closing the gate." However, inhibitory modulation can take place locally within the dorsal horn and as a result of descending modulatory systems originating in the brain (see Chapter 6).

Local mechanisms of central sensitization

Dorsal horn neurons of origin of pain-related pathways also undergo central sensitization during tonic impulse input from C nociceptive afferent neurons. This phenomenon, in turn, is closely related to a mechanism of slow temporal summation termed "wind-up." This mechanism is also envisioned as a form of "opening the gate." Wind-up has been elucidated in electrophysiological experiments involving microelectrode recordings of neurons of the dorsal horn (Mendell 1966; Price et al. 1978). A single brief nociceptive stimulus that activates Aδ and C nociceptive afferents results in a brief-latency and long-latency impulse discharge in both WDR and NS dorsal horn neurons. The characteristics of the long-latency C response help to explain the psychophysical property of temporal summation of second pain (described in Chapter 2). During a train of 51°C heat pulses, for example, the long-latency, C-fiber-mediated responses of spinothalamic neurons and the sensation of second pain all increase progressively over a similar time course (Fig. 8, right). This temporal summation is dependent on CNS mechanisms, specifically those within the dorsal horn of the spinal cord (Dickenson and Sullivan 1987, 1990; Kelstein et al. 1990; Thompson and Woolf 1990; Woolf and Thompson 1991). The most compelling evidence that responses of first-order afferents are not the basis for wind-up is that the responses of C primary nociceptive afferents do not temporally summate in response to trains of heat pulses. In fact, their responses are progressively suppressed, as is the case for Aδ heat nociceptive afferents (Fig. 8). However, the summation of C-afferent-induced responses of spinothalamic tract neurons to repeated heat pulses was similar in both magnitude and time course to the summation of second pain in psychophysical experiments that used the same type of stimulation. As can be seen in Fig. 8, both second pain and C-fiber spinothalamic tract neuronal responses in-

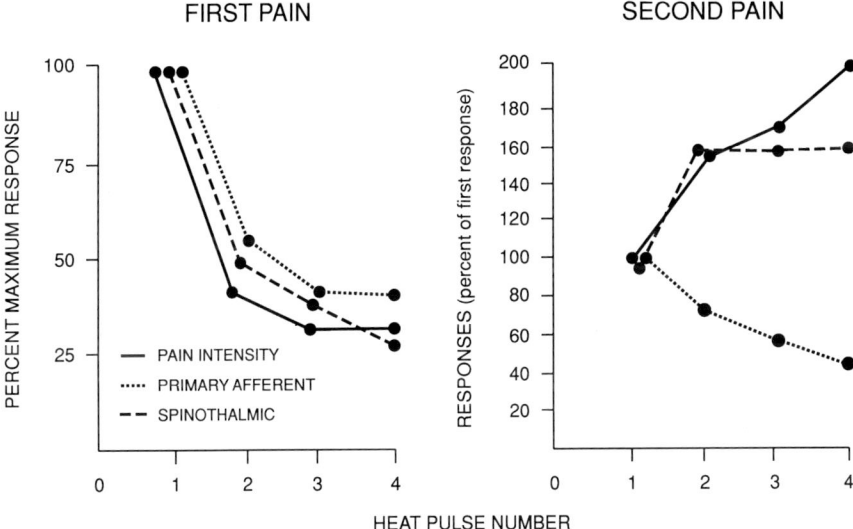

Fig. 8. Different effects of repetitive heat pulses on first and second pain. Repeating a 51°C heat pulse produced a striking decrement in the neural responses of primary afferents and spinothalamic neurons, as well as the judged intensity of first pain (left). However, the same stimuli produced very different results for second pain (right). In this case only the long-latency primary afferent activity (associated with second pain) decreased with repetitive stimulation. Long-latency spinothalamic activity and judgments of second pain sensation intensity increased in this situation. Apparently, a CNS mechanism exists for amplifying second pain with repetitive noxious stimuli. Adapted from Price et al. (1978), with permission.

crease over time—even when the responses of C-polymodal nociceptive afferents become progressively reduced.

Wind-up of long-latency C responses of dorsal horn WDR and NS neurons and second pain also occur when electrical shocks are used to activate C afferents, but only if the stimulus frequency is greater than once every 3 seconds (Mendell 1966; Dickenson and Sullivan 1987, 1990). This critical frequency is likely to mimic the natural frequency of peripheral C nociceptors that discharge at about once every 2–3 seconds at stimulus intensities that are likely to be minimally painful (Torebjork and Hallin 1974). Tonic impulse input over C nociceptive afferents is critical for inducing and maintaining central hyperalgesic states that accompany persistent pain conditions, including inflammatory and neuropathic pains (Dubner 1991; Gracely et al. 1992).

Neural mechanisms critical for wind-up and temporal summation of second pain exist at the level of synaptic interactions between C-polymodal nociceptive afferents and dorsal horn neurons. These synaptic interactions are now known to involve long-duration excitatory processes related to release of neurotransmitters such as glutamate/aspartate and neuromodulators such as substance P. These agents respectively activate receptors of N-methyl-D-aspartate (NMDA) and neurokinin 1, leading to prolonged depolarizations (see Thompson and Woolf 1990 for review). Thus, NMDA-receptor antagonists block both temporal summation of second pain and the wind-up responses of dorsal horn neurons to repeated C-fiber input (Dickenson and Sullivan 1987, 1990; Price et al. 1994a; Arendt-Nielson 1997). To some extent, and as would be predicted from the wind-up theory, NMDA-receptor antagonists also reduce hyperalgesic states that are produced experimentally or that occur in pathophysiological pain states such as postherpetic neuralgia (Dubner 1991; Eide et al. 1994). Indeed, slow temporal summation has long been considered a central neural mechanism that has a critical role in pathophysiological pain (Noordenbos 1959).

A second factor that appears to be related to temporal summation mechanisms involves the breakdown of the inhibitory mechanisms of Aβ afferents (Price et al. 1989b, 1992a). Under some pathophysiological circumstances, such as may occur in individuals with complex regional pain syndrome (CRPS), repetitive stimulation of Aβ afferents evokes not the usual inhibition of pain but rather an abnormal triggering of the wind-up mechanism. For example, repeated electrical stimulation of Aβ axons at one stimulus every 3 seconds evokes a progressive increase in burning pain (Price and Bennett 1989). This temporal summation is strikingly similar to that observed in normal individuals whose C fibers are stimulated at the same rate. This phenomenon suggests an abnormal triggering of physiological mechanisms that exist in normal pain-free individuals. Temporal summation of mechanical allodynia can be blocked with NMDA antagonists such as ketamine (Eide et al. 1994).

Regardless of whether wind-up is normally or abnormally triggered, its relationship to central hyperalgesic states is explained by the long-term consequences of this mechanism (Dubner 1991; Palecek et al. 1992). Wind-up is accompanied by a progressive membrane depolarization to the point that dorsal horn neurons remain partially depolarized afterwards. This partial depolarization is likely to be accompanied by an increase in "spontaneous" impulse discharge and by greater responsiveness to peripheral somatic stimuli. Thus, somatic stimuli within the receptive field become more effective, and those outside the previously mapped receptive field start to become effective. In other words, the receptive field of the neuron becomes more sensitive and expanded in size. Direct evidence for this explanation is provided by a study that examined the relationship between wind-up and central sensitization (Li et al. 1999). Wind-up was produced in WDR neurons by a train of 12 electrical pulses to receptive fields. The intensity of each pulse was above threshold for C nociceptive afferents. This train of pulses simultaneously resulted in a progressive enhancement of the C-fiber-mediated central responses and in expansion of receptive fields of WDR neurons. Moreover, the enhanced C-fiber-mediated responses could subsequently be maintained by a very low frequency of C-fiber stimulation, one stimulus every 10 seconds. This result suggests that once central sensitization occurs, the sensitized state can be maintained by extremely low frequencies of tonic peripheral input from nociceptors.

The expanded receptive fields and enhanced responsiveness of dorsal horn nociceptive neurons result in a *greater number* of neurons responding to a nociceptive or non-nociceptive stimulus. Given the role of receptive field size in neuronal recruitment, larger receptive field size implies that a given stimulus would activate even more dorsal horn nociceptive neurons than would occur otherwise. Increased activation of greater numbers of dorsal horn nociceptive neurons along the rostrocaudal axis of the spinal cord may be associated with exaggerated pain and with enhanced spatial radiation of the painful sensation. In support of this prediction, 2-DG metabolic mapping of neural activity in rats with chronic constrictive injury of the sciatic nerve (to simulate neuropathy) revealed extensive rostrocaudal elevations in neural activity of the dorsal horn extending from L1 to L5 (Mao et al. 1992; Fig. 9). Thus, temporal summation interacts with spatial summation mechanisms to recruit neurons across several spinal segments. Expanded receptive fields, increased responses to somatic stimuli, and increased spontaneous impulse discharge result behaviorally and perceptually in hyperalgesia, allodynia, and ongoing pain.

Descending modulatory mechanisms

Dorsal horn neurons can undergo inhibition and facilitation from pathways that descend from the brain to the spinal cord (see Chapter 6 for further details). However, these descending systems are likely to engage many of the local mechanisms discussed in the preceding section. Thus, the receptive fields of NS and WDR neurons can be expanded or contracted by activity in various descending pathways under different behavioral conditions.

Descending modulatory influences and the behavioral conditions with which they are associated have been demonstrated in experiments in awake trained monkeys (Hayes et al 1981; Hoffman et al. 1981). These studies showed that responses of WDR and NS neurons of the medullary dorsal horn could be modulated by different attentional sets and different conditions of stimulus relevance. The receptive fields of these neurons expanded

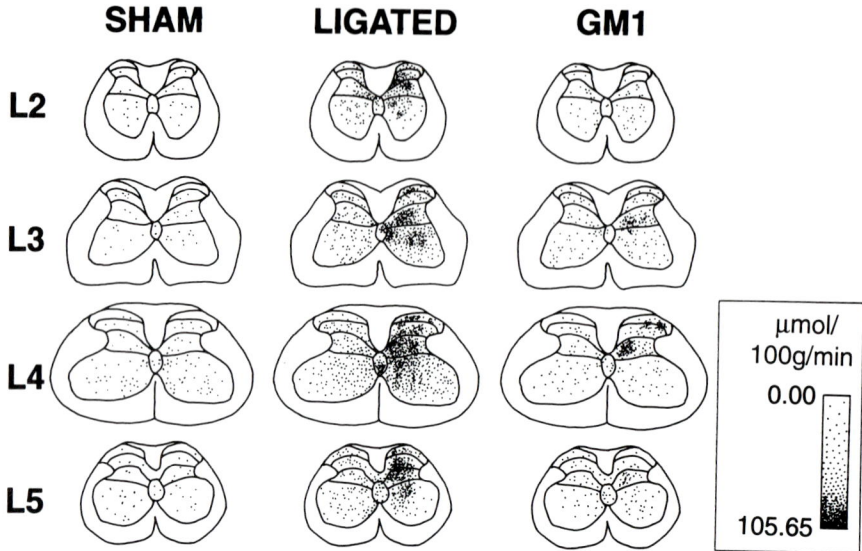

Fig. 9. Patterns of elevated neural activity (measured by 2-DG metabolic mapping) in rats with chronic constrictive injury of the right sciatic nerve. The spinal cord sections at left are from a rat whose right sciatic nerve was surgically exposed but not ligated. The spinal cord sections in the middle are from a rat whose right sciatic nerve was loosely ligated in four places and which displayed behaviors indicative of a persistent pain condition. The spinal cord sections at the right are from a rat with similar sciatic nerve constriction that was treated with an agent (GM1 ganglioside) that greatly reduced behavioral indications of persistent pain. The ipsilateral dorsal horn is shown at right in all spinal sections. Based on data from Mao et al. (1992).

or contracted, depending on the attentional set of the animal. In particular, the receptive field areas from which nociceptive temperatures (45°–49°C) elicited neural responses expanded during a task in which the monkey discriminated a temperature change in the nociceptive range and contracted during a visual discrimination task. Given the importance of receptive field size in the spatiotemporal recruitment concept of encoding nociceptive intensity, these results suggest that a stimulus-relevant attentional set (i.e., thermal discrimination) would recruit more dorsal horn sensory projection neurons in comparison to a nonrelevant attentional set (i.e., visual discrimination). This effect, in turn, should increase the perceived intensity of pain during thermal as compared to visual discrimination. A psychophysical study by Miron et al. (1989) confirmed this prediction.

The impulse frequencies evoked in NS and WDR neurons by the same range of nociceptive temperatures (45°–49°C) also can be modulated by attentional set and stimulus relevance. Impulse frequencies were higher when a warning light preceded nociceptive stimuli as opposed to when the stimuli occurred unexpectedly. Therefore, the slope of the stimulus-response relationships, the number of dorsal horn neurons activated, and hence the composition of centrally activated neurons are all under dynamic modulatory control and may play as direct a role in determining pain perception as do the peripheral stimulus events themselves.

The psychological factors that modulate nociceptive processing at the first synapse in the dorsal horn of the spinal cord need to be further related to their neuroanatomical and physiological substrates. Likewise, the anatomical structures that have been implicated in modulation of dorsal horn neural responses need to be further related to the psychological contexts under which they are activated. For example, are these modulatory influences manifested during placebo analgesia, during hypnotic analgesia, or in contexts where pain is enhanced by psychological factors?

THE BIOLOGICAL ROLES OF TEMPORAL AND SPATIAL SUMMATION AND CENTRAL SENSITIZATION

The central sensitization and summation mechanisms just described are likely to serve the function of maintaining a persistent pain state over a time when tissue is injured. Injured tissue needs protection in order for healing to take place. Protection includes avoidance of somatic stimulation of the injured area as well as general quiescence. The central mechanisms that maintain a persistent pain state result in allodynia, hyperalgesia, and ongoing pain, which serve such protective functions and evoke the chronic phase of pain behavior described in Chapter 1. These phenomena are sustained by tonic input in nociceptive afferents that have not been destroyed by the initial injury. Most critically, they appear to override decrements in primary afferent nociceptive input. For example, temporal summation of C responses occurs even in the presence of a progressive decrease in input from C nociceptors (Fig. 9). Similar decrements in primary afferent input are likely to occur after injury or partial injury.

Another functional consequence of these mechanisms is that adaptation to a sustained nociceptive stimulus would be expected to be very limited. Consistent with results of psychophysical studies described in Chapter 2, dorsal horn WDR neurons have limited adaptation in response to intradermal capsaicin injection (Simone et al. 1991) or to a repetitive nociceptive heat stimulus (Coghill et al. 1993b). In contrast, NS neurons respond vigorously to such stimuli during the first minute or two but have substantially decreased responses thereafter. The much greater responses of NS neurons and the somewhat enhanced responses of WDR neurons in the first minute or two may relate to the immediate phase of pain behavior characterized by strong escape and autonomic responses (see Chapter 5).

CONCLUSIONS

The neural mechanisms described in this chapter further explain the fundamental psychophysical attributes of pain discussed in Chapter 2. The biological roles of these mechanisms and their related psychophysical attributes are to promote initial escape behaviors followed by quiescence and protection of injured tissue so that healing takes place. Pain intensity is encoded by primary and secondary neurons that respond in a highly discriminative manner to different intensities of nociceptive stimulation. However, the capacities of spinal dorsal horn neurons to encode distinctions between non-nociceptive and nociceptive sensory input as well as those between different nociceptive intensities are likely to require additional central integrative mechanisms of neuronal recruitment. These central mechanisms are likely to underlie psychophysical attributes of spatial summation and spatial radiation of pain sensations.

Neural mechanisms underlying psychophysical attributes of pain sensation intensity, intensity differences, spatial summation, radiation, and temporal summation are important for the sensory-discriminative dimension of pain. The afferent system for pain is exquisitely sensitive to very small differences in stimulus intensity, yet has mechanisms for enhancing sensitivity once tissue is injured. However, the sensory-discriminative attributes of pain are equally important for the affective-motivational dimension. As pointed out in Chapters 1–3, the sensory features of nociceptive sensations dispose us to perceive them as unpleasant. Nociceptive sensations often spread, summate, radiate, and outlast the stimulus that evoked them. Consequently, they are likely to be perceived as intrusive and hence threatening in most contexts. The following chapter will discuss the central processing of pain in relation to these psychophysical attributes and to various dimensions of pain.

Psychological Mechanisms of Pain and Analgesia, Progress in Pain Research and Management, Vol. 15, by Donald D. Price, IASP Press, Seattle, © 1999.

5

Brain Processing of Pain

Beyond the level of primary afferents and spinal cord neurons, information has until recently been scant and controversial concerning the processing of nociceptive information and the representation of different dimensions of pain within the brain. Most of the available data on pain mechanisms in the brainstem and cerebral cortex have come from human studies evaluating the effects of destructive lesions or electrical stimulation. Within the last 10 years, however, considerable neurophysiological and neuroanatomical information about brain mechanisms of pain has accumulated from animal experiments, human experiments involving microstimulation and microelectrode recordings within the brain, and animal and human neural imaging studies.

In this chapter I synthesize information from diverse sources of knowledge in an attempt to explain the underlying neural and psychological mechanisms of pain. First, I explain the ascending pathways for pain and functional types of nociceptive neurons and their central target brain structures. Second, I describe animal and human studies that identify cerebral cortical areas activated during different pain states. Third and finally, I discuss the brain networks that underlie the representation and processing of different dimensions and stages of pain. The schematic in Fig. 1 serves as an initial guide to the relevant anatomical pathways and brain structures.

ASCENDING PAIN-RELATED PATHWAYS

In general, the characteristics of classes of neurons observed at the level of the spinal cord dorsal horn appear to be preserved within brain areas that receive input from these spinal cord neurons. Thus, both wide-dynamic-range (WDR) and nociceptive-specific (NS) neurons occur at several brainstem and cortical levels, and their physiological characteristics in many ways resemble those of dorsal horn nociceptive neurons. Nevertheless, important differences emerge at higher levels; some brain regions that are involved in pain appear to contain nearly exclusive input from spinal WDR neurons, while others have greater input from spinal NS neurons. The central destinations and physiological characteristics of different pain-

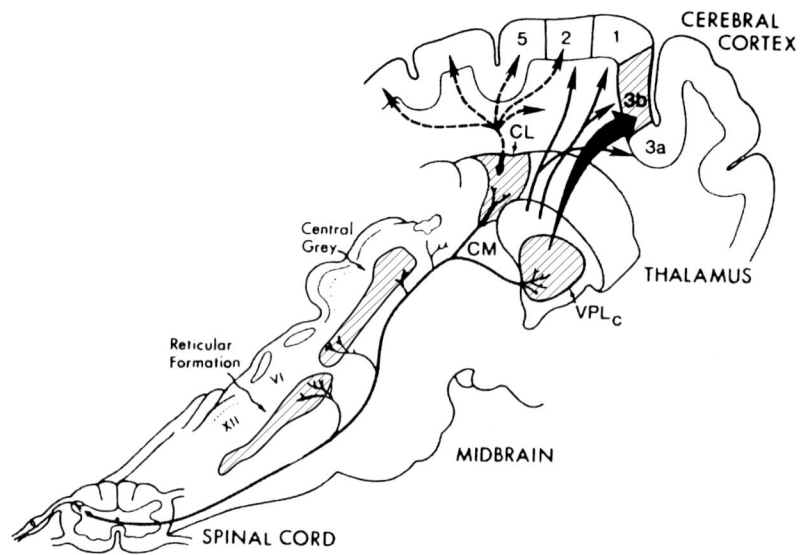

Fig. 1. Schematic representation of major ascending "pain pathways" showing spinoreticular, spinothalamic, and thalamocortical connections.

related ascending pathways have definite bearing on differential processing of components of pain and pain-related behavior. These components include (1) somatic reflexes (spinal cord); (2) autonomic nervous system and neuroendocrine responses (parabrachial nucleus, central gray, and hypothalamic connections); (3) arousal (spinoreticular connections): (4) integrated postural adjustments and orientation toward the nociceptive stimulus (connections to deep layers of the superior colliculus); (5) sensory discrimination of the intensity, location, and qualities associated with the evoking stimulus (spinothalamic connections); and (6) affective-motivational dimensions (spinothalamic, spinohypothalamic, spinopontoamygdaloid, spinomesencephalic, and spinoreticular connections and their subsequent central projections). I will discuss each of the major ascending pathways in terms of anatomical connections, physiological characteristics of neurons at each level, and possible functions in pain processing.

SPINOTHALAMOCORTICAL PATHWAYS

The spinothalamic tract and its continuation from thalamus to cerebral cortex has been considered the major ascending central pathway for pain (Willis 1985). This system has been anatomically and physiologically characterized in great detail in several animal species, including humans. A major impetus for investigating its role in pain has been the observation that its interruption at spinal levels results in profound, though sometimes temporary, analgesia in humans (White and Sweet 1966). Electrical stimulation of the spinothalamic tract at spinal levels or at its thalamic target sites often evokes pain sensations in humans, though other types of somatosensory sensations can also result from stimulation of this pathway (White and Sweet 1966; Mayer et al. 1975).

The origin of the spinothalamic tract is mainly the dorsal horn of the spinal gray matter and to a much lesser extent, neurons within the ventral horn (Willis 1985). Dorsal horn WDR and NS neurons both have axons that cross over to the contralateral white matter of the spinal cord and then project to the thalamic ventroposterior lateral (VPL) nucleus and to certain medial thalamic nuclei. However, individual spinothalamic neurons often project to multiple levels of the brain, and the same WDR or NS neuron often has collateral axonal branches projecting to several brainstem sites (Fig. 1). These central targets include reticular formation nuclei of the lower brainstem and midbrain, deep layers of the superior colliculus, the periaqueductal gray, parabrachial nuclei, hypothalamus, and various ventrolateral and medial thalamic nuclei. To some extent, these multiple projections reflect the diverse functional consequences of nociceptive input and increase the likelihood that spinothalamic neurons contribute to several different components of pain behavior and experience.

Thus, the spinothalamocortical pathway transmits nociceptive information to multiple brain sites that are related to several functions. The overall experience of pain is synthesized from multiple consequences of ascending input rather than from activation of a single discrete "pain center" of the brain. Moreover, this ascending pathway transmits information about a wide variety of somatosensory events, including those related to touch, pain, and possibly innocuous temperature sensibility. For example, the power functions describing both human judgments and dorsal horn WDR responses to mild mechanical indentation of the skin are very similar and have exponents close to 0.7 (McHaffie et al. 1994). The view that ascending spinal neurons involved in pain convey information about multiple types of somatosensory modalities contrasts sharply with specificity theory, which assumes that pain-related neurons only transmit nociceptive information along a single point-to-point projection pathway for pain.

Individual spinothalamic neurons can be anatomically and physiologically traced to the VPL nucleus. In primates, the WDR and NS spinothalamic neurons projecting to this nucleus originate in laminae I and IV–VII of the contralateral spinal cord, as shown in Fig. 1. The caudal ventroposterior lateral nucleus, termed VPLc, is a major locus of spinothalamic axon termination. Other major thalamic nuclei receiving input from the spinothalamic tract include the ventral posterior inferior nucleus (VPI), the ventrocaudal part of the medial dorsal nucleus (MDvc), and the central lateral (CL) nucleus. Thalamic VPLc (and ventroposterior medial nucleus [VPM] in the case of trigeminal or facial input) projects to S-1 and S-2 somatosensory areas of the cerebral cortex in a restricted and somatotopically organized manner (Willis 1985). Spinothalamic and trigeminothalamic axonal projections within the VPLc and VPM and the corresponding thalamocortical projections within cortical somatosensory areas S-1 and S-2 are somatotopically organized. In contrast, CL and other medial thalamic nuclei (MDvc) and the ventromedial part of the posterior nuclear complex (VMpo) appear to have less somato-topic organization; they project more diffusely to other regions of the cere-bral cortex involved in more complex functions related to attention, cogni-tion, and emotions (Willis 1985; Craig 1995). For example, CL projects diffusely to wide regions of the parietal cortex, VMpo to the anterior insular cortical region, and MDvc to the anterior cingulate cortex (Craig 1995). In sum, these anatomical facts support the hypothesis that the lateral thalamic nuclei (VPLc and VPM) have a greater role in sensory-discriminative as-pects of pain, while the medial thalamic nuclei (CL, MDvc, and VMpo) are more involved with other components of pain processing.

Ventroposterior lateral (VPL) nociceptive neurons

Until recently, the characterization of neurons within the mammalian VPL has emphasized the responses of neurons to gentle mechanical stimuli. Sporadic reports of nociceptive neurons within VPL, combined with well-established spinothalamic terminations there, have spurred persistent efforts to identify nociceptive neurons in this nucleus and to determine whether it contains a subregion specialized to process nociceptive input.

Kenshalo et al. (1980) systematically characterized nociceptive neurons in VPL, using methods similar to those used to characterize spinothalamic nociceptive neurons. The nociceptive neurons identified were greatly out-numbered by cells activated optimally by innocuous mechanical stimuli. However, nociceptive neurons appeared to be concentrated in the caudal portion of the VPLc and were located in somatotopically appropriate re-gions of the nucleus. These thalamic neurons could be antidromically acti-vated from somatosensory S-1 cortical regions. Their response characteris-tics were in many ways similar to those of spinothalamic tract neurons. For example, their responses to graded nociceptive heat stimuli were similar to those of spinothalamic tract and primary afferent nociceptive neurons (Fig. 2). The cells could easily be divided into WDR and NS (high-threshold) categories, similar to spinothalamic tract neurons. An important feature of

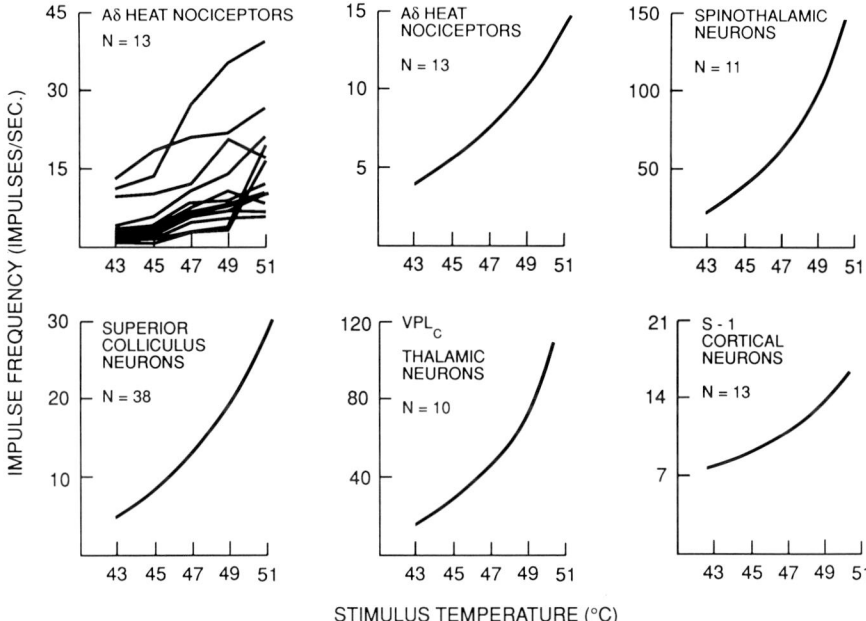

Fig. 2. Stimulus-response curves for nociceptive neurons at different levels of the peripheral and central nervous system. At upper left are the functions of 13 individual Ad primary afferent nociceptive neurons and to the immediate right is the population function (i.e., mean responses) of this same population. Note that for all areas of the nervous system, the response is characterized as a positively accelerating and is generally similar at all levels. Reprinted with permission from Price, D.D., McHaffie, J.G., Stein, B.E. The psychophysical attributes of heat-induced pain and their relationships to neural mechanisms. *Journal of Cognitive Neuroscience* 1992; 4:1–14. © The Massachusetts Institute of Technology.

these thalamic WDR neurons was that their receptive field organization was very similar to that of spinothalamic tract WDR neurons (see Fig. 5 of Chapter 4). In a small central zone, the neuron responded with graded impulse frequency over a very broad range of mechanical stimulus intensity, extending from very gentle touch to painful squeeze or noxious heat (i.e., 52°C). Surrounding this zone was a much larger area in which firm pressure or nociceptive stimuli could evoke impulse discharge. NS neurons had smaller, more uniform receptive fields within which only strong mechanical or nociceptive stimuli were effective, similar to NS spinothalamic tract neurons.

One difference between primary afferents, spinothalamic tract neurons, and VPLc neurons involves their rates of adaptation to graded, long-duration nociceptive temperatures. VPLc neurons have a distinctly slower rate of adaptation in response to long-duration nociceptive temperatures as compared to spinothalamic tract neurons. This difference suggests a mechanism that transforms nociceptive information at this level; similar transformations likely occur at other levels of this pathway.

VPM, VMpo, and Pf/MDvc neurons in monkeys trained to detect temperature differences

Bushnell and colleagues (Bushnell and Duncan 1989; Bushnell et al. 1993; Bushnell 1995) have conducted a series of elegant studies of nociceptive and thermoreceptive thalamic neurons in awake behaving monkeys. They compared the physiological characteristics of these neurons to determine whether they subserve sensory-discriminative or affective-motivational functions related to pain. The thalamic nuclear regions they compared included the trigeminal ventroposterior medial nucleus (VPM), the ventrocaudal part of the medial dorsal nucleus and parafascicular nucleus (Pf/MDvc), and the ventromedial part of the posterior nuclear complex (VMpo). These three regions receive somewhat different ascending spinothalamic tract inputs and have distinctly different connections to the cerebral cortex. VPM receives major input from the ventral portion of the contralateral dorsal horn (WDR neurons of laminae V–VI), whereas Pf/MDvc and VMpo receive major input from the superficial dorsal horn (lamina I NS neurons and neurons responsive to innocuous cooling of the skin). VPM, like VPLc, projects mainly to the primary somatosensory cortex (S-1). VMpo projects to the rostral insular cortex and to a lesser degree to the somatosensory cortex. Pf/MDvc projects to area 24 of the anterior cingulate cortex (ACC) (Vogt et al. 1993). Bushnell and colleagues proposed that VPM neurons would be more involved in sensory-discriminative aspects of pain as a result of connections to primary somatosensory cortical regions, whereas VMpo and Pf/MDvc would more likely subserve affective-motivational functions because they project to limbic cortical regions.

Of considerable interest is Bushnell's finding that nociceptive neurons within all three nuclear regions could differentially respond to graded nociceptive skin temperatures (43°–50°C) and could discriminate very small differences in stimulus intensity (i.e., 0.2°–0.3°C). This is not surprising, since both sensory-discriminative and affective-motivational functions are likely to require differential responses to nociceptive stimuli of increasing intensity. On the other hand, receptive field sizes of nociceptive and thermoreceptive neurons of the three regions differed considerably, as shown in Table I. Receptive field sizes of VPM neurons were usually restricted to less than 3 cm diameter, whereas those of VMpo were more evenly distributed among areas defined as restricted (<3 cm diameter), medium, large (greater than most of the contralateral face or limb), and bilateral. Pf/MDvc neurons had either large or bilateral receptive fields. Modality specificity likewise differed among these nuclear groups. Whereas VPM neurons were

Table I
Comparison of receptive field size distribution (%) in the
medial, lateral, and posterior thalamus

Nucleus	Small	Medium	Large	Bilateral
VPM ($n = 19$)	89%	11%	0%	0%
VMpo ($n = 73$)	48%	26%	15%	11%
Pf/MDvd ($n = 6$)	0%	17%	50%	33%

Note: Small = less than 3 cm, large = most of contralateral face or limb. VPM = ventroposterior medial nucleus; VMpo = ventromedial part of the posterior nuclear complex; Pf/MDvd = ventrocaudal part of the medial dorsal nucleus and parafascicular nucleus.

almost all WDR, the large majority of VMpo (80%) and Pf/MDvc (88%) neurons were either specifically nociceptive (NS) or thermoreceptive. Finally, responses of Pf/MDvc neurons to changes in nociceptive stimulus intensity, such as an increase from 47° to 48°C, were enhanced when monkeys were rewarded for detecting this change, but not when they were rewarded for detecting changes in light intensity. VPM neurons were less affected by these conditions of stimulus relevance.

Taken together, differences in cortical projection, receptive field size, relative modality specificity, and modulation by behavioral state led Bushnell and colleagues to conclude that lateral and medial thalamic nuclei subserve different physiological functions related to pain. They reasoned that thalamic regions that are most heavily influenced by conditions of behavioral relevance (e.g., VMpo and Pf/MDvc) may be important for affective and motivational reactions to pain and would be expected to project to motor and limbic regions of the cerebral cortex. They believed that VPM nociceptive neurons encoded sensory-discriminative features such as stimulus intensity and location, although they acknowledged that these neurons were slightly modulated by the same attentional manipulations that influenced medial thalamic nociceptive neurons. The involvement of VPM in sensory aspects of pain has been further confirmed by the observation that correct detection of noxious heat stimuli was considerably reduced after a double injection of 2% lidocaine into the VPM of awake monkeys (Duncan et al. 1993).

However, these lines of evidence do not warrant a completely separate representation of sensory and affective functions between lateral and medial thalamic nuclear groups. In fact, a human psychophysical study of similar design to the thalamic electrophysiological studies showed that the same conditions of attention modulate ratings of pain sensation intensity and pain unpleasantness in parallel (Miron et al. 1989). Ratings of *both* pain intensity and unpleasantness increased slightly when subjects attended to small temperature shifts in the nociceptive range in comparison to when they attended to shifts in light intensity. Thus, although different cortical projections of

VPM, VMpo, and Pf/MDvc indicate differential involvement in sensory and affective dimensions of pain, it is likely that lateral and medial thalamic nuclear groups are involved to different degrees in *both* sensory discriminative and affective-motivational dimensions of pain. Studies described below support this possibility.

Studies of thalamic mechanisms of pain in humans

The results of neurophysiological studies of thalamic nociceptive neurons within the spinothalamocortical system may help us to interpret the effects of lesions of specific thalamic nuclei and of electrical stimulation of these nuclei in humans. The effects of lesions provide further insight into the specialization of thalamic neural systems that mediate different aspects of the total pain experience. Evidence is provided by clinical studies in which surgical lesions of the thalamus were made in order to alter some or all aspects of pain, and by classic studies of patients with stroke-induced damage to the lateral thalamus. Lesions that are directed toward the entire ventrobasal complex provide poor pain relief and have the undesirable side effect of creating a large mechanoreceptive sensory deficit (White and Sweet 1969). This deficit does not appear to occur when the lesion is confined to the portion of the ventrocaudal nucleus (Vc) that corresponds to VPLc in other mammalian species. Lesions of the Vc, similar to lidocaine block of VPM in monkeys, produce a distinct though temporary reduction in perception of acute pain. Better and longer-lasting relief has been observed when using ventroposterior medial nucleus lesions to treat facial pain, possibly because such lesions may also interrupt projections to medial intralaminar thalamic nuclei (White and Sweet 1969). For similar reasons, medial thalamic lesions have been combined with Vc lesions to produce more permanent pain relief. Lesions within the intralaminar thalamic complex or the anterior and medial dorsal nuclei of the thalamus also may produce temporary reduction of pain. However, such relief appears to result from an interference with generalized, thalamically mediated, diffuse cortical activation, consistent with animal anatomical and physiological studies showing widespread projections from these thalamic nuclei to the cerebral cortex (Mark et al. 1960; White and Sweet 1969).

Results of a classic study by Head and Holmes (1911) were consistent with those of the animal physiological studies described above. The authors conducted sensory testing and extensive neurological examination of 22 patients with damage to the lateral thalamus as well as postmortem examination of the patients' brains when possible. Histological examination in one case showed damage confined mainly to the ventrobasal complex. Nine pa-

stimuli. The most positive statement that we can make is that some neurons of the midbrain and medullary lateral reticular formation appear to be accessed by nociceptive input. Such input could be related to arousal, aversive, motor, or less likely, to sensory-discriminative functions.

Deep layers of the superior colliculus

The superior colliculus, particularly the deeper laminae, may well play a role in pain. Neurons of this region receive ascending afferent connections from the anterolateral quadrant and lateral cervical nucleus (Larson et al. 1987). Neurons of deep layers of the superior colliculus have been physiologically characterized in hamsters as WDR and NS neurons (Larson et al. 1987). Their responses to peripheral somatosensory stimuli and their receptive field organizations were strikingly similar to WDR and NS neurons of the dorsal horn.

Larson et al. (1987) suggest that neurons of deep layers of the superior colliculus are involved in alerting and orienting an animal toward a source of nociceptive stimulation. A wealth of data implicates the deep layers of the superior colliculus in orienting an animal toward a source of peripheral stimulation. Clearly, this neural mechanism has significant survival value.

Human studies of midbrain regions involved in pain

The most striking effect of electrical stimulation of periaqueductal structures in humans is the resulting emotional complex of unpleasantness and fear that often causes the subject to forbid further stimulation (Nashold et al. 1969, 1974; White and Sweet 1969). At higher stimulation intensities, reports of frankly painful sensations occur. The pain is typically diffuse, deep, and localized to midline structures, particularly the face (Nashold et al. 1969), in contrast to midbrain spinothalamic stimulation, which produces sharp, well-localized pain referred to the contralateral body surface (White and Sweet 1969). The emotional complex of unpleasantness, fear, and sometimes intense dread that results from stimulation of periaqueductal structures is consistent with animal data that implicate these structures in fear responses. For example, lesions of the periaqueductal central gray matter reduce fear responses of rats (Mayer and Price 1976).

In summary, the available evidence from lesion and recording studies in animals and electrical stimulation studies in humans suggests that distinct medullary and midbrain regions receive input from spinoreticular and spinomesencephalic nociceptive neurons. These regions appear to be preferentially involved with the arousal, autonomic, and somatomotor escape and orienting responses associated with pain. These studies are consistent with classic physiological studies of "high" decerebrate animals (Bard 1928). Cats with brain transections just above the superior colliculus exhibit elaborate behavior in response to a nociceptive stimulus (Bard 1928). The behavior, termed "sham rage," consists of intense autonomic and somatomotor responses suggestive of escape or defense. Clearly, even at medullary and midbrain levels a complex and highly organized neural circuitry mediates emotional and behavioral responses associated with pain in human and other mammalian species.

DORSAL COLUMN POSTSYNAPTIC AND SPINOCERVICAL PATHWAYS

A pathway originating from neurons of layers III and IV of the spinal cord dorsal horn projects to both dorsal column nuclei and the spinocervical tract nucleus (Willis 1985; Lu 1989). Most of the nociceptive neurons of origin are WDR neurons (Giesler and Cliffer 1985; Willis 1985; Lu 1989). Somatosensory information from both dorsal column nuclei and the spinocervical tract nucleus is then relayed to the ventroposterior lateral nucleus (VPL) of the thalamus and thence to somatosensory cortical areas. The role of this pathway in pain, particularly in humans, is questionable. Both human clinical data and rat experiments provide some evidence that this pathway signals pelvic visceral pain, yet lesioning of this pathway appears to produce no deficit in cutaneous pain (Hirshberg et al. 1996). This is somewhat perplexing, because neurons of this pathway have cutaneous receptive fields and respond differentially to mechanical nociceptive stimuli applied to the skin. However, based on rats' lack of neural response to nociceptive thermal stimulation, even in sensitized skin, Giesler and Cliffer (1985) concluded that the dorsal column pathway is minimally involved in nociception. The involvement of the spinocervical tract in human pain is also questionable, given that this nucleus is marginally present or absent in humans (Willis 1985).

SPINOHYPOTHALAMIC CONNECTIONS

Both anatomical and electrophysiological studies of the last 13 years have demonstrated a spinohypothalamic pathway in rats, cats, and primates (Burstein et al. 1987; Giesler 1995). The total number of spinothalamic and spinohypothalamic neurons is similar, at least in the rat, and this pathway may make an important contribution to nociceptive processing. This possibility is of considerable interest because the hypothalamus may well contribute to autonomic responses to painful stimulation, such as increased blood flow to the heart and skeletal muscles, decreased blood flow to the skin and viscera, decreased gastrointestinal motility, piloerection, and sweat secretion (Giesler 1995). Retrograde tracers have located the neurons of origin of the spinohypothalamic tract in rats and cats (Burstein et al. 1987; Giesler 1995). These neurons exist in high concentrations in lamina I (the superficial layer of the dorsal horn), the ventral layers of the dorsal horn (layers V–VI), and the area around the central canal. These areas are strikingly similar to regions of origin of spinothalamic tract neurons. In fact, double labeling studies have shown that many spinohypothalamic tract neurons are also spinothalamic tract neurons; that is, the same neurons project to both places (Giesler 1995). The spinal cord areas of spinohypothalamic tract neurons (layers I, V–VI, and X) receive direct input from primary nociceptive afferent neurons.

Consistent with their locations in the spinal gray matter and the likelihood of their anatomical connections with nociceptive afferents, spinohypothalamic tract neurons fit into the same physiological categories as spinothalamic tract neurons; most can be classified as WDR or NS neurons (Giesler 1995). Dado et al. (1994) further characterized responses of these neurons to graded noxious heating or cooling of their cutaneous receptive fields. Similar to spinothalamic tract neurons and human psychophysical judgments of pain, their responses to temperatures in the nociceptive range were easily fit to a positively accelerating power function with an exponent of 3.5 for heat pain and had a nearly linear function with an exponent of 1.2 for cold pain. Thus, spinohypothalamic tract neurons appear capable of encoding precise information about nociceptive stimulus intensity; they convey this information simultaneously to several brain structures, including the hypothalamus.

Although considerable evidence supports projection of pain-related pathways to the hypothalamus, little has been done to characterize nociceptive neurons within hypothalamic nuclei. Pretel and Piekut (1991) found expression of c-*fos*-like immunoreactivity in the periventricular nucleus (PVN) of the hypothalamus after stimulation of nociceptive afferents in the hindpaw of the rat. C-*fos* expression is a presumed marker of nociceptive-related neural activity. Clearly, further studies are needed to determine the extent to which specific hypothalamic nuclei contain neurons that process pain-related information. Hypothalamic nuclei that receive nociceptive input also are likely to receive information about innocuous temperature and are probably involved in both nociceptive responses and responses related to temperature regulation. To the extent that such nuclei participate in autonomic and neuroendocrine responses to painful stimuli, they may play an important role in affective-motivational components of pain.

SPINOPONTOAMYGDALOID AND
SPINOPONTOHYPOTHALAMIC PATHWAYS

Beginning in 1989, Bernard and colleagues have characterized two novel pathways for pain, termed the spino-parabrachio-amygdaloid and the spino-parabrachio-hypothalamic pathways (Bernard et al. 1989; Bernard and Besson 1990). These pathways are of considerable interest for understanding processing of pain because their target brain structures are heavily involved in autonomic processes and behaviors related to fear and defense. These brain structures include the parabrachial nucleus of the dorsolateral pons (pontine PB or pPB), the central nucleus of the amygdala (Ce), and the hypothalamus. The parabrachial nucleus of the midbrain and pons is involved in numerous autonomic processes such as cardiovascular and respiratory modulation, adrenocortical responses, and visceral responses to stress (e.g., pupil dilatation and micturition). For example, microstimulation of pBP induces strong cardiovascular responses (Bernard et al. 1989). Similarly, the Ce has been strongly implicated in fear, emotional memory and behavior, and autonomic and somatomotor responses to threatening stimuli (reviewed in Damasio 1994). Various hypothalamic nuclei have also been implicated in these functions, as described above.

A most remarkable and consistent feature of neurons within these two pathways is that they are either unresponsive to peripheral stimulation or responsive only to nociceptive stimulation. That is, responsive neurons within these pathways consist almost entirely of nociceptive-specific (NS) neurons. Consistent with this unique feature is the finding that spinal cord neurons of origin of these pathways are exclusively within layer I of the dorsal horn, a region that is dominated by NS neurons (Willis 1985; Craig 1995). Neurons within these pathways appear to encode nociceptive stimulus intensity with some degree of precision. For example, parabrachial-amygdaloid NS neurons respond with positively accelerating stimulus-response curves to nociceptive cutaneous temperatures of 44°–50°C and to graded painful colorectal distension pressures of 25–125 mm Hg (Bernard and Besson 1990). Their target neurons within the Ce also encode stimulus intensities within these ranges.

The schematic diagram of Fig. 3 summarizes the anatomical connections within these two interrelated pathways. Similar to other ascending spinal pathways, their projections are mostly contralateral. However, a definite ispilateral projection exists as well. Considering the circuitry of these pathways and their target brain structures, this system appears designed to produce a coordinated behavioral response to acute painful stimuli, consisting of autonomic responses, fight-or-flight defensive behaviors, and emotional responses of fear or aggression.

In light of the possible functional roles of these pathways, the fact that their central origin consists almost entirely of NS neurons takes on further significance. As pointed out in Chapter 4, NS neurons respond vigorously to an acute nociceptive stimulus for about the first 2 minutes and show greatly reduced responses thereafter. This raises the possibility that NS neurons in these two pathways play a major role in the immediate phase of affective-

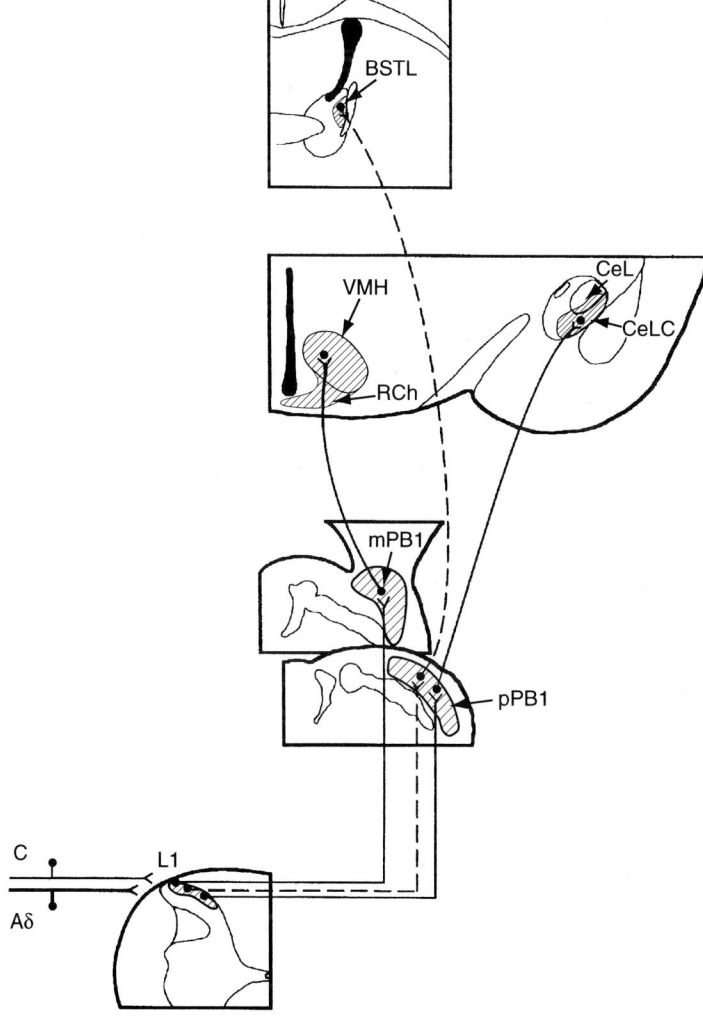

Fig. 3. Schematic representation of spinopontoamygdaloid, spinopontohypothalmic, and spinohypothalamic pathways. LI = layer I of dorsal horn; pPBI = posterior parabrachial nucleus; mPBI = medial parabrachial nucleus; CeL and CeLC = central nuclei of the amygdala; RCh = retrochiasmatic area; VMH = ventromedial hypothalamic nucleus; BSTL = bed nucleus of the stria terminalis.

motivational responses to nociceptive stimuli (Chapter 1) and a lesser role in the affective responses that attend persistent pain states. Such a possibility would be consistent with strong escape and affective behaviors of mammals for the first few minutes that follow an acute nociceptive stimulus as well as the lack of strong responses of the autonomic nervous system, escape behavior, and emotional feelings of fear during chronic pain states.

Several functionally distinct ascending pathways subserve pain, and numerous brain regions receive inputs from them. To some extent, these pathways serve different components of pain experience and pain-related behavior. This complexity is appropriate, because both the experience of pain and the behaviors that are associated with pain are complex and diverse.

Cerebral cortical representations of pain are likely to heavily depend on the multiple and diverse subcortical processing of nociceptive input. However, the cortical representations offer the greatest challenge in explaining the experiential aspects of pain because these aspects depend on the interrelationship of several functions, including somatosensory processing, cognition, memory, sensorimotor integration, and the generation of emotional feelings.

CEREBRAL CORTICAL REPRESENTATIONS OF PAIN

Much of the human cerebral cortex appears to be involved in the different dimensions of pain. The cortical representations of these dimensions are still somewhat of a mystery. The problem, as pointed out by Willis (1985), is that it is far more likely that the cerebral cortex has multiple representations of pain than that it has none. These multiple representations are likely to be at least partly related to multiple dimensions of pain, including sensory discrimination, arousal, cognitive evaluation, affect, and organized motor responses.

STUDIES OF CEREBRAL CORTICAL SOMATOSENSORY REGIONS INVOLVED IN PAIN

Knowledge about pain representation and nociceptive processing within cerebral cortical somatosensory areas was derived initially from clinical observations of effects of lesions or damage to these areas, subsequently from electrophysiological recordings of neurons within these areas, and most recently from neural imaging studies conducted in human and other mammalian species. The combination of results from these diverse types of studies is beginning to reveal at least some principles that explain how these areas participate in different dimensions of pain experience.

Early evidence for the role of the cerebral cortex
in sensory-discriminative aspects of pain

Evidence for involvement of the human cerebral cortical areas in pain is limited by the fact that few systematic studies have addressed this topic, especially with regard to sensory-discriminative aspects. However, two types of clinical and experimental observations implicate the postcentral somatosensory cortex in pain perception. First, lesions of the postcentral gyrus produce a temporary reduction in ongoing clinical pain intensity (Lewin and Phillips 1952; White and Sweet 1969). Second, electrical stimulation of sites within this region elicits pain. Penfield and Boldrey (1937) found 11 out of 426 stimulation sites at which electrical stimulation of the exposed postcentral gyrus in awake patients produced painful sensations, although they did not perform a systematic search for cortical sites involved in pain. These reports were such rare occurrences that the investigators concluded that appreciation of pain was not represented in the cerebral cortex. However, the fact that stimulation of at least some postcentral gyrus sites produced pain is evidence in favor of its role in sensory-discriminative aspects of pain. As with electrical stimulation of other CNS structures, such as the anterolateral quadrant, evoking specific pain sensations by cortical stimulation may require higher current intensities for sufficient spatial recruitment of neurons as compared to intensities required for tactile sensations (see Chapter 4). The paucity of specific pain-related cortical sites therefore could partly reflect the technical limitations of Penfield and Boldrey's approach. Another attempt to evoke pain by stimulation of the postcentral gyrus found that intense and unpleasant pains can be consistently elicited by stimulation of these sites (Echols and Cogclough 1947). The problem with this study is that it enlisted patients suffering from phantom limb pain, a condition that may have potentiated pain or lowered the cortical threshold for pain.

Thus, the effects of lesions and electrical stimulation of the human postcentral gyrus, though producing somewhat equivocal results, tend to be consistent with animal neuroanatomical and neurophysiological studies that provide evidence for a role of the primary somatosensory cortical area in sensory aspects of pain.

Animal electrophysiological studies
of cortical somatosensory areas

To date, four cerebral cortical somatosensory regions have been studied using electrophysiological techniques of single neuron recording. These include somatosensory areas S-1 and S-2, infraparietal area 7b, and the anterior cingulate cortex. All of these regions contain nociceptive-specific (NS) neurons that respond exclusively to nociceptive stimuli as well as wide-dynamic-range (WDR) neurons. Therefore, many of the physiological characteristics of nociceptive neurons at spinal and thalamic levels are preserved within somatosensory regions of the cerebral cortex.

Primary (S-1) and secondary (S-2) somatosensory regions. Kenshalo and Isensee (1983) characterized different types of nociceptive neurons in monkey S-1 cortex, using a method similar to that used to characterize caudal ventroposterior lateral nucleus (VPLc) and spinothalamic tract neurons. As might be expected, nociceptive neurons could be characterized as WDR (multireceptive) cells or as NS (high-threshold) cells. Among 68 classified neurons, 37 were WDR and 31 were NS. However, unlike neurons of the VPLc, S-1 cortical nociceptive neurons had either restricted contralateral receptive fields (34 of 68) or very large receptive fields that included most of the body's surface. Neurons with these two types of receptive fields were located side by side near the boundary between areas 3b and 1. Interestingly, Kenshalo and Isensee (1983) found this cortical region to be the site from which the majority of nociceptive VPL neurons could be most effectively antidromically activated.

The receptive field organization and other physiological response characteristics of S-1 neurons with restricted receptive fields were in many respects similar to those of VPLc and spinothalamic tract neurons. The WDR neurons showed increasing responses to gentle tactile stimuli, firm pressure, and pinching of the skin. They responded maximally to nociceptive stimuli and to both thermal and mechanical noxious stimulation. Their increased responses to a second series of nociceptive heat stimuli reflected the sensitization that occurs for primary mechanothermal nociceptive afferents as well as the hyperalgesia that can be measured psychophysically. NS cells responded only to intense pressure and nociceptive mechanical and thermal stimuli. The receptive field sizes of these NS neurons could be as small as a fraction of a single toe. S-1 neurons with restricted contralateral receptive fields are likely to subserve the capacity to recognize the location and quality of a nociceptive stimulus.

The receptive field organization and other physiological response characteristics of S-1 neurons with large receptive fields resembled some spinothalamic tract neurons that project to the medial thalamus and were similar to neurons of the ventromedial part of the posterior nuclear complex (VMpo) and of the ventrocaudal part of the medial dorsal nucleus and parafascicular nucleus (Pf/MDvc) described earlier. For this reason, Kenshalo and Isensee (1983) proposed that cortical nociceptive neurons with large receptive fields could receive information from the projection of the spinothalamic tract via medial thalamic nuclei. The latter are known to project diffusely to the somatosensory cortex. It also is possible that these types of cortical nociceptive neurons receive excitatory effects from other thalamic nuclei such as VMpo and Pf/MDvc, which have large receptive fields. The large-field cortical nociceptive neurons appear to represent the end stage of an ascending afferent system involved in widespread cortical activation.

The detailed analysis of responses of cortical nociceptive neurons with both restricted and large receptive fields to graded nociceptive temperatures sheds further light on the functional roles of these two neuronal populations. The nociceptive temperature-response relationships of both types of neurons were found to be positively accelerating functions (Price et al. 1992; see Fig. 2, lower right panel). Thus, similar to primary nociceptive afferents, spinothalamic tract neurons, and VPLc neurons, cortical nociceptive neuronal responses to graded nociceptive temperatures are consistent with ratings of nociceptive temperature pain intensity in several human psychophysical studies (Chapter 2). Therefore, both large-field and restricted-field nociceptive cortical neurons can provide precise information about nociceptive sensation intensity.

S-1 WDR neurons with restricted receptive fields exhibited almost no adaptation to a 30-second temperature stimulus of 47°C or greater. S-1 WDR neuron responses more closely parallel human pain perception. During similar prolonged thermal stimulation, human subjects report almost no adaptation to continued stimulus intensities above 45°C (Chapter 2). Thus, S-1 WDR cortical nociceptive neurons are most likely responsible for sustained, nonadapting pain that results from long-duration nociceptive stimuli. The adaptation rate of S-1 nociceptive cortical neurons, which presumably receive input from VPLc neurons, is even slower than that of VPLc neurons. The slower adaptation rate of S-1 neurons suggests a transformation mechanism similar to that which occurs at thalamic and dorsal horn levels. Such mechanisms may extend the nociceptive signal well beyond the duration of the stimulus and counter the effects of adaptation at the receptor level, and may have survival value in providing a warning signal that does not decline over time.

Physiological characteristics of nociceptive neurons at lower levels of nociceptive processing are preserved within the cortical S-1 area. However, additional integrative mechanisms occur in the S-1 cortex, as demonstrated by Tommerdahl and colleagues (1996, 1998). They analyzed subregions of S-1 cortex of anesthetized squirrel monkeys, comparing responses to vibrotactile stimuli (mechanical skin tapping) and brief repeated heat pulses (e.g., 52°C applied to the skin once every 2.4 seconds), similar to stimuli that evoke first and second pain (see Chapter 2). They used both intrinsic optical signal imaging (IOS) to analyze neural population responses and microelectrode recordings of single neurons. Maximum neural responses were evoked in areas 3b/1 by vibrotactile stimulation and in area 3a by repeated heat pulses. Neural responses of area 3a increased progressively throughout the train of heat pulses and remained above prestimulus levels for several seconds afterwards. These response characteristics match those of second pain in response to similar trains of heat pulses (Chapter 2). The spatial extent of the IOS was greater for painful stimuli than for vibrotactile stimuli, which supports the spatiotemporal recruitment mechanism described in Chapter 4. The heat-evoked increase in neural activity in area 3a was accompanied by decrease in neural activity in surrounding regions, including 3b, consistent with psychophysical studies showing that painful stimulation inhibits perception of tactile stimuli. These studies show the preservation of nociceptive neural integrative mechanisms at lower levels of processing and additional inhibitory interactions intrinsic to the S-1 cortical area. These latter interactions suggest that nociceptive processing within S-1 is related to discriminating nociceptive from non-nociceptive stimulus events and to other sensory-discriminative features of pain.

The secondary somatosensory area S-2 and neighboring areas 7b and retroinsular cortical regions also contain nociceptive neurons, although they have been characterized in much less detail than those in S-1 (Robinson and Burton 1980; Dong et al. 1989). At least some neurons of these regions can encode the intensity of nociceptive heat stimulation, suggesting a possible role in sensory-discriminative aspects of pain. Clearly, the roles of these areas in sensory and affective dimensions of pain need to be clarified.

Infraparietal cortical area 7b. Beyond the immediate processing of pain sensation intensity, it seems reasonable that further processing of pain requires an evaluation of the pain sensation in relationship to the overall context in which the nociceptive stimulus occurs. This evaluation may indeed represent part of the interface between sensory and affective dimensions of pain. Thus, we might expect that neurons involved in such a function would integrate sensory inputs from multiple sources; that is, they would be multisensory. For example, if the perceived degree of threat of a bee sting is enhanced by hearing and seeing the stinging bee, then such enhancement could occur among multisensory neurons and could be verified in neurophysiological experiments that use combinations of visual, auditory, and nociceptive stimuli.

In direct support of this possibility, some neurons of the infraparietal cortex in area 7b in the monkey respond optimally to nociceptive stimuli, yet also respond to visual stimuli (Dong et al. 1989, 1994). Dong et al. (1994) found that the responses of 7b neurons to mildly noxious heat stimuli (44°–45°C) were enhanced by prior or concurrent visual stimuli. However, this enhancement only occurred if the target location or direction of motion within the visual receptive field was spatially aligned with the cutaneous receptive field. The enhancement was much greater for mild nociceptive stimuli (44°–45°C) than for stronger stimuli (47°C). Thus, it appears that this region of the posterior parietal cortex integrates nociceptive inputs with other sensory inputs to convey information about the overall degree of threat presented to an organism (i.e., seeing a bee while feeling its sting). This integration is especially critical at the low end of the nociceptive stimulus range, where an organism must make a behaviorally relevant decision about the extent of a perceived threat. This interpretation is based on principles of multisensory integration that have been elaborated in great detail by Stein and Meredith (1993).

Further support for this interpretation is derived from observations of effects of lesions to this area, both in monkeys and human patients. Dong et al. (1992) found that focal damage to this area in the monkey eliminated escape responses to normally painful temperatures (i.e., 51°–52°C), although the animals could still detect the offset of noxious thermal stimuli. When an area comparable to area 7b is damaged in humans, a syndrome of pain asymbolia results, where patients no longer appreciate the destructive significance of pain. They do not withdraw from pain stimuli or threatening gestures, despite their capacity to detect the sensory features of nociceptive stimulation (Rubins and Friedman 1948; Weinstein et al. 1995). Therefore, this region of the infraparietal cortex may be a critical interface between the sensory-discriminative and the immediate affective-motivational dimension of pain.

Anterior cingulate cortex. Finally, nociceptive neurons in the ACC have large receptive fields that usually include the whole body surface and yet exhibit the capacity to differentially respond to increasing levels of nociceptive stimulation (Sikes and Vogt 1992). The receptive fields resemble those of neurons in Pf/MDvc medial thalamic nuclei described earlier, as well as those of some types of spinothalamic tract neurons projecting to the medial thalamus (Willis 1985). Thus, the preservation of these physiological characteristics in the ACC has relevance to its proposed role in affective components of pain. A general function of this medial system may to monitor the overall state of the body, a role reflected by neurons with whole-body receptive fields (Craig 1995).

ROLE OF THE CEREBRAL CORTEX IN AROUSAL DURING PAIN

The involvement of the human cerebral cortex in arousal associated with pain is unquestionable. It has long been known that pain is a potent means of producing arousal and widespread cortical activation. This effect has been observed as widespread electroencephalographic changes and increases in brain metabolism over wide areas of the cerebral cortex, especially the frontal cortex (Willis 1985). Similarly, synchronous and repetitive nociceptive stimuli produced by tooth-pulp stimulation or laser beam heat stimulation evoke cortical potentials that can be recorded over the human somatosensory cortex but are maximal at the vertex (Chatrian et al. 1975; Carmon et al. 1976). This result indicates widespread cortical involvement in nociceptive stimulation, possibly mediated by mechanisms of the ascending reticular activating system and medial thalamocortical pathways described earlier. Potent widespread cortical activation by noxious stimulation fits generally with the well-known observation that pain tends to dominate consciousness and takes priority over other ongoing sensory inputs. This arousal mechanism may well be associated with the immediate affective dimension of pain, because the domination of consciousness would likely contribute to the overall sense of intrusion that occurs during pain.

FRONTAL CORTICAL AREAS INVOLVED IN "HIGHER-ORDER" PAIN PROCESSING

The involvement of the prefrontal cortical lobes in complex aspects of cognitive-evaluative and hence secondary affective dimensions of pain is supported by detailed observations of patients before and after prefrontal lobotomy. Hardy et al. (1952) found that prefrontal lobotomy produced no overall change in heat-induced experimental pain thresholds in eight patients tested. Nevertheless, perceived intensity of clinical pain decreased somewhat in four of five patients studied. However, the most striking changes were in patients' attitudes, emotional reactions, and cognitive processing of pain. The lobotomized patients were emotionally indifferent to low-intensity pains, which though perceived, evoked few affective reactions. A statement that epitomized this attitude was "Yes, I feel the pain, but it doesn't bother me." Moderate- to high-intensity pains sometimes evoked overreactions, manifested by grimacing and agitation when direct questions forced patients to focus on the pain. When patients were left alone, however, they had few thoughts about pain and showed little spontaneous concern about its negative implications in terms of damage to the body or threat to life. White and Sweet (1969) have corroborated these observations. Evidently, lobotomy somehow interferes with the spontaneous ongoing cognitive evaluations that are related to the long-term implications of having a persistent pain condition. It is possible that lobotomy selectively reduces the secondary stage of pain affect described in Chapter 3, a stage that is partly based on reflective processes related to memory of past consequences of having pain as well as future implications. The lack of spontaneous pain-related suffering in patients with prefrontal lobotomy differs from pain asymbolia (Rubins and Friedman 1948; Weinstein et al. 1995). Lobotomized patients appear to perceive the immediate threat of pain once it is brought to their attention (Hardy et al. 1952), whereas patients with pain asymbolia appear incapable of perceiving the threatening nature of nociceptive stimuli under any circumstances.

NEURAL IMAGING STUDIES OF PAIN

Within recent years, neural imaging studies of pain have confirmed increases in neural activity within the pain-related pathways and brain regions discussed so far. These studies provide a three-dimensional view of multiple CNS regions activated during pain. Two types of neural imaging experiments involve mapping pain-related neural activity in animals with a persistent pain condition and studying regional cerebral blood flow (rCBF) in experimental pain in human subjects. The results from both types of studies are complementary.

2-Deoxyglucose mapping studies and cerebral blood flow studies in rats

Regional increases in brain neural activity were examined in rats with painful peripheral mononeuropathy produced by chronic constrictive injury (CCI) of the sciatic nerve by using the ^{14}C-2-deoxyglucose (2-DG) autoradiographic technique to measure local glucose utilization rate and hence neural activity (Mao et al. 1993). The extensive activation of brain regions of a CCI rat in comparison with a sham-operated control is shown in Fig. 4. The pattern of activation shown here is representative of that based on statistical analysis of group data. Significant increases in neural activity were found in virtually all of the ascending pain-related pathways and their target brain structures. Thus, increases in neural activity were found in the hypothalamic nuclei (VPM and arcuate nucleus), ventral posterior lateral nucleus, posterior thalamic nucleus, central gray matter, deep layers of the superior colliculus, pontine reticular formation, pontine parabrachial nucleus, medullary nucleus gigantocellularis, and paragigantocellular nucleus. The hindlimb region of S-1 and S-2 somatosensory areas, representing the cortical endstage of the spinothalamocortical pathway, had the greatest increase in activity within the parietal cortex. As expected, thalamic VPL/posterior nuclear complex nuclei and S-1/S-2 somatosensory areas contralateral to the injured nerve showed larger increases in neural activity than did corresponding ipsilateral brain regions. However, significant bilateral increases occurred within these regions. In addition, cortical areas heavily interconnected with subcortical limbic structures also were activated. These included the ACC (within frontal lobes), retrosplenial granular cortex, and amygdala. Finally, small increases in neural activity occurred throughout the parietal cortex, suggesting widespread cortical activation. However, this diffuse increase was not present in cortical areas unrelated to somatosensory processing, such as the auditory or visual areas. Thus, sciatic nerve injury induced increases in neural activity within extensive brain regions previously implicated in sensory and affective-motivational dimensions of pain. These increases are likely to reflect neural representations of spontaneous pain as well as activation of brain areas involved in the modulation of pain.

These patterns of increased brain neural activity following CCI are similar in many respects to those induced by acute noxious heat or formalin stimulation. Porro et al. (1991) observed similar brain metabolic activity in response to subcutaneous formalin injection, and Morrow et al. (1998) have shown very similar patterns of rCBF in CCI rats as well as rats injected with intradermal formalin. Both studies found increases in activity of cortical areas involved in somatosensory processing and areas heavily interconnected with subcortical limbic structures. The correspondence between results using 2-DG autoradiography and rCBF mapping is important because it helps us to validate and interpret the results of human rCBF studies.

Neural imaging studies in humans that identify cortical regions involved in pain

Similar to these metabolic mapping studies of pain in rats, several neural imaging studies using either positron emission tomography (PET) or functional magnetic resonance imaging (fMRI) have shown increases in neural activity, as measured by rCBF, in several areas of the human cerebral cortex and thalamus. Table II summarizes the main structures activated across five PET studies of human pain (but see Hsieh et al. 1996 for a much more comprehensive list of pain imaging studies). Although these five studies had modest differences in the PET techniques and forms of experimental pain, results were fairly consistent. Cerebral cortical areas most commonly activated included the S-1 and S-2 somatosensory cortex, anterior insular cortex, anterior cingulate cortex (ACC) (particularly area 24), and supplementary motor areas. Not all of these structures were activated in every study, but the combined results of neural imaging studies conducted to date strongly implicate all of these cerebral regions in pain processing. There is also evidence that the number of brain areas activated and their overall areas of activation increase as a function of the intensity of pain. Casey et al. (1996) demonstrated the influence of pain intensity on the number of cortical regions activated. They compared the activation pattern of the scans taken during the first 60 seconds of a noxious heat stimulation session of repetitive 50°C pulses with scans from the last 55 seconds of the stimulation period. Although the stimulus intensity was the same for both periods, both perceived pain intensity and the number of brain areas dramatically increased from early to late periods. Brain areas activated during the early period included the contralateral primary sensorimotor cortex, ACC, and thalamus. These same areas plus the contralateral premotor cortex, insular cortex, S-2, ipsilateral insula, and ipsilateral medial thalamus were activated during the late period. Furthermore, the regions activated during the early period showed increased responses during the late period. Taken together, these results demonstrate that multiple forebrain structures encode the increasing intensity and unpleasantness of pain under conditions where the physical stimulus intensity remains constant.

A PET study by Hsieh et al. (1996) identified the largest number of brain structures activated during pain. This study was unique in using an intracutaneous injection of a minute amount of ethanol to produce both pain and minor dermal injury. In this respect, the study modeled acute clinical pain. Brain areas activated included the primary somatosensory/motor areas, ACC areas 32 and 24, the supplementary motor area, insular cortex, cerebellum, posterior parietal cortex, prefrontal cortex, hypothalamus, and central gray. This study is noteworthy because the activated brain regions are the targets of central pathways discussed in this chapter and because the pain was produced by mild traumatic injury.

Hsieh and colleagues suggested that the traumatically evoked pain is additionally associated with central processing at the levels of the hypo-

Table II
Regions showing significant increases in regional cerebral blood flow in
five PET studies of normal subjects

Structure	Study 1	Study 2	Study 3	Study 4	Study 5
Somatosensory area S-1	+	+	+	+	+
Somatosensory area S-2	+	+	+	+	+
ACC area 24	+	+	+	+	+
Anterior insular cortex	+	+	+	+	+
Thalamus	n.a.	+	+	+	n.a.
Premotor cortex	n.a.	0	+	+	+

Note: Study 1 = Talbot et al. (1991), using heat; 2 = Coghill et al. (1994), heat; 3 = Casey et al. (1994), heat; 4 = Casey et al. (1996), cold; 5 = Hsieh et al. (1996), cutaneous ethanol; ACC = anterior cingulate cortex; n.a. = not applicable.

thalamus and central gray, regions that are involved in autonomic and automatic affective responses associated with sudden acute pain. However, cortical regions that are likely to be involved in "higher-order" processing related to pain affect also were activated by the same injurious stimulus. The posterior parietal cortex contains representations of intra- and extrapersonal space, including a body schema on which humans establish a physical sense of the self (Anderson 1987; Heilman et al. 1987; Stein 1989). As discussed earlier, this region contains neurons that may combine nociceptive inputs with those of other sensory modalities to provide an integrated output related to a sense of intrusion or threat to the physical body (Dong et al. 1994). The concomitant activation of the prefrontal cortex may be related to a part of a feedback network related to attention, cognitive evaluation, and self-awareness (Cohen 1993). This possibility is consistent with the effects of damage to this brain region, which include impairments in planning, behavioral control, affective attachment, and ability to direct or sustain attention. The ACC may well be a part of a network to facilitate attention to and evaluation of pain. Finally, the pain-related activation of the anterior insular cortex may reflect mechanisms and circuits that integrate sensory input from somatosensory areas with limbic structures involved in memory, motivation, and affective functions (Mesulam 1999).

CHARACTERIZATION OF CORTICAL NETWORKS INVOLVED IN DIFFERENT STAGES AND DIMENSIONS OF PAIN

The ascending neural pathways and brain regions involved in neural processing of pain, as well as their interconnections, are summarized in Fig.

Fig. 4. Topographic presentation of coronal sections showing local glucose utilization in the brain of a chronic constriction injury (CCI) rat (right column) and a sham-operated rat (left column). Sciatic nerve ligation produced substantial increases in metabolic activity within cortical hindlimb (HL) and forelimb (FL) area, retrosplenial granular cortex (RG), cingulate cortex (CG), parietal area (PA), caudate-putamen complex (CP), amygdala (AG), ventral posterolateral thalamic nucleus (VPL), ventral posteromedial thalamic nucleus (VPM), and ventral medial thalamic nucleus (VM), as compared to corresponding regions of sham-operated rats. This increase was more pronounced on the contralateral side (left side of an image) of CCI rats than on the ipsilateral side. Other activated structures include the lateral paragigantocellular nucleus (LPG), posterior thalamic nucleus (PO), parabrachial nuclei (PB), parvocellular reticular nucleus (PCR), superior colliculus (SC), and spinal vestibular nuclei (SV). The anteroposterior coordinates of each coronal section (from pair A to pair E) are –0.80 mm, –3.14 mm, –7.80 mm, –9.80 mm, and –11.96 mm, respectively, based on Paxinos and Watson (1986). The color bar represents the calibration of the local glucose utilization rate ($\mu mol \cdot 100$ $g^{-1} \cdot min^{-1}$) for these images. Reprinted from Mao et al. (1993), with permission. $\longrightarrow$

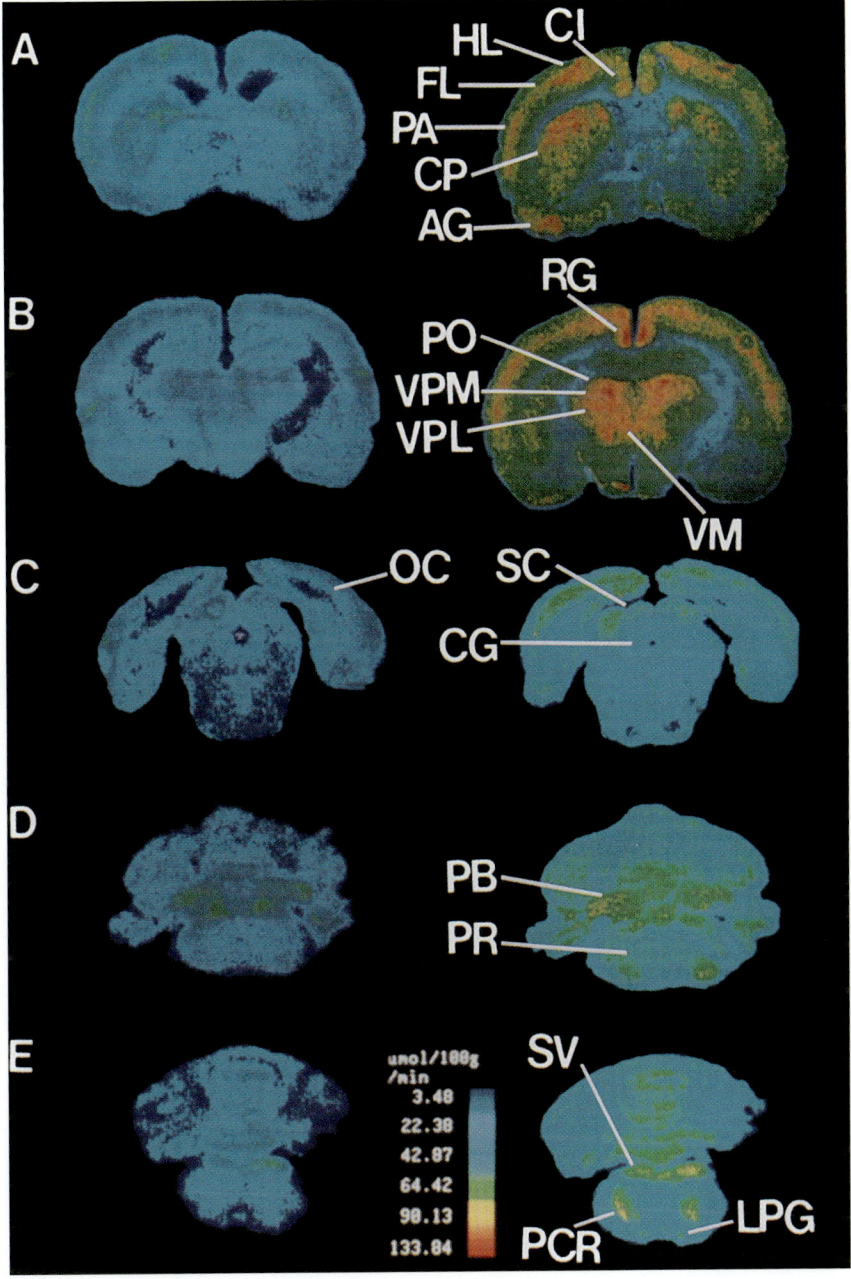

5. These pathways and brain regions have three notable characteristics. First, pain-related somatosensory information is transmitted over multiple parallel ascending pathways to subcortical and cortical regions. Second, an elaborate cortical network is involved in pain. Third, this network contains many reciprocal interconnections to areas involved in somatosensory processing and other areas involved in attention, memory, cognitive evaluation, affect, and motivation. The collective results of human cerebral cortical studies of pain have allowed us to identify the multiple anatomical sites of pain-related activation. A major challenge remains: to determine how this distributed network processes different components of pain experience and behavior. For example, how can neural imaging studies be extended to demonstrate the differential involvement of these various cortical regions at the sensory-discriminative stage and the immediate and secondary stages of pain-related affect? How do these various brain regions encode the magnitudes of these pain dimensions?

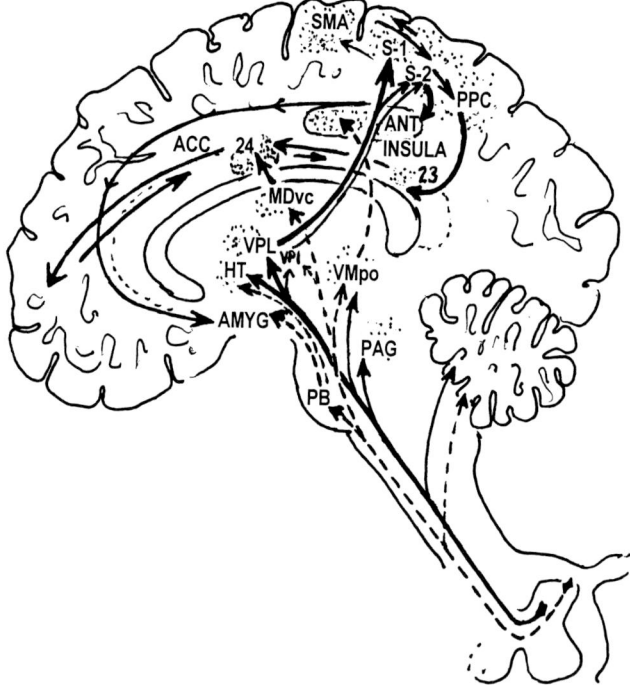

Fig. 5. Schematic of ascending pathways, subcortical structures, and cerebral cortical structures involved in processing pain. ACC = anterior cingulate cortex; HT = hypothalamus; MCvc = ventrocaudal part of the medial dorsal nucleus; PAG = periaqueductal gray; PB = parabrachial nucleus of the dorsolateral pons; PPC = posterior parietal cortex; SMA = supplementary motor area; VMpo = ventromedial part of the posterior nuclear complex; VPI = ventral posterior inferior nucleus.

In recent years, human neural imaging studies and other types of human neurological studies have moved beyond functional neuroanatomical identification of brain structures activated during pain. Such studies now represent dynamic analyses of changes in pain intensity and unpleasantness in relationship to changes in neural activities of various brain areas. Two types of studies represent efforts to answer the questions posed above. The first type have examined temporal and spatial factors that encode the intensity of pain. The second type have used psychological strategies of differentially modulating the affective or sensory dimension of pain and then examining how neural activity in different cortical regions covaries with these differential effects.

HUMAN STUDIES SUPPORTING CEREBRAL CORTICAL SPATIOTEMPORAL CODING OF PAIN

Porro and colleagues (1998) used a high-resolution fMRI technique to demonstrate cortical areas showing changes in neural activity related to the time profile of pain intensity produced by subcutaneous injection of dilute ascorbic acid into the foot. This stimulus produced pain with a mean intensity of 48 on a scale of 100 and a mean duration of about 12 minutes. Both the *magnitudes* of the fMRI signals and the *spatial extents* of these signals within S-1 and ACC areas were strongly and positively correlated with pain intensity. These results corroborate those of Tommerdahl et al. (1996, 1998) described earlier. The authors further demonstrated that these observed spatial and temporal responses were specifically related to pain intensity and duration and not to nonspecific arousal or emotional aspects of the experimental context.

This evidence that the magnitude and spatial extent of the signals within S-1 and ACC contribute to the overall perceived intensity of pain confirms and extends the spatiotemporal hypothesis outlined in Chapter 4, which states that impulse frequency and the total number of neurons activated combine to encode pain intensity. The magnitude and spatial extent of the fMRI signal would reflect the former and latter, respectively. This pain-encoding mechanism would be expected, given that the spatial organization of receptive fields of WDR neurons at thalamic VPLc and cortical S-1 areas is precisely similar to that of dorsal horn WDR neurons. The receptive field includes a central zone that is differentially responsive to innocuous and nociceptive stimulation and a much larger surrounding zone that is responsive mainly to nociceptive stimuli. Taken in light of neuronal recruitment mechanisms proposed for dorsal horn neurons in Chapter 4, a nociceptive stimulus would be expected to activate more VPLc and more S-1 WDR noci-

7). Ratings of stimuli presented contralateral to the responding hemisphere were normal. This pattern of responses suggests that at high enough nociceptive levels, recruitment of pathways other than the classical crossed spinothalamic-cortical pathway may make up for the pain sensory deficit that occurs when one cerebral hemisphere is no longer able to share nociceptive information with the other via the corpus callosum. A similar pattern of results was reported in a patient with a lateral thalamic lesion (Greenspan et al. 1997), and the findings are also consistent with observations of Head and Holmes (1911) described earlier. Higher levels of nociceptive stimulation increase both the areas of activated brain regions and the number of regions activated (Fig. 6). This spatiotemporal recruitment is relevant for all dimensions of pain experience and behavior.

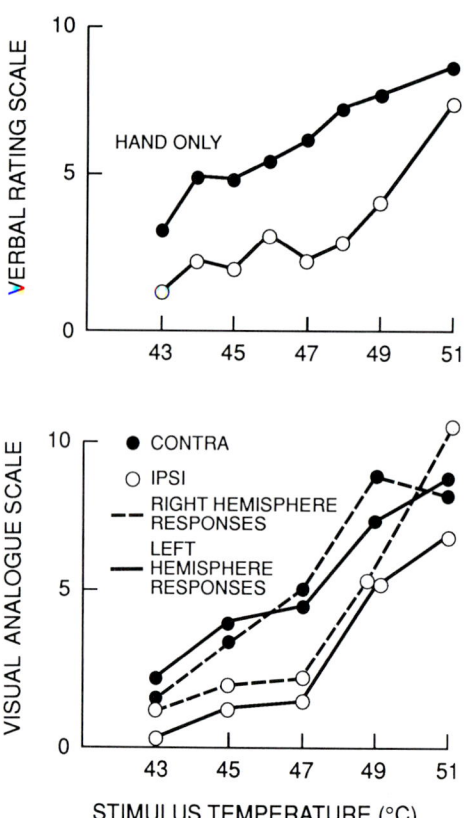

Fig. 7. Perceived pain intensity in a split-brain patient. The ipsilateral hemisphere perceived low-intensity nociceptive stimuli (43°–47°C) poorly, as indicated by VAS ratings, but readily perceived high-intensity stimuli (49°–51°C), which the patient rated as both very intense and very unpleasant. This pattern of responses indicates that "ipsilateral" pathways can contribute to pain dimensions at high enough stimulus levels. Adapted from Stein et al. (1989), with permission.

NEURAL IMAGING OF SENSORY AND AFFECTIVE REPRESENTATIONS OF PAIN WITHIN THE HUMAN CEREBRAL CORTEX

A further step in analysis of cerebral cortical representations of pain is to determine which structures are most closely related to the different dimensions of pain. Two recent PET studies revealed significant activation in somatosensory area S-1, anterior cingulate cortex (ACC) area 24, and the anterior insular cortex both before and during hypnosis. In the first study, hypnotic suggestions were given to selectively alter the affective dimension of pain without changing the perceived intensity of the painful sensation (Rainville et al. 1997). The experimental conditions included immersion of the left hand in moderately painful water (47°C) without hypnosis, with hypnosis but without suggestions, with hypnosis with suggestions for *increased* unpleasantness, and finally with hypnosis with suggestions for *decreased* unpleasantness. Unpleasantness ratings were much higher during the high compared to the low unpleasantness condition, but pain sensation ratings were the same. High and low unpleasantness conditions also had no difference in effect on somatosensory area S-1, a region considered to process sensory-discriminative components of pain (Fig. 8). In striking contrast, and consistent with unpleasantness ratings, activity in ACC area 24 was much greater in the high than the low unpleasantness condition. A separate regression analysis, controlling for factors such as individual differences in global cerebral blood flow and pain sensation intensity ratings, showed that pain unpleasantness ratings were significantly associated *only* with ACC activity in a specific region of area 24 ($R = 0.55$, $P < 0.001$). These results indicate that hypnotic modulation of the affective dimension of pain is at least partly reflected by changes in cortical limbic regional activity (i.e., in ACC area 24). As stated above, the ACC may be a part of a network of attention, evaluation, and affect that establishes negative emotional valence to pain. It also may coordinate inputs from parietal areas involved in perception of bodily threat with frontal cortical areas involved in plans and response priorities for pain-related behavior. Thus, the role of the ACC in pain-related affect is likely to be both pivotal and complex.

The second, similarly designed study used hypnotic suggestions that were selectively targeted toward the sensory-intensive dimension of pain (Hofbauer et al. 1998). However, the suggestions were effective in modulating both sensory and affective dimensions of pain experience, as rated by the subjects. Unlike the first study, both activity in somatosensory area S-1 and pain sensation ratings were higher in the high than the low sensory intensity condition. A similar but nonsignificant trend occurred in the ACC. The most important result of the Hofbauer study is that it provides a confir-

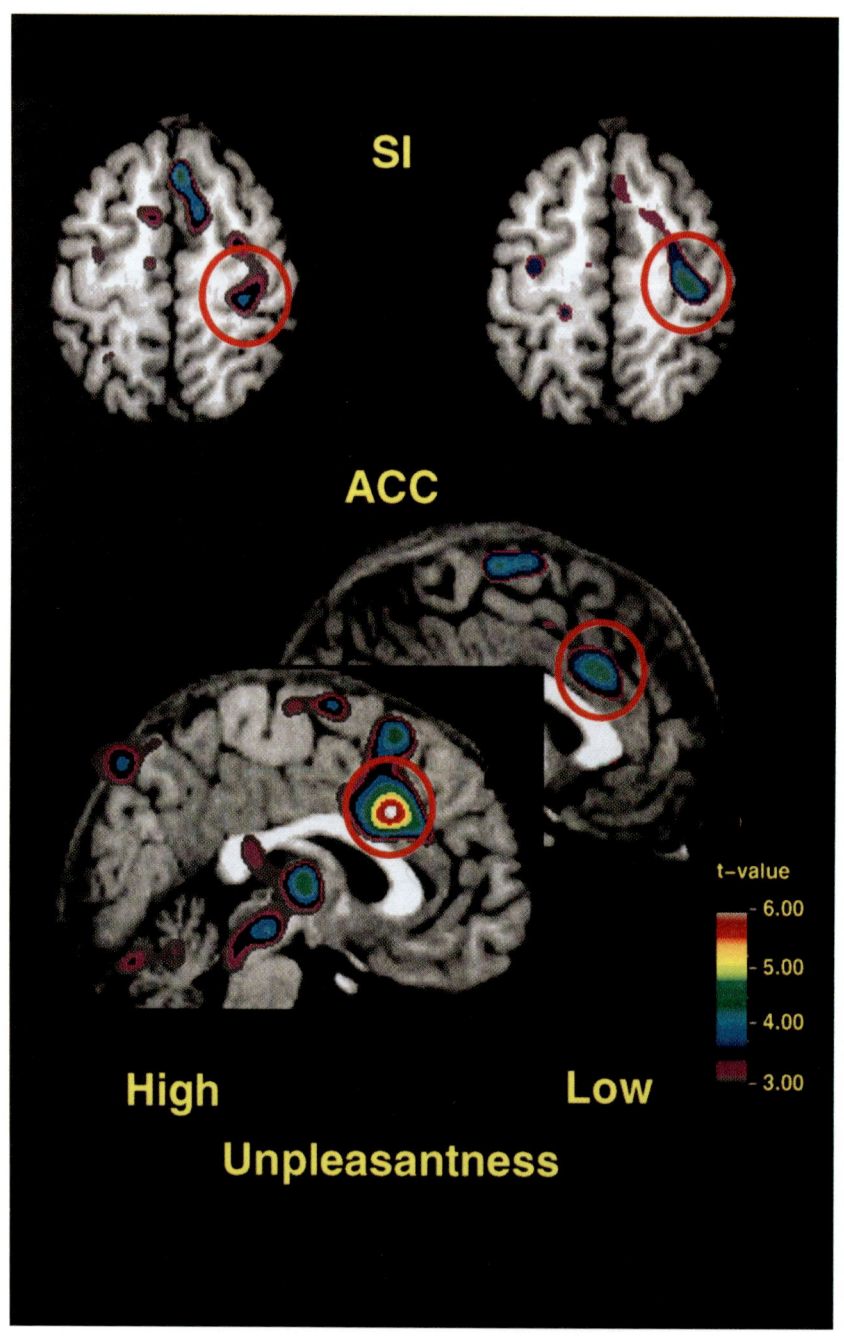

mation of the role of the S-1 somatosensory cortex in the sensory-discriminative dimension of pain.

Tolle et al. (1999) used a different experimental approach to dissociate sensory from affective pain dimensions, using PET to examine cortical regions differentially associated with the two dimensions. Using noxious heat and successive experimental pain trials, the authors evoked lower ratios of pain unpleasantness to pain sensation intensity on the first two trials and higher ratios on the second two trials. Their regression analysis revealed that somatosensory cortical area activity coded the intensity of pain sensation, as did the periventricular gray and posterior cingulate cortex (PCC). Pain unpleasantness was mainly encoded in the posterior sector of the ACC. These results confirm those of Rainville et al. (1997) and extend them by showing pain intensity coding in the PCC, which is known to receive input from posterior parietal areas that are likely to be involved in multisensory processing of pain (Neal et al. 1987; Dong et al. 1994). The PCC may be a link between somatosensory processing of pain and affective processing related to the ACC (Vogt et al. 1979, 1993; Hsieh et al. 1996). Other PET studies of human pain, including that of neuropathic pain, have shown activation within the PCC (Hsieh et al. 1996).

These experiments suggest strategies for the preliminary characterization of different dimensions of pain and their underlying neural mechanisms. Clearly, further studies using similar approaches must be conducted. Already, however, the view that cortical representation of pain is impossible or that it is limited to a single region has been replaced by the concept that a complex network of cortical areas processes the different components of pain.

Returning to the schematic of Fig. 5, we can at least speculate about the general mechanisms by which multiple ascending pathways and brain regions participate in the various stages of pain processing and in the different dimensions of pain experience. First, it is clear that direct pathways lead from the spinal cord to brain structures that are involved in rudimentary aspects of escape, motor orientation, arousal, and fear. These include medullary and midbrain structures such as reticular formation nuclei, deep layers of the superior colliculus, and the central gray, and also limbic structures

---

← **Fig. 8.** Hypnotic suggestions for high and low pain unpleasantness produce corresponding increases (left sagittal scan) or decreases (right sagittal scan) in neural activity (measured by rCBF) in the anterior cingulate cortex (ACC), but no change in S-1 somatosensory cortex (SI), similar to respective effects on unpleasantness and sensation intensity ratings. The colored areas are those with statistically significant increases in rCBF (and hence neural activity). The *t* values for those increases are shown to the right of the color key. Reprinted with permission from Rainville, P., Duncan, G.H., Price, D.D., Carrier, B., Bushnell, M.C. Pain affect encoded in human anterior cingulate but not somatosensory cortex. *Science* 1997; 277:968–971. © 1997, American Association for the Advancement of Science.

such as the amygdala and hypothalamus. Activation of these structures
is likely to occur somewhat automatically during the *immediate* and perhaps
even during the *acute* phase of pain behavior described in Chapter 1. Thus,
fear, defensive behavior, and autonomic responses associated with fight or
flight would be associated with activation of these structures. These responses would involve a minimum amount of reflection or cognition.

Superimposed on this level of integration would be that related to perceptual aspects of pain processing, such as the appreciation of the intensive
and qualitative aspects of pain sensation. Primary and secondary somatosensory cortical areas would be involved at this level. For example, evidence
suggests that the S-1 cortex is involved in discriminating nociceptive from
non-nociceptive stimulus events. A closely associated but higher level of
processing in more posterior parietal regions would include mechanisms
that integrate somatosensory nociceptive input with other multisensory contextual inputs to provide an overall sense of intrusion and threat to the
physical body and self. Both posterior parietal and insular cortical regions
would be involved at this level. Friedman et al. (1986) similarly suggested a
ventrally directed corticolimbic pathway that integrates somatosensory input with learning and memory. The somatic perceptual features of pain would
then be integrated with cognitive-evaluative and attentional mechanisms
that, in turn, establish emotional valence and response priorities. Response
priorities would be closely related to premotor functions (represented in the
supplementary motor area, for example) that are integrally related to motivation and emotions. The ACC may have a pivotal role in interrelating
attentional and evaluative functions with the task of establishing emotional
valence and response priorities. Response priorities may be associated with
immediate efforts to cope with, escape, or avoid the pain and pain-evoking
situation and therefore with cortical activity in premotor areas. In this way,
cortical areas involved in the sensory-discriminative dimension of pain are
at least partly *in series* with the immediate affective-motivational dimension
of pain. As discussed in Chapter 3, this is also true at a psychological level.

However, the response priorities change over an extended period of
time. Pain unpleasantness endured over time engages prefrontal cortical areas involved in reflection and rumination over the long-term consequences
and future implications of a persistent pain condition. The ACC may also
coordinate somatosensory features of pain with cerebral mechanisms involved in the secondary stage of pain-related affect discussed in Chapter 3.
Importantly, cerebral cortical mechanisms of pain affect may also engage
many of the same subcortical limbic structures that are involved in rudimentary aspects of emotional feelings. This possibility is consistent with
Damasio's (1994) general view of neural mechanisms of human emotions.

Thus, activation of subcortical and limbic cortical structures by ascending input from pain-related pathways produces autonomic and somatomotor activation and at the same time provides a background of afferent input from the body that is part of the felt sense of emotional feeling. However, this background is juxtaposed with the content provided by pain-related somatic perceptions, perceptions that are integrated with contextual factors. The "background" and pain-related somatic perceptions converge within common cortical areas and contribute to pain-related emotional feelings.

Therefore, the affective-motivational dimension of pain is likely to involve both "bottom-up" and "top-down" processing. Rudimentary aspects of pain affect are processed by direct spinal inputs to limbic structures and medial thalamic nuclei involved in affect. These structures provide direct input to cortical regions involved in monitoring the overall state of the body and in directing attention. However, the same structures can also be accessed by cortical structures that add greater or lesser degrees of cognitive evaluation to pain affect (Fig. 5). This explanation is consistent with psychological evidence that pain unpleasantness comprises multiple components, including one that is directly related to the sensations and others that require greater degrees of evaluation (Chapter 3). The relationships among brain regions involved in processing the various dimensions of pain are both in parallel and in series, and are reciprocal.

Psychological Mechanisms of Pain and Analgesia, Progress in Pain Research and Management, Vol. 15, by Donald D. Price, IASP Press, Seattle, © 1999.

6

General Mechanisms of Pain Modulation

Anyone who has witnessed several athletic events or has visited many patients in hospital knows that the relationship between stimulus intensity and magnitude of pain perception often is not simple. Two kinds of observations support the complexity of this relationship. The first is clinical: pain often occurs without any apparent precipitating pathology. The second is the common observation that pain may not be experienced in the presence of factors that should produce it; that is, under various circumstances, partial or total analgesia can occur. Earlier theoretical models of pain perception (Noordenbos 1959; Melzack and Wall 1965) recognized that the nervous system possesses intrinsic pain-inhibitory mechanisms, although only indirect supporting evidence was available.

Considerable progress has been made in the past 35 years toward identifying and characterizing the neural circuitry that underlies the inhibition of pain. Many of the ascending pain-related pathways discussed in the previous two chapters terminate within cortical and subcortical structures that represent origins of pain-modulatory pathways, such as the hypothalamic nuclei, amygdala, and midbrain periaqueductal gray (PAG). Interestingly, these brain structures are related to three currently active areas of psychology and neuroscience relevant to pain inhibition, which involve learning and memory, threat-elicited defensive behavior, and pain modulation. For example, threat and pain modulation interact during the production of conditioned fear (Faneslow 1984, 1991; Helmstetter and Tershner 1994). Furthermore, our knowledge of the circuitry underlying each of these general phenomena is increasing. These three research areas relate in turn to questions about general neural mechanisms of pain inhibition. First, under what psychological and environmental circumstances do analgesic systems operate—that is, what triggers analgesic systems? Second, once these systems are triggered, by what mechanisms do they produce the analgesic effect? Third, what is the evidence that these psychological and physiological mechanisms of pain inhibition exist in humans?

This chapter provides a mechanistic foundation to explain both simple and complex forms of psychologically mediated analgesia in humans. It discusses the general mechanisms of analgesia and the biological conditions under which they are triggered. The schematic of Fig. 1 serves as a general guide to the general neural circuitry involved in analgesia mechanisms. This chapter emphasizes mechanisms that modulate *both* sensory and affective dimensions of pain (for a discussion of psychological mechanisms that selectively modulate the affective-motivational dimension of pain, see Chapter 3).

ANIMAL STUDIES OF LEARNING ANALGESIA

Activation of analgesic mechanisms requires an extrinsic environmental cue or condition. In humans, cues associated with past relief of pain may be visual (the pill or syringe), auditory (the nurse's voice), or tactile (the prick of the needle associated with intravenous morphine). These cues may be effective for evoking endogenous analgesic mechanisms because they were present during previous effective treatments for pain or because they have symbolic meaning: for example, if the phrase "this is a powerful painkiller" accompanies an intravenous injection, analgesia may be enhanced. The po-

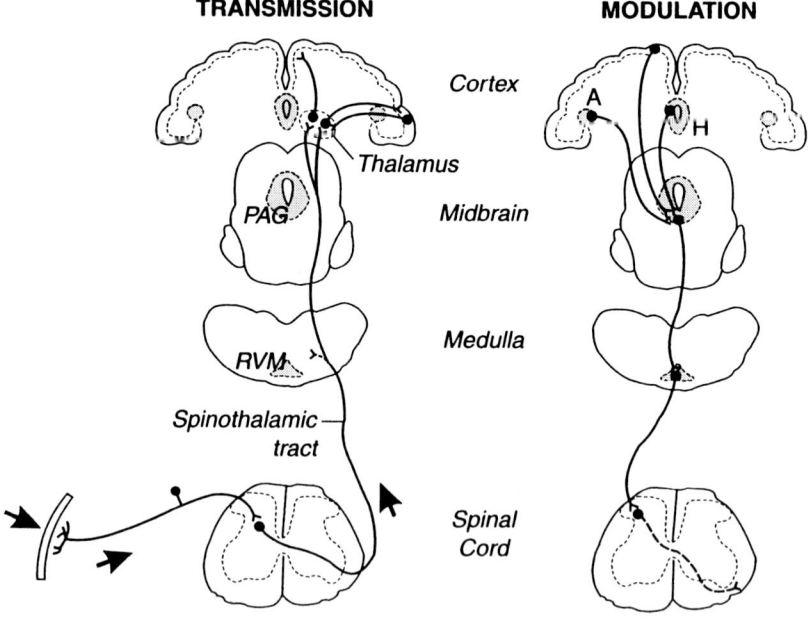

Fig. 1. Transmission and modulation of pain transmission pathways. Note that the origin of pain-modulatory pathways includes the cerebral cortex, hypothalamus, amygdala, periaqueductal gray (PAG), and rostroventral medulla (RVM). Many of these structures are also central targets of ascending nociceptive pathways discussed in Chapter 5. From Fields and Price (1997), with permission from Harvard University Press.

tential neurobiology of how symbolic meaning can elicit analgesia is much more problematic than that of simple forms of learning, such as classical conditioning.

Nevertheless, animal models of learning analgesia are useful and may be partly applicable to analgesia evoked by complex meanings. Conditioned analgesic responses in animals can be robust; they can be elicited in ways that are relevant to analgesia in humans, particularly placebo analgesia. The most extensively studied form of conditioned analgesia involves fear-evoked defense responses. In studies of this phenomenon, rats are subjected to an inescapable noxious footshock that causes stress and analgesia (Watkins and Mayer 1982a; Watkins et al. 1983; Faneslow 1984, 1991; Helmstetter and Tershner 1994). The stress analgesia subsides, but when the rats are later returned to the apparatus in which the noxious stimulus was administered, the environmental context is sufficient to produce an analgesic effect. The inescapable footshock serves as the unconditioned stimulus, and the environmental cues associated with the footshock are conditioned stimuli. Several trials of inescapable footshock result in a classically conditioned analgesia that can be evoked when rats are placed within the apparatus. Such analgesia can be blocked by the opioid antagonist naloxone or by lesions of a specific neural circuit implicated in the production of defense behaviors in response to threat (Helmstetter and Tershner 1994). Watkins and Mayer (1982a) proposed this type of conditioned analgesia as a general model for placebo analgesia.

Specific central nervous system (CNS) circuitry has been implicated in conditioned analgesia in animals. Therefore, to the extent to which these animal models of learned analgesia are applicable to humans, they could be important in determining the underlying neural mechanisms of psychologically mediated analgesia. The extent to which conditioning, fear, and anxiety contribute to such analgesia in humans is of particular interest, because such factors are likely to contribute both to placebo analgesia and to analgesia caused by threatening circumstances. The following discussion will focus on endogenous pain-inhibitory circuitry and its role in psychologically mediated analgesia. In the chapters that follow I will refer to this discussion in order to link neurobiological and psychological explanations of pain inhibition.

ENDOGENOUS OPIOID PAIN-INHIBITORY SYSTEMS

Information about tissue damage is not passively received by the nervous system; rather, it is modulated even at the first synapse within the dorsal horn by complex inhibitory and facilitatory control systems, as discussed in Chapter 4. The discovery of these systems has fostered, and has in turn been fostered by, the notion that the CNS contains endogenous substances—endorphins—that possess analgesic properties virtually identical to opioids of plant and synthetic origin. In this section, I examine the development of these concepts and consider opioid and nonopioid CNS pain-modulatory mechanisms that are activated by environmental and psychological circumstances.

The earliest work indicating that opiates produce analgesia, at least in part, by activation of endogenous pain-inhibitory systems was done by Irwin and colleagues (1951). They demonstrated that morphine was not effective in inhibiting the spinally mediated tail-flick response in rats whose spinal cords were transected at mid-thoracic levels. Based on this result, they reasoned that morphine must activate supraspinal neural circuitry that has an output to the spinal cord and modulates the processing of nociceptive information at the spinal level. This work was largely ignored until the early 1970s.

The first impetus for the detailed study of pain-modulatory circuitry was the observation that electrical stimulation of the PAG region could powerfully suppress the perception of pain (Reynolds 1969; Mayer et al. 1971). Further investigation of brain-stimulation-produced analgesia (SPA) provided considerable detail about the neural circuitry involved (see Mayer and Manning 1995 for a detailed review). Significantly, at that time, several similarities were recognized between these observations and information emerging from a concomitant resurgence of interest in the mechanisms of opioid analgesia (Mayer et al. 1971). Two important parallel facts were discovered. First, effective loci for both opioid microinjection analgesia (Tsou and Jang 1964) and SPA (Mayer et al. 1971) reside within the periaqueductal and periventricular gray matter of the brainstem (Fig. 1). Second, opioid analgesia and SPA are both mediated in part by the activation of a centrifugal control system that descends from the brain and modulates pain transmission at the level of the spinal cord dorsal horn (Mayer et al. 1971) (Fig. 1). Thus, the ultimate inhibition of the transmission of nociceptive information occurs, at least in part, at the initial processing stages in the spinal cord dorsal horn and homologous trigeminal caudal nucleus by selective inhibition of nociceptive neurons (Satoh and Takagi 1971).

In addition, studies of SPA have provided direct evidence that the CNS has mechanisms that depend upon endogenous opioids. Subanalgesic doses of morphine were shown to synergize with subanalgesic levels of brain stimulation to produce behavioral analgesia (Saminin and Valzelli 1971). Analgesic tolerance, a phenomenon invariably associated with repeated administration of opioids, occurred in response to repeated trials of brain stimulation, and cross-tolerance occurred between the analgesic effects of brain stimulation and of systemic opioids (Mayer and Hayes 1975). Finally, SPA was at least partially antagonized by naloxone, a specific narcotic antagonist (Akil et al. 1972, 1976). This last observation, in particular, could be most parsimoniously explained if electrical stimulation of the PAG releases an endogenous opioid-like factor. Indeed, naloxone antagonism of SPA was a critical impetus for the eventual discovery of enkephalin (Hughes 1975).

Coincidental with work on SPA, another discovery was of critical importance for our current concepts of endogenous analgesia systems. Several laboratories, almost simultaneously, reported stereospecific binding sites for opioids within the CNS (Hiller et al. 1973; Pert and Snyder 1973; Terenius 1973). Opioid receptor sites were subsequently shown to be localized to neuronal synaptic regions (Pert et al. 1974) and to overlap anatomically with loci involved in the neural processing of pain (Pert et al. 1975). The existence of an opioid receptor again suggested an endogenous compound with opioid properties to occupy it.

In 1975, Hughes reported the isolation from neural tissue of enkephalin. An immense amount of subsequent work has characterized this and other neural and extraneural compounds with opioid properties. As with the opioid receptor, the anatomical distribution of endogenous opioid ligands shows overlap with sites involved in pain processing (see Mayer and Price 1994 for a review).

NEURAL CIRCUITRY ACTIVATED BY EXOGENOUS OPIOIDS

We now have considerable data on the sites and mechanisms involved in the modulation of pain following the administration of exogenous opioids. Two primary lines of experimentation have been conducted. The first has been to map several areas in the CNS and identify specific sites at which administration of opioids results in analgesia and that of opioid antagonists blocks analgesia. The second has been to determine brain locations where lesions block the analgesic effects of exogenous opioids.

Opioid microinjection mapping studies determined that periaqueductal and periventricular regions of the mesencephalon and diencephalon contain critical sites at which microinjection of opioids results in analgesia (Tsou and Jang 1964; Jacquet and Lajtha 1973, Pert and Yaksh 1974; Yaksh et al. 1976). The resurgence of interest in these particular sites of opioid action probably resulted from work showing that electrical stimulation of the PAG causes analgesia (Mayer et al. 1971). Overall, these and other studies confirmed the importance of the periaqueductal and periventricular regions in opioid analgesia and provided impetus for analysis of other brain areas.

A second brain area that has proved to be of considerable importance for opioid action is the anatomically complex region of the ventromedial medulla (Fig. 1). This region consists of at least three distinct nuclei: the medially located nucleus raphe magnus (NRM), the more laterally situated nucleus reticularis paragigantocellularis (NRP), and the dorsolaterally located nucleus reticularis gigantocellularis (NRG). Microinjection of morphine into these brain areas results in analgesia, though with some differences in sensitivity (Takagi et al. 1976; Takagi 1980; Azami et al. 1982; Zorman et al. 1982). Opioids produce analgesia when injected into several other brain areas, including the amygdala (Rodgers 1977, 1978), the medial lemniscus (VanRee 1977), nucleus medialis dorsalis of the thalamus (VanRee 1977), the mesencephalic reticular formation (Pert and Yaksh 1974; Haigler and Spring 1978), and the nucleus of the solitary tract (Oley et al. 1982).

A final region of critical importance is the spinal cord dorsal horn (Fig. 1). Although Tsou and Jang (1964) reported no analgesia from direct spinal application of morphine, subsequent work has consistently demonstrated relatively potent effects of intrathecal morphine microinjection (Yaksh and Rudy 1976; Oley et al. 1982). This observation has clinical importance as direct intrathecal application of opioids can have analgesic effects without the concomitant psychoactive effects observed with systemic administration.

Therefore, several general areas of the CNS are involved in opioid analgesia: the central nucleus of the amygdala, the periaqueductal and periventricular gray matter, the ventromedial medulla, and the spinal cord dorsal horn (Fig. 1). The analgesic effects of a systemically administered opioid may produce analgesia by acting at any, all, or some combination of these distinct regions. The microinjection of narcotic antagonists has at least partially answered questions as to whether activation of each of these structures is necessary or sufficient for opioid analgesia.

Several early studies concluded that supraspinal sites were active in opioid analgesia because analgesia from systemically administered opioids was antagonized either by intracranioventricular or intracerebral microinjection of narcotic antagonists (Tsou 1963; Albus et al. 1970; Jacquet and Lajtha 1974). Later work, however, demonstrated that naloxone administered intrathecally could antagonize the analgesia resulting from even relatively high doses of systemically administered opioids (Yaksh and Rudy 1977). These studies have led to the paradoxical conclusion that both supraspinal and spinal sites of opioid action are important in analgesia.

This apparent paradox was resolved in a series of complex but unusually important studies by Yeung and Rudy (1980a,b). The authors demonstrated that simultaneous administration of various doses of morphine intrathecally (into the spinal cord) and intraventricularly (into the brain) resulted in a multiplicative dose-response function. That is, simultaneous spinal and supraspinal morphine caused much greater analgesia than did the same total dose administered at either location alone, with the multiplicative factor being as much as 45 under certain circumstances (Yeung and Rudy 1980b). Therefore, supraspinal and spinal sites of opioid mechanisms probably interact synergistically

Another approach to understanding the neural circuitry participating in opioid analgesia is to selectively destroy nuclei and pathways suspected to be involved in opioid analgesia (see Mayer and Price [1994] and Mayer and Manning [1995] for reviews). Opioids are administered systemically or at discrete sites in the nervous system, and the effect of particular lesions is examined. An overview of this work supports the conclusion of Yeung and Rudy. Apparently several brain areas, including the central nucleus of the amygdala, PAG, NRM, and NRP must be intact for the full expression of opioid analgesia.

Manning and Mayer (1995a,b) have provided evidence that the central nucleus of the amygdala (Ce) is an integral component of this endogenous pain-modulatory circuit. This nucleus is critical for systemic morphine-induced suppression of formalin-induced nociceptive behaviors (Manning and Mayer 1995a) and for morphine-induced suppression of the tail-flick nociceptive reflex (Manning and Mayer 1995b). Bilateral NMDA-induced lesions of the Ce but not other amygdala nuclei abolished the antinociception produced by 2.5 mg/kg morphine sulfate in the noxious heat tail-flick test. These results relate to other evidence linking the Ce to several forms of conditioned and unconditioned antinociception that occur under circumstances aversive to rats (Helmstetter and Tershner 1994). Manning and Mayer's results suggest that the Ce should be incorporated into current models of endogenous pain control circuitry, as shown in Fig. 1.

The endogenous opioid analgesic system appears to be activated by several types of external conditions, particularly those related to perceived threat or fear. Thus, as shown in Fig. 1, the cerebral structures, amygdala, PAG, and hypothalamus all project to the rostroventral medulla (RVM), which in turn projects to the spinal cord dorsal horn. The latter is an ultimate site of action of descending modulation of nociceptive transmission. At least some of these structures, including the amygdala, hypothalamus, and PAG, receive direct input from ascending pain-related pathways, as discussed in Chapter 5. Thus, the circuitry for pain modulation is to some extent a feedback loop, in which stimuli that are likely to induce perceived fear or threat, such as painful stimuli, activate limbic, cortical, and subcortical structures involved in fear-related defensive behaviors. The outputs of these structures converge on a common output region of the RVM, which in turn projects to and modulates neurons of origin of central pain pathways.

OUTPUT NEURONS OF OPIOID DESCENDING MODULATORY SYSTEMS

We now have detailed knowledge of the neural mechanisms by which opioids act at the sites within the pain-modulatory circuitry just described. Neurons at all of these levels are densely innervated by other neurons containing endogenous opioid peptides (Atweh and Kuhar 1977; Delfs et al. 1994). Furthermore, we know the neural mechanisms by which opioids act at some of these sites to produce analgesia (see Fields et al. 1991 for review). To take just one of these sites, the RVM has two distinct classes of pain-modulating neurons. One class is the *on cell,* which *increases* its impulse frequency just before withdrawal from a nociceptive stimulus. On cells are directly inhibited by endogenous opioids, and they appear to have a facilitatory influence on pain and withdrawal reflexes. The second class is the *off cell,* which *decreases* its impulse frequency just before withdrawal from a nociceptive stimulus. Although off cells are not directly affected by opioids, they are inhibited by on cells. Since opioids inhibit on cells, off cells increase their activity as a consequence of opioid inhibition of on cells. In other words, off cells become disinhibited (Fig. 2).

The existence of on cells and off cells within the RVM and elsewhere within the pain-modulating system (e.g., PAG) has important implications for how pain is modulated by various psychological conditions (Fields and Price 1997). First, the modulation of pain and pain behavior is bidirectional; pain can be enhanced or inhibited by these descending controls. Similar to local mechanisms within the dorsal horn that produce hyperalgesia, allodynia, and antinociception, there are descending controls that produce and enhance or inhibit the same phenomena. Pain sensitivity can be enhanced under certain psychological conditions, and it is even possible that pain can be generated in the complete absence of a peripheral nociceptive signal—a "virtual" pain. Second, the somewhat phasic nature of on-cell and off-cell responses suggests that the descending control of ascending nociceptive information may be more dynamic and dependent on moment-by-moment contingencies than previously acknowledged. For example, as discussed in Chapter 7, placebo responses can be traced to a specific area of the body and can be quickly initiated and terminated, features that would be consistent with a phasic control system. Other types of descending controls may be more tonically active, such as when analgesia is produced by environ-

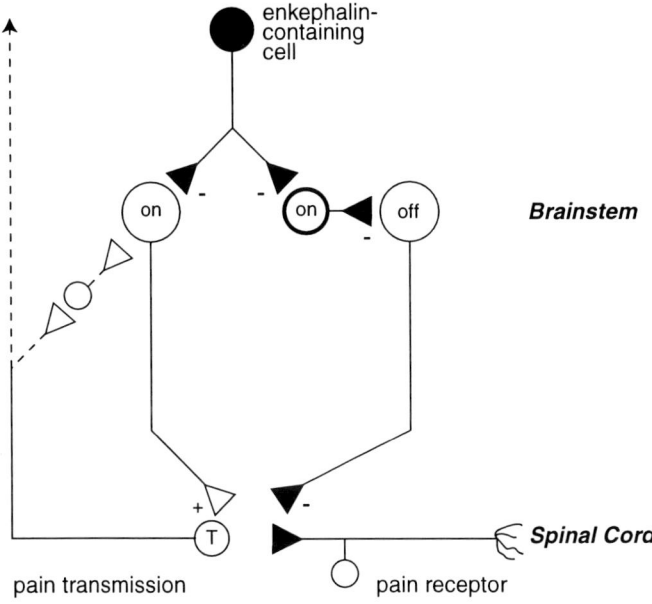

Fig. 2. Opioid-mediated pain-modulatory circuit. From Fields and Price (1997), with permission from Harvard University Press.

mental stress or by prolonged somatosensory stimulation. Further tonic forms of analgesia may be activated by central modulatory neurons other than off cells, for example, by serotonergic "neutral" cells of the RVM or by a combination of neutral and off cells.

THE PSYCHOLOGICAL AND PHYSIOLOGICAL ACTIVATION OF ENDOGENOUS ANALGESIA SYSTEMS

ENDOGENOUS ANALGESIA SYSTEMS IN ANIMALS

The demonstration that opioids activate well-defined neural systems capable of blocking pain transmission suggests, but by no means proves, that the function of this system is to dynamically modulate the perceived intensity of noxious stimuli. If, in fact, this system has such a physiological role, then we might expect its activity level to increase during various psychological circumstances. Evidence that such circumstances produce analgesia would give credibility to the idea that invasive procedures, such as brain stimulation or narcotic drugs, inhibit pain by mimicking the natural activity within these pathways.

Hayes et al. (1978a,b) initiated the first systematic search for the physiological conditions that activate pain-inhibitory systems. They observed that potent analgesia could be produced by such diverse stimuli as brief footshock, centrifugal rotation, and injection of intraperitoneal saline. Subsequent research from several laboratories has catalogued numerous types of external conditions that evoke analgesia in animals (see Mayer and Manning 1995 for review). From these experiments emerged the important finding that naloxone blocks some *but not all* forms of externally induced analgesia (Hayes et al. 1978a,b). Therefore, nonopioid systems must exist in addition to the endogenous opioid system.

Of considerable interest is that some forms of analgesia produced by aversive conditions can be classically conditioned. For example, repeated pairings of footshock with associated cues induces conditioned analgesia; that is, the cues alone evoke an analgesic response (Watkins et al. 1982a). This response must involve an opioid analgesia system, since conditioned analgesia is eliminated by systemic and intrathecal naloxone, morphine tolerance, and lesions of descending pathways of the endogenous pain-modulatory circuit (Watkins et al. 1982b). In addition, as would be expected, higher structures are involved in such analgesia since it is eliminated by decerebration and reduced by lesions of the PAG (Watkins et al. 1982a).

At the level of the spinal cord dorsal horn, complex neurotransmitter or neuromodulatory mechanisms are also involved in learned analgesia. For example, cholecystokinin (CCK) appears to modulate endogenous opioid systems. Intrathecal application of CCK antagonizes analgesia from application of exogenous opioids as well as that elicited by activation of endogenous opioids (Faris et al. 1983; Watkins et al. 1984). Also, CCK antagonists applied intrathecally potentiate these analgesias and reverse opioid tolerance (Watkins et al. 1984). These findings suggest that other transmitters and modulators may interact with opioids to form complex circuits. These circuits relate, in turn, to the complexity of psychological factors that regulate pain and analgesia. For example, stimuli that signal safety reduce the analgesic effects of morphine in rats (Wiertelak et al. 1992). Furthermore, this anti-opioid effect occurs because the safety signal leads to the release of CCK in the spinal cord. A similar CCK neuromodulatory mechanism may be involved in placebo analgesia in humans (see Chapter 7 for discussion).

In sum, a review of the animal data provides strong evidence for endogenous pain-modulatory circuitry and for at least some of the circumstances under which this circuitry is activated. These circumstances largely involve environmental threats or aversive stimulation, including pain itself. Knowledge of this circuitry and the conditions under which it is activated has clear and important implications for understanding general principles of pain inhibition in humans.

EVIDENCE FOR ENDOGENOUS ANALGESIA MECHANISMS IN HUMANS

It is difficult to directly determine whether pain-modulatory circuitry similar to that characterized in animal experiments exists in humans. Nevertheless, several independent, albeit indirect, lines of evidence support the likelihood we have a similar pain-modulatory system. First, the brainstem-to-spinal-cord circuitry implicated in endogenous opioid analgesia is highly conserved in a variety of mammalian species, including marsupials, rodents, carnivores, and primates (Fields and Price 1997). Importantly, the locations and extent of neurotransmitters, including opioid peptides, in this circuitry appears to be similar in several species, including humans (Emson et al. 1984; Pittius et al. 1984). The homogeneity of pain-modulatory circuitry across such a diversity of species leaves little doubt that such circuitry is present in humans. Second, opioid drugs that significantly reduce clinical pain are effective in inhibiting various measures of nociceptive processing in other animal species, including nociceptive reflexes, more integrated escape behaviors, and nociceptive afferent neuron responses to painful stimuli (Fields et al. 1991). In these species, analgesic effects of opioids are exerted in part through actions upon the brainstem-to-spinal-cord circuitry that mediates learned analgesia.

In addition to these indirect lines of evidence, other literature describes more direct determinations of endogenous opioid pain-modulatory circuitry in humans. At this point, parallels can be drawn between the work described above and experimental and clinical studies in humans. These parallels highlight the potential relevance of this work to the difficult problem of treating human pain syndromes. Throughout this discussion, it will be important to bear in mind that several distinct modulatory systems have been identified under controlled laboratory conditions. In the more naturalistic circumstances of clinical research, more than one of these systems could be active at any given time, which may account for the variability and controversy in the clinical literature.

There are at least two situations in which endogenous pain-modulatory systems may be active in humans. The first involves the basal, tonic activity within these systems and allows the experimenter to assess whether pain inhibition occurs continuously, at least to some degree. The second involves clinical manipulations that attempt to activate pain-inhibitory systems.

Evidence for tonic pain-modulatory mechanisms

Attempts have been made to determine whether pain-modulatory systems are tonically (i.e., continuously) active. The assumption has been that administration of opioid antagonists should alter the perception of pain if opioid systems are tonically active. This change in pain perception would be recorded either as a decreased pain threshold or an increased level of ongoing pain. In general, naloxone has failed to affect pain thresholds of normal human volunteers (El-Sobky et al. 1976; Grevert et al. 1978). On the other hand, Buchsbaum et al. (1977) found that naloxone lowered the thresholds of subjects with naturally high pain thresholds, yet had no effect in subjects with low pain thresholds. This observation is consistent with reports that the high pain thresholds seen in some cases of congenital insensitivity to pain can be lowered by naloxone (Dehan et al. 1977; Cesselin et al. 1984). However, it is difficult to demonstrate analgesic or hyperalgesic effects of drugs in human subjects. These studies, taken together, suggest that endogenous opioid pain-modulatory circuits may not always be tonically active in all people. Such a conclusion is supported by a replication of Buchsbaum et al.'s study showing that naloxone decreased the higher pain thresholds more in the morning than in the afternoon (Davis et al. 1978).

Naloxone appears to be more consistently effective in persons who are experiencing some level of clinical pain. In this regard, the results of human studies are consistent with the animal studies described above in which pain was observed to be a powerful activator of endogenous analgesia systems. Thus, Levine et al. (1979) and Gracely et al. (1983) report that naloxone can increase the reported intensity of postoperative pain. In conclusion, under normal circumstances, endogenous opioid pain-inhibitory systems apparently have little spontaneous activity. However, when some level of pain is present for a critical amount of time, these systems seem to be activated.

Conditions that may trigger endogenous analgesia mechanisms in humans

Research on the involvement of endogenous opioids in pain modulation also has examined several environmental manipulations known to reduce clinical or experimental pain. This research has followed two primary experimental strategies. The first reasons that if a particular physiological or psychological condition induces analgesia by releasing endogenous opioids, that analgesia should be antagonized by a narcotic antagonist, usually naloxone. The second strategy holds that if endogenous opioids are involved in these forms of analgesia, then changes should be observed in the levels of these compounds in plasma or in the CNS. Endogenous opioid peptides and opioid receptors exist at CNS sites involved in pain modulation, and exogenous opioids, which potently inhibit pain in humans, are likely to act at the same receptor sites. If these two assumptions are correct, there should be physiological and psychological conditions under which endogenous opioids reduce pain, and administration of an opioid receptor antagonist should block the resultant analgesia. For similar reasons, the release of endogenous opioid peptides should be detectable under psychological or physiological conditions that activate endogenous pain-inhibitory circuitry.

Brain-stimulation-produced analgesia (SPA) in humans. As early as 1973, Richardson and Akil reported the use of periventricular gray (PVG) stimulation to treat pain syndromes. Over 20 reports describing various studies of this technique were published between 1973 and 1983 (see Young et al. 1984 for review); the number of studies has greatly diminished since then. Most studies observed analgesic effects, thereby corroborating animal studies of SPA (see Duncan et al. 1991 for review). However, the numerous published studies indicate that the efficacy of this procedure is highly variable, and the vast majority of clinical studies had poor outcome measures. Nevertheless, the studies are useful in providing some evidence that a central neural substrate of endogenous pain-inhibitory mechanisms exists in humans and that it is generally similar to that of other mammalian species.

Several lines of evidence indicate a likely but not unequivocal role for endogenous opioids in SPA in humans. Opioid antagonists reduce SPA (Adams 1976; Hosobuchi et al. 1977), tolerance develops to it (Hosobuchi 1978), and dependence has been reported (Hosobuchi et al. 1977). Somewhat controversial evidence suggests that endogenous opioids, primarily β-endorphin, are released by electrical stimulation of PAG in humans (Richardson and Akil 1973). It seems likely that endogenous opioids mediate, at least in part, the analgesia elicited by PAG or PVG stimulation in humans, but the particular endogenous opioid and its site and mechanism of action have not been established.

Counter-irritation analgesia in humans. The observation that an acute painful stimulus can alleviate ongoing pain has been known since antiquity and is known as counter-irritation. Counter-irritation has characteristics in common with acupuncture and some forms of transcutaneous electrical nerve stimulation (TENS): all use somatic stimuli, either noxious or innocuous, to obtain relief from pain. Relief often persists beyond the period of treatment when the treatment itself is intense or painful. The site of treatment in relation to the painful area is highly variable, ranging from the painful dermatome itself to the theoretical constellation of points in classical Chinese acupuncture. Similar to acupuncture, the efficacy of counterirritation procedures most likely depends on multiple factors, including those related to parameters of stimulation as well as placebo effects. Lastly, the duration of treatment varies from less than a minute to hours. These factors are important determinants of the effects produced by footshock in animals (Mayer and Manning 1995). Thus, the highly variable effects observed in the clinic would be predicted from animal research. Nevertheless, human data suggest the involvement of the same systems described in the animal literature.

Several studies have examined the effect of naloxone on acupuncture analgesia in humans. Many of these have also measured acupuncture-induced changes in β-endorphin or enkephalin levels in plasma or cerebrospinal fluid (CSF) (see references in Price and Mayer 1995). It is important to note that "acupuncture" is not always a well-defined procedure. Among sixteen studies that measured the effect of naloxone on clinical or experimental analgesia produced by acupuncture, 11 reported that naloxone reduced analgesia while 5 found no effect; no study to date has found that naloxone increases analgesia (Price and Mayer 1995). Thus, most results are consistent with an endogenous opioid mechanism. The effects of acupuncture on CSF and plasma endorphin levels present a somewhat less consistent picture, but this is not surprising, considering the complexities of these types of data (see references in Price and Mayer 1995). Among eight studies that have examined plasma endorphin levels, only one reported endorphin increases. We could question the entire concept of plasma endorphin levels since they are only indirectly indicative of CNS level. Nevertheless, all five studies that examined cerebrospinal levels of either β-endorphin or enkephalin showed increased levels of these agents during acupuncture analgesia. Even CSF endorphin levels are likely to be ambiguous because the site of their release probably varies with the particular type of acupuncture stimulation. Nevertheless, an overview of these studies is consistent with an involvement of endogenous opioids in at least some forms of acupuncture analgesia.

The literature concerning the involvement of endogenous opioids in TENS analgesia is considerably more complicated than that associated with acupuncture analgesia. This may reflect the greater variability in the intensity, frequency, duration, location, and other parameters of TENS. Despite this diversity of experimental paradigms, some general consistencies have emerged. Four of seven studies of TENS analgesia reported naloxone antagonism for low-frequency, high-intensity TENS, while none demonstrated naloxone antagonism for high-frequency, low-intensity TENS (references in Price and Mayer 1995). The effects of TENS on endorphin levels have been less well studied. Three of the six reported studies found an increase in endorphin levels, while the remainder found no effects (Price and Mayer 1995). Such results should be interpreted with the caveats discussed above in mind. Overall, these results are strikingly consistent with reports in the animal literature and suggest that certain types of somatosensory stimulation either inactivate opioid analgesia systems or activate opioid hyperalgesia systems. In particular, the combined results support the hypothesis that low-frequency, high-intensity, acupuncture-like TENS invokes endogenous opioid mechanisms.

In conclusion, acupuncture and transcutaneous nerve stimulation appear to be forms of counter-irritation that activate both opioid and nonopioid systems. The variable clinical outcomes observed following these treatments probably result from differential recruitment of segmental, extrasegmental, opioid, and nonopioid pain-inhibitory systems, all of which are now known to be activated by these types of stimulation in animals.

Stress analgesia in humans. A phenomenon that is related to, but not identical with, counter-irritation analgesia is *stress analgesia.* Studies of stress analgesia have used environmental manipulations that are either severe physical or psychological stressors (see references in Mayer and Price 1994). The stressors include surgery, labor and childbirth, application of overtly painful stimuli (such as cold pressor pain or ischemic pain), chronic pain, anticipation of pain, and chronic stressful states (such as life-threatening disease).

Studies of analgesic effects of these types of stressors have strikingly consistent outcomes. For all eight studies in which a "stressful" manipulation increased nociceptive thresholds, naloxone at least partially reversed this increase. One of these studies (Janal et al. 1984) used vigorous exercise, at least a possible stressor, to increase pain threshold; the results also showed naloxone reversibility. Not surprisingly, since β-endorphin is co-released with adrenocorticotropic hormone (ACTH), stress increased plasma β-endorphin levels in all five studies that measured these agents. Although such a result is not convincing alone, it is certainly consistent with the notion that endogenous opioids may underlie changes in pain threshold produced by stress. In addition, such results are consistent with the findings of counter-irritation studies discussed above in that naloxone reversibility is more likely to occur with high-intensity peripheral stimulation.

Analgesic effects of vaginal stimulation and sexual arousal. In a study designed to confirm and parallel studies of analgesic effects of vaginal stimulation in rats (Komisaruk and Wallman 1977), Whipple and Komisaruk (1985) measured thresholds and tolerances to painful stimulation produced by calibrated finger compression, in relation to self-application of vaginal mechanostimulation. In two studies with 10 women each, they found that nonpleasurable vaginal self-stimulation significantly increased both the threshold to detect (47.4% increase) and tolerate (40.3% increase) painful finger compression, but did not significantly affect the threshold to detect innocuous tactile stimulation. These analgesic effects were significantly greater when vaginal stimulation was pleasurable. Under these conditions, pain threshold and tolerance increased by 74.6% and 106.7%, respectively. Again, tactile thresholds were unchanged. Thus, it appears that the analgesic effect of vaginal stimulation is mediated partly by somatosensory-induced inhibitory mechanisms independent of the affective-motivational state produced by such stimulation. This component of the analgesia is consistent with studies in rats showing that analgesia from vaginal stimulation is partly mediated by spinal-inhibitory mechanisms (Komisaruk and Wallman 1977). Whipple et al. (1992) subsequently determined that sexual imagery accompanied by sexual arousal was sufficient to raise pain threshold and pain tolerance levels in women. Thus, sexual arousal and somatosensory input from vaginal stimulation apparently make separate contributions to analgesia during sexual activity.

   Summary. Considering the diversity of stimulation conditions that result in pain modulation in humans, a generally convincing picture of mechanisms of pain modulation emerges. The same types of somatosensory stimuli that result in analgesia in several mammalian species also reduce pain in humans, and many of them activate endogenous opioid systems. Important questions about the nature of this involvement remain unanswered: What is the particular endogenous opioid involved? What is its site of action? Answers to such questions are unlikely to come from human studies alone since invasive procedures are probably necessary to acquire such information. The consistency of the animal and human studies, however, indicates that such questions can be studied with animal models and verified in humans.

CONCLUSIONS

   This chapter has presented a brief overview of the evidence for endogenous pain-inhibitory circuitry that is activated in all mammals under various physiological and psychological circumstances. This pain-modulatory system uses opioid peptides at several levels of the neuraxis. There are good reasons to conclude that exogenous opioids activate this system at all of these levels to result in the inhibition of pain. However, the most important aspect of research on endogenous pain-inhibitory systems pertains to the demonstration of such a system in human beings and the development of ways to identify the psychological and physiological conditions under which this system operates.

   The strategy for characterizing these types of analgesia as opioid related has consisted mainly of antagonizing the analgesic effects of these manipulations with a narcotic antagonist, such as naloxone, or measuring plasma or CSF levels of opioid peptides. As I will discuss in the next two chapters, the test of naloxone reversibility represents a powerful and feasible approach to determining involvement of endogenous opioid systems. Naloxone is fairly specific for opioid receptors and is undetectable when given on a double-blind basis. A major limitation to this approach is that it cannot determine the exact CNS sites of these opioid-related mechanisms.

However, several additional technologies and experimental approaches allow us to study neural mechanisms of analgesia more directly in human participants. These include single neuron recordings in the human somatosensory thalamus, functional imaging methods such as PET or fMRI, and measures of spinal nociceptive reflexes. For example, the R-III is a spinally mediated withdrawal reflex that can be noninvasively measured in human volunteers and correlates well with reported pain intensity. Inhibition of this spinal reflex during some type of psychologically mediated analgesia, such as hypnotic analgesia, would support the hypothesis that a brainstem-to-spinal pathway is involved in this type of analgesia.

In the next two chapters, I will discuss several types of experiments that have characterized the general psychological and neural mechanisms of placebo and hypnotic analgesia. As an important consequence of this approach, we have evidence that hypnotic and placebo analgesia depend on different general neural mechanisms, which is appropriate as they probably depend on different psychological mechanisms as well.

Psychological Mechanisms of Pain and Analgesia, Progress in Pain Research and Management, Vol. 15, by Donald D. Price, IASP Press, Seattle, © 1999.

7

Placebo Analgesia

The previous chapter provided an overview of psychological factors that modulate pain intensity and of the neural circuitry that is involved in pain modulation. The emphasis was on relatively simple environmental or stimulus factors that modulate pain. However, among human beings, complex and subtle psychological factors are among the most powerful modulators of pain. Under certain circumstances, beliefs, expectations, changes in consciousness, and various forms of symbolic meaning can strongly influence pain perception.

If a patient experiences a strong need for pain relief and expects to obtain relief from a treatment, part of the relief may result from psychological factors. This constitutes the placebo analgesic response, and may occur when the treatment situation reproduces in some way a previously effective treatment or when a patient is told about the potential effectiveness of the treatment. To better understand how placebo manipulations such as saline injections work, we must determine which dimensions of pain are most affected by such manipulations and what are the most important psychological factors that contribute to the placebo effect. In this chapter I explore the psychological mechanisms and some of the neural mechanisms by which placebo effects take place. First I address the methods and problems inherent in measuring placebo analgesic effects and responses. This background is necessary for the second point of discussion, which deals with the alternative psychological mechanisms that could mediate placebo effects and responses. Finally, I relate these alternative psychological mechanisms to neurobiological mechanisms to extend explanations of placebo analgesia.

MEASURING PLACEBO EFFECTS AND IDENTIFYING PLACEBO RESPONSES

PROBLEMS OF MEASURING PLACEBO EFFECTS AND RESPONSES

The placebo analgesic effect is the measured mean reduction in pain for a group of individuals given a placebo treatment, and the placebo analgesic response is the reduction in pain that occurs in an individual as a result of placebo administration (Fields and Price 1997). Measurement of both pla-cebo effects and responses requires estimates of pain intensity under both untreated baseline and placebo treatment conditions. The difference in pain intensity between these two conditions provides a measure of the placebo effect for groups and of the placebo response for individuals. The untreated baseline pain in experimental studies usually results from a controlled pain stimulus. Experimental studies have an enormous advantage because the stimulus can be repeated at different times in relationship to the placebo manipulation, and pain intensity can be controlled to some extent by stimu-lus parameters. Using multiple trials of stimuli at baseline and after placebo administration, we could identify and measure a placebo response in an individual participant.

Measuring a placebo response in one person is not nearly as feasible in the case of clinical pain. In clinical studies, investigators must rely on the "natural history" of pain intensity, that is, the temporal profile of pain inten-sity that occurs without any treatment whatsoever (Fields and Price 1997). Natural histories of pain vary according to type of clinical pain and circum-stances. For example, the natural history of most postoperative pains is a slow increase in intensity over time, whereas that of migraine headaches is often a gradual rise in pain intensity to a severe level followed by a decline to no pain at all. Natural histories of pain also vary considerably across patients. As a result of both of these sources of variation, any treatment may be followed by a reduction in pain level as a result of the natural history rather than as a result of the treatment itself. To attribute a reduction in pain to any antecedent treatment, including placebo, is therefore an inference. Without a natural history control condition, we would not know what change in pain intensity would have occurred without the treatment. For this reason, the mean magnitude of a placebo analgesic effect in a group of patients can only be assessed by comparing a no-treatment condition with a placebo treatment condition. Since few studies of placebo analgesia have included an untreated comparison group or condition (in crossover studies), we know little about the magnitude and time course of placebo effects or the fre-quency of placebo responses among individuals. Indeed, without a no-treat-ment group or condition, it is difficult to know whether a placebo treatment has produced any effect at all.

Disregard for the influence of multiple psychological factors and failure to consider the natural history of the pain condition have resulted in the frequently unwarranted conclusion that a placebo response has occurred if a patient's pain is observed to decrease following placebo treatment. Over-looking the importance of an untreated comparison group remains a major source of confusion in the current literature on placebo (Wickramasekera

1985; Wall 1994). Without a natural history control comparison, we can neither exclude the possibility that a placebo response is absent nor confirm that it has occurred. The two types of pain mentioned above can serve as examples. A placebo treatment at the peak of a migraine headache would most likely be followed by a reduction in pain, regardless of whether the placebo had any effect; the reduction does not establish a placebo response, however. Likewise, a postoperative pain that steadily increased in intensity may continue to increase in intensity despite any small reduction in pain produced by a placebo treatment; the absence of an overall reduction in pain does not mean that a placebo response did not occur. In both examples, the placebo response of individual patients is the measured difference between the level of pain with and without the placebo treatment. Where there is a strong placebo response, it may be difficult or impossible to determine anything about the effects of the test agent, as illustrated below for a group comparison between immediate effects of local anesthetics and saline.

Because of the variability in the natural histories of different individuals and different types of clinical pain, group comparisons are usually the only reliable way to assess the magnitude and time course of placebo analgesia. However, as pointed out above, experimental pain studies may be able to establish the presence and magnitude of a placebo response by exposing an individual to multiple trials. Theoretically, it should also be possible to establish an individual's placebo response in clinical studies, but this requires much more extensive analysis and more complex procedures than are used by most clinical investigators, who too readily claim to identify placebo responders and nonresponders. An individual occurrence of the placebo analgesic effect could be determined by comparing the patient's post-placebo pain level at any given time with a group-derived mean. If the patient's response were significantly below the group mean, we could infer (at a defined level of confidence) that a response to placebo had occurred. Alternatively, we might administer multiple placebo treatments and compare the patient's mean analgesic response to these treatments with the same patient's response to multiple untreated occurrences of the same pain condition. This approach has practical, theoretical, and ethical problems. It requires extensive experimentation on the same patient, which may be costly, time consuming, and greatly discomforting and stressful to the patient. It could also produce long-term increases in the natural history of pain, particularly in neuropathic pain patients.

Given the difficulty in identifying an individual placebo response, the assumption that an individual placebo responder can be identified does not seem to be warranted, nor can the fraction of placebo responders can be identified within a given study. Although the figure of 33% is commonly quoted in papers and textbooks, it is extremely misleading because that "fraction" varies enormously (from close to 0% to 100%), depending on the exact circumstances of the study and probably on considerable within-subject factors (see Wall 1994 for review). Closely allied with the fixed fraction myth is the notion that the tendency to respond to a placebo represents a stable personality trait. Based on a review of 36 studies by Turner et al. (1994) and another review by White et al. (1985), most papers report no significant correlation between placebo response and personality, and the remainder are contradictory. Given the problems of these studies, the question of whether placebo responsiveness is a personality trait remains open.

HOW LARGE AND HOW PREVALENT IS THE PLACEBO ANALGESIC EFFECT?

Given the problems involved in measuring placebo analgesia, it is nearly impossible to arrive at any meaningful generalization about the magnitude or prevalence of placebo analgesia in clinical studies. Part of the reason for this uncertainty is that natural histories of pain and the psychological circumstances under which placebo treatments are given vary enormously across studies and are rarely assessed. One productive approach would be to consider the factors that may contribute to placebo analgesia and to examine specific studies in light of these factors. Two extreme examples serve to illustrate circumstances under which placebo analgesic effects can be very large or negligible; they emphasize the need to analyze the basis for the wide variation in responses to placebo.

The first example, shown in Fig. 1, demonstrates a very large placebo effect in a group of seven patients with complex regional pain syndrome, type I (CRPS-I) (Price et al. 1998). Pain-relieving effects of local anesthesia of sympathetic ganglia were compared with saline placebo and with natural history on a double-blind, crossover basis. Each patient received two injections into the sympathetic ganglia. The interval between treatment blocks was long enough to permit an assessment of natural history. The patients rated their pain on visual analogue scales (VAS) before and after blocks, and also rated their pain intensities in diaries four times a day throughout the study. Immediate reductions in pain intensity from the baseline or natural history control condition were 69% and 74% for saline and local anesthetic injections, respectively. Thus, saline injection had a powerful *initial* placebo effect, which was unlikely to be related to active effects of saline; Haddox and Kettler (1987) had previously shown that saline injections do not produce significant physiological effects on sympathetic ganglia in human subjects. However, the analgesic effect lasted statistically longer for

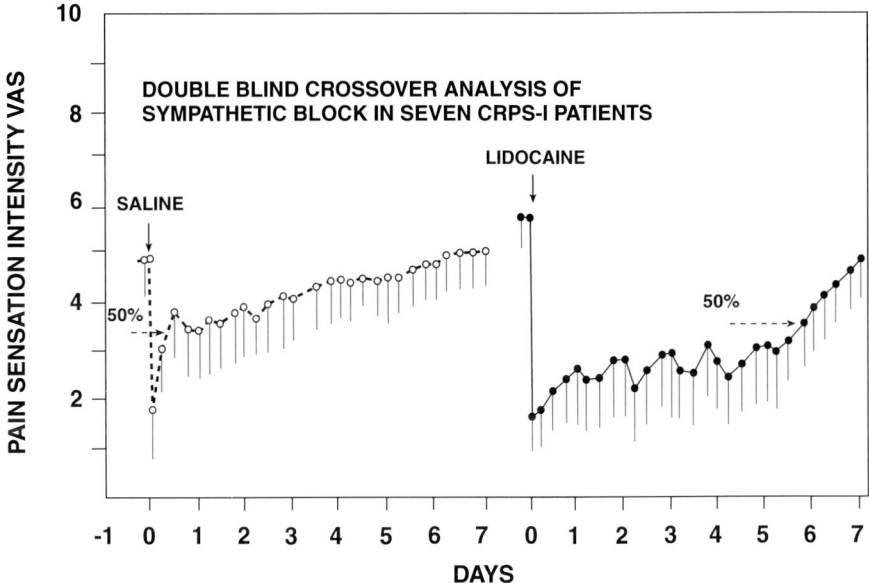

Fig. 1. Mean VAS ratings of pain sensation intensity after saline and lidocaine anesthetic blocks of sympathetic ganglia in seven CRPS-I patients. Standard errors are indicated by vertical lines. Reprinted with permission from Price, D.D., Long, S., Wilsey, B., Rafii A. Analysis of peak magnitude and duration of analgesia produced by local anesthetics injected into sympathetic ganglia of complex regional pain syndrome patients. *Clinical Journal of Pain* 1998; 14(3):216–226.

active local anesthetic injection and outlasted the placebo effect.

This somewhat extreme example illustrates the complexity of measuring the placebo effect in a group of patients and presents a set of circumstances under which a large placebo effect can occur. The comparison of natural history and placebo treatment conditions in the same patients provided a measure of the placebo effect. The immediate placebo effect was quite large, probably because all the factors suspected of contributing to the placebo effect were present. These patients had a strong need or desire to be relieved of pain because their pain was nearly always present and was fairly high in intensity (between 5 and 6 on the VAS). Their expectations for pain relief were likely to be high because of the elaborate and invasive procedure and because they had all experienced pain relief from previous local anesthetic injections into sympathetic ganglia. Although not overtly painful, the procedure may have been stressful enough to result in some degree of analgesia. Patients may have been anxious prior to the procedure, which may have increased their sympathetic outflow at the time, and the decrease in anxiety afterwards may have reduced it. If the pain was at least partially maintained by sympathetic efferent activity, then pain relief may have reflected changes in sympathetic outflow before and after injection. Many possible contributing factors could have converged to produce a large placebo effect. This effect can be conceptualized as resulting from all nonspecific aspects of the treatment (aspects that are unrelated to the active effects of the therapeutic agent) and from psychological factors, such as stress, anxiety, expectancy, and desire for relief.

The second example is the absence of a placebo effect in a group of 12 musculoskeletal pain patients receiving an intravenous saline placebo injection (Price et al. 1986b). Mean VAS ratings of both clinical pain and experimental pain were nearly identical before and after the injection. Unlike the patients of the first example, these patients had never experienced this specific type of pain-relieving procedure, which was less invasive than that used in the first example. Pain-free participants tested with brief heat pulses also had negligible placebo effects from intravenous placebo injection (Price et al. 1985b). Small or negligible placebo effects are common in studies that use brief experimental pain stimuli. Effects are larger in studies in which the experimental pain simulates the persistence and severity of some types of clinical pain (Jospe 1978, Gracely 1979). The large difference in placebo analgesic effect between these different studies is likely to be the result of several factors, including the experienced need for relief, expectations, and anxiety. Clearly, there is a drastic need to determine exactly which specific psychological factors contribute to the magnitude of placebo analgesia.

GENERAL PSYCHOLOGICAL MECHANISMS
OF PLACEBO ANALGESIA

Many of the same strategies for understanding placebo analgesia apply at least in a general way to other psychologically mediated forms of analgesia, such as hypnotic analgesia. Psychological explanations of placebo analgesia have evolved from proposed environmental causes to identifying mediating factors within human experience. For example, classical conditioning and more recently, the experiential factors of expectancy and desire for pain relief have been advanced to account for some forms of placebo analgesia. In this section, I compare environmental and experiential hypotheses of placebo analgesic mechanisms.

THE POTENTIAL ROLE OF CLASSICAL CONDITIONING

A major hypothesis considers placebo analgesia to be a function of classical (Pavlovian) conditioning. Indeed, several psychologists have independently proposed this idea (Korcyn 1978; Watkins and Mayer 1982b; Wickramasekera 1985). Wickramasekera suggested that active agents that reduce pain (e.g., morphine and aspirin) serve as unconditioned stimuli (UCS) and that neutral stimuli associated with reduction of unpleasant symptoms (due to spontaneous remission or delivery of an active drug) or with the onset of therapeutic action serve as conditioned stimuli (CS). CS can come to be associated with the therapeutic agent and its efficacy, such as syringes, health care professionals who appear authoritative, and elaborate medical equipment.

Consistent with the classical conditioning hypothesis, a landmark study of patients clearly showed that prior treatments with effective analgesic drugs enhanced the analgesic effectiveness of a subsequent placebo (Laska and Sunshine 1973). A second medication, always placebo, followed graded doses of propoxyphene HCl (three dose levels), propoxyphene napsylate (three doses), or placebo. Seven groups each had 14–20 patients. The results showed convincing evidence of a dose-response relationship between the dose of the first medication and the analgesic response to the subsequent placebo, though the effects of placebo were weaker than those of corresponding doses of the active drug. Placebo was more effective when it followed a more potent analgesic, whereas following another placebo it continued to have the same slight analgesic effect as the first administration. These results support learning and even classical conditioning as major factors in placebo analgesia, but do not distinguish between the relative contributions of conditioning and expectation.

PROBLEMS WITH THE CLASSICAL CONDITIONING HYPOTHESIS

There have been challenges to the classical conditioning explanation of placebo effects, particularly the stimulus-substitution model[1] of classical conditioning. In particular, Kirsch (1990) pointed out that various studies of placebo effects have failed to fulfill criteria used to determine whether a phenomenon can be attributed to classical conditioning in the following respects: (1) conditioning trials with tranquilizers weaken rather than produce the predicted strengthened placebo effect; (2) contrary to the criterion that the magnitude of placebo effect should be directly related to the strength of the active tranquilizer, it is *inversely related*; (3) placebo effects are often not specific to the pharmacological properties of the active drug (e.g., alcohol, caffeine) but depend heavily on context and suggestion; (4) placebos

---

[1] The stimulus-substitution model of classical conditioning posits that repeated exposure to a conditioning stimulus (CS) paired with an unconditioned stimulus (UCS) is both necessary and sufficient for a conditioned response (CR). This model of learning does not require a conscious association between the CS and UCS.

often fail the extinction test, (wherein the conditioned response decreases with repeated presentations of the conditioning stimulus alone), as in the case of placebo treatment for panic disorder; and (5) placebo effects sometimes can be stronger (not weaker) than the effects of an active drug. On the other hand, except for the demonstration of extinction, all criteria for classical conditioning are fulfilled by the Laska and Sunshine study discussed above. Moreover, Fedele et al. (1989) demonstrated a loss of analgesic effectiveness of placebo with repeated administration (i.e., extinction). Thus, the exceptions stated above (1–5) may be related to global psychological therapeutic effects, such as reductions in panic or anxiety, or effects such as caffeine-induced arousal or alcohol-induced sedation. The specific effects observed, such as increased motor performance, could then be attributed largely to contextual factors and suggestion. These effects may thus have less application to placebo analgesia, at least to its sensory-discriminative dimension.

DO COGNITIVE FACTORS CONTRIBUTE TO PLACEBO RESPONSES?

The study of cognitive factors could increase understanding of how learning influences the placebo effect and how factors not directly related to classical conditioning influence placebo responses. First of all, conditioning stimuli (e.g., syringes, doctors in white coats) and conditioned responses (e.g., pain relief) may well have concomitant dimensions within human experience. For example, conditioning stimuli, such as pills and syringes, become associated with active pharmacological agents (i.e., unconditioned stimuli), as well as with the reduction in pain (unconditioned responses), and indicate that relief and healing are imminent.

Secondly, while the consideration of experiential factors extends and supports the role of learning and even classical conditioning in placebo analgesia, it also helps to resolve some of the limitations and inconsistencies of older stimulus substitution models of classical conditioning as an explanation for placebo analgesia. Although there is ample evidence that prior exposure to an effective treatment enhances placebo effects, it is questionable whether such prior exposure is necessary for a placebo response. Meanings, attributions, imagery, and information have important roles in mediating beliefs, desires, and expectations. Thus, it is plausible that the placebo response is more directly controlled by these cognitive factors than by the immediate and direct association of a specific treatment with pain reduction, as required for classical conditioning. An example would be a patient receiving an unknown pain medicine for the first time from the family doctor. The patient's general life experience with doctors, trust in this specific doctor, and the nature of the communication between the doctor and this patient all may codetermine this patient's level of expectation that this specific (and unknown) pain medicine will provide significant pain relief.

Indeed, the nature of suggestions inherent in placebo manipulations might lead us to hypothesize that suggested meanings influence and even determine the nature and magnitude of the placebo analgesic response. The suggestion in placebo analgesia is typically that pain relief is being provided by an authoritative source (e.g., pain medicine prescribed by a knowledgeable professional). Implicit in the overall suggestion inherent to a placebo analgesic manipulation is the credibility of this outside agent. Thus, a tacit assumption in the administration of placebo analgesics is that patients will expect them to relieve pain.

The role of expectation

This possible role of expectation in placebo responses is supported both by alternative models of learning (Mowrer 1960; Reiss 1980; Rescorla 1988) and by studies showing that it mediates placebo effects (Montgomery and Kirsch 1996b; Price et al. 1999). Classical conditioning itself may lead to the acquisition of expectancies. Thus, Reiss argues that what is learned in Pavlovian conditioning is an expectation regarding the occurrence or non-occurrence of an unconditioned response onset. In fact, contemporary theories of Pavlovian conditioning emphasize the role of expectancies (Rescorla 1988). However, although classical conditioning is one way to change one's expectation, other types of learning can contribute. For example, expectation can reflect knowledge about the therapeutic agent, the circumstances under which it is administered, and the condition to be treated. Classical conditioning could result in increased knowledge about the efficacy of the therapeutic agent by producing a memory of past effects. On the other hand, as indicated by the hypothetical example given above, expectation also could be critically influenced by information that is independent of one's previous direct experience with a specific therapeutic agent. For example, the patient could read a book about the agent's therapeutic efficacy. In either case, increased information indicating an agent's effectiveness could increase the patient's expectation of relief. What all of this implies for placebo analgesia is that expectation for relief may cause a placebo response without prior exposure to a similar therapeutic agent, though such exposure does increase expectation (e.g., Laska and Sunshine 1973).

Until recently, the effects of expectation on placebo analgesia have not been convincingly distinguished from those of conditioning. In the first attempt to test these two possible factors simultaneously, Voudouris et al. (1990) compared effects of *conditioning* (exposure to a "pain-reducing treatment") and explicit *expectation* manipulations (written suggestions for pain reduction) within the same experiment on placebo analgesia. The conditioning manipulation consisted of providing subjects an experience of topical cream-induced analgesia by surreptitiously lowering painful stimulation intensity after administering the "analgesic cream." There were four groups in the study: group 1 received a combined expectancy and conditioning manipulation; group 2, expectancy treatment alone; group 3, conditioning alone; and group 4, a control group, neither treatment. All subjects' VAS ratings of pain were compared with and without a placebo cream, using iontophoretic pain stimulation. Their results showed an enhanced placebo effect from conditioning but not from verbally induced expectancy, and found no interaction between the two different types of manipulations. The authors suggest that conditioning may be a more powerful factor than verbal cues in inducing a placebo response.

This study was the first attempt to assess the differential role of conditioning and expectancy in evoking placebo analgesia and had several problems specifically related to the expectancy manipulation and its assessment. In the first place, the expectancy manipulation itself was questionable because it consisted of simply providing different consent forms for the expectancy groups and the conditioning alone group, one stating that they would receive a powerful analgesic and the other stating that they were in a control group. Whether this approach was actually effective among the university students who participated, given their possible knowledge of psychology experiments, is open to question. Secondly, the expectancy manipulation check was simplistic, and analyzed responses to a single question (embedded in a series of other irrelevant questions) asking "whether they expected this cream to be effective." Finally, the authors asked this question only once, *prior* to the conditioning manipulation. Thus, the effect of conditioning on expectancy was never assessed. As is appropriate given these problems, the authors indicate that their results by no means exclude a role of expectation in evoking placebo responses. Rather, they suggest that expectations may be more strongly shaped by previous experience (such as that provided by conditioning) than by verbal persuasion. The authors admit that it would have been more revealing to have directly assessed the expectation levels of subjects who received only conditioning rather than simply assume that expectation was successfully increased only by the expectancy manipulation. Direct measures of expectation by means of continuous scales or questionnaires with multiple questions about expectation clearly need to be incorporated into studies of placebo effects. These measures may account for more of the variance in placebo effects than do the manipulations intended to produce changes in expectation.

A useful approach would be to obtain measures of expectation and introduce an experimental manipulation that dissociates the factor of expectancy, for example, from that of conditioning. This was precisely the approach taken by Montgomery and Kirsch (1996a). They tested opposing models of classical conditioning (the stimulus substitution variant) and expectancy by using an experimental paradigm similar to that used by Voudouris et al. in the study described above. They provided two conditions of UCS/CS pairings by informing one group of subjects about the lowering of painful stimulus intensity and not informing the other group. The uninformed group was thereby provided with an experience of cream-induced analgesia during conditioning, and as expected, subjects demonstrated placebo analgesia in the subsequent test trials. In contrast, the group that was informed of reduction of stimulus intensity during the conditioning trials had both lowered expectations of analgesia and no overall analgesia (i.e., placebo effect) during test trials. Furthermore, although conditioning trials significantly enhanced placebo response, this effect was eliminated by adding expectancy values of the subjects to the regression equation, indicating that the effect of pairing trials on placebo response was mediated completely by expectancy (Baron and Kenny 1986). Finally, the magnitude of the placebo effect increased significantly over 10 extinction trials, a result opposite to that predicted by a stimulus substitution model of classical conditioning. This experiment is important because it demonstrates that conditioning is not sufficient for placebo effects, and it supports the hypothesis that high expectation of a therapeutic effect is necessary for placebo effects. Indeed, this experiment provides multiple lines of evidence against the stimulus substitution model of classical conditioning and for the mediating role of expectancy. Thus, according to Baron and Kenny (1986):

> To establish mediation, the following conditions must hold: First, the independent variable must affect the mediator. Second, the independent variable must affect the dependent variable. Third and finally, the mediator must affect the dependent variable. Perfect mediation holds if the independent variable has no effect when the mediator is controlled.

By these criteria, Montgomery and Kirsch established that the effect of conditioning on responses to placebo is mediated perfectly by expectancy, consistent with contemporary theories of classical conditioning.

Perhaps the most intriguing and unexpected result of the Montgomery and Kirsch study is that not only did the placebo effect fail to become extinguished, it actually increased across the 10 extinction trials. This pattern of results is inconsistent with a stimulus substitution model but supports an informational model of classical conditioning. If placebo produces a powerful effect the first time it is given, then the perception of placebo as pain relief is bolstered and strengthens the effect of subsequent placebo treatments. In this study, pain stimulation without placebo produced a progressive increase in reported pain with repeated trials, and the possibility was raised that the magnitude of the placebo effect is proportional to the magnitude of pain without the placebo. The magnitude of pain, in turn, may relate to a second factor in placebo analgesia, namely that of the perceived need or desire for pain relief.

These results of Montgomery and Kirsch (1996a) were replicated and extended in a subsequent study that used a similar paradigm of surreptitious lowering of stimulus intensity during conditioning trials (Price et al. 1999). The experimental design of this study is shown in schematic form in Fig. 2. Noxious skin temperature stimuli were applied to three areas of the forearm and intensities of these stimuli were surreptitiously reduced in conditioning trials. Intensities were lowered by 67%, 17%, and 0% in areas A, B, and C respectively. Participants were told that two analgesic creams (applied to areas A and B) were being compared on a double-blind basis and that area C was a control area. Using an approach similar to that of Voudouris et al. (1990) and Montgomery and Kirsch (1996a), the investigators assessed placebo effects in subsequent trials in which stimulus intensities were re-established to their original baseline values (Fig. 2). Just prior to the placebo trials, participants rated the pain intensities and pain unpleasantness they expected to experience in areas A, B, and C and their desire for pain reduction. Expectancy was then analyzed as a possible mediator of placebo analgesia.

The results confirmed and extended those of previous studies in clarifying the roles of conditioning and expectancy as mediators of placebo analgesia. First, placebo analgesic effects during test trials were graded according to the extent of surreptitious lowering of stimulus intensity during conditioning trials; these effects occurred for both pain intensity and pain unpleasantness (Fig. 3). These graded effects provide a constructive replication of the study by Laska and Sunshine (1973) described earlier. In both studies, stronger prior analgesic effects resulted in stronger subsequent placebo effects. However, for the results presented in Fig. 3, these graded placebo analgesic effects were associated with corresponding graded differ-

FAMILIARIZATION TRIALS (N = 4) (44°, 45°, 47°, 49°C)	CALIBRATION TRIALS (N = 8) (44°, 45°, 47°, 49°C)	MANIPULATION TRIALS (N = 30) (C = 6; B = 5; A = 2)	POST-MANIPULATION TRIALS (N = 6) (A, B, C = 4)

Fig. 2. Time course of experimental conditions and experimental design of the Price et al. (1999) study of responses to placebo in experimental heat pain trials.

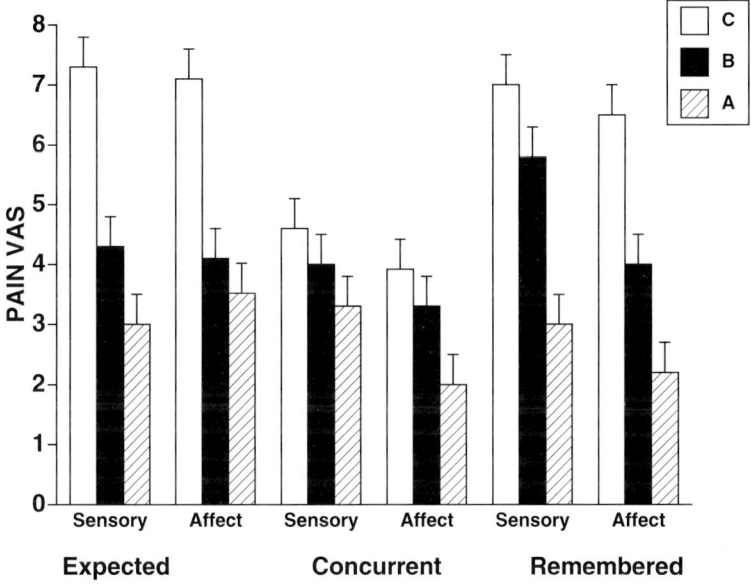

Fig. 3. Pain sensation intensity and pain unpleasantness ratings of 40 participants for three areas of skin (A, B, and C) in the Price et al. (1999) placebo study. Area C was untreated with conditioning trials, area B was treated with weak placebo conditioning trials, and area A was treated with strong placebo conditioning trials. These ratings are for (1) expected pain within areas C, B, and A, (2) pain just after placebo conditioning trials for these areas, that is, concurrent pain, and (3) remembered pain about 2 minutes after post-test trials for the same areas. Adapted from Price et al. (1999), with permission.

ences in expectancy levels. More importantly, placebo analgesic effects were strongly associated with expectancy *within* each of areas A and B ($R = 0.5$ and 0.6 for areas A and B, respectively). The combination of these results, like those of Montgomery and Kirsch (1996a), show that although conditioning may be sufficient for placebo analgesia, it is likely to be mediated by expectancy.

The same experiment assessed placebo analgesia based on *remembered* pain intensities. When participants were asked to remember and rate pain intensities and unpleasantness levels within each of the three areas during post-conditioning trials, their ratings closely followed their *expected* but not *actual* pain levels associated with postmanipulation trials (Fig. 3). As shown in Fig. 3, participants remembered the untreated pain within control area C as being much more intense and unpleasant than it actually was. This distortion was less for area B and minimal for area A. Selective distortions, in turn, resulted in large placebo effects for *remembered* pain, effects that were over three times larger than those based on *concurrent* ratings of pain (Fig. 3). Moreover, these large placebo effects occurred for both areas A and B and for both sensory and affective dimensions. However, similar to concurrent placebo effects, they were strongly associated with expectancy ratings made just prior to test trials (Fig 3). Furthermore, ratings of these expected pain levels were similar to participants' ratings of remembered pain intensities (Fig. 3). Expectations and memory distortions thus mediate large placebo effects based on retrospective ratings of pain or pain relief.

The selective exaggeration of remembered pain intensity within untreated area C and the consequent enhancement of placebo analgesia are consistent with previous studies that show that memory distortion of pretreatment pain contributes to exaggerated self-reports of pain relief (Mathias et al. 1995; Feine et al. 1998). Feine et al. found that pain relief scores based on memory were over three times higher than those based on pretreatment minus present pain VAS ratings, consistent with the results of Price et al.'s (1999) study of placebo analgesia.

As pointed out by Feine et al., patients' reports of relief following treatment are often used to establish the effectiveness of treatments. To the extent that such measures are used in clinical studies of pain treatments, estimates of magnitudes of analgesic effects from both placebo and active treatments are likely to be significantly enhanced when reports are made retrospectively. We must wonder to what extent commonly quoted magnitudes of placebo analgesia (Beecher 1955, 1959; Turner et al. 1994) as well as reported magnitudes of analgesia from active treatments have been based on retrospective judgments of pain relief. To take a relevant example, decisions as to whether and to what extent patients with chronic nonmalignant pain should rely on opioid analgesics are likely to be critically determined by whether their efficacy is assessed concurrently or retrospectively by clinicians who prescribe them and by researchers who study them. These considerations also apply to the growing literature on expectancy and placebo effects in clinical medicine (Montgomery et al. 1998). Future research should determine whether the findings of studies of placebo analgesia generalize to treatments of clinical problems other than pain (e.g., nausea, distress, and fatigue).

The role of desire for relief

An approach similar to that used to analyze expectancy must be used to evaluate the additional role of motivation or desire for pain relief. Placebo effects are commonly observed in circumstances wherein subjects not only expect but also strongly desire therapeutic effects. The potential role of this factor is consistent with literature showing that analgesia is a common consequence of threatening or fearful circumstances in animals (see Chapter 6).

Although desire for relief (or motivation, which is not quite the same thing) has been directly or indirectly implicated in the placebo response, less explicit recognition has been given to this factor than to expectation. Evaluation of the role of desire for pain relief in placebo analgesia could be accomplished in part by systematically varying the degree of pain or degree of threat presented in an experiment or by using the natural variability of patients' desire for pain relief in clinical settings. The interrelationship between expectation and desire for relief also needs to be evaluated.

Although direct evidence for the mediating role of desire for relief has yet to be obtained, some indirect evidence supports the possible contribution of this factor to placebo analgesia. First, the magnitude of placebo analgesia seems to be influenced by the degree of threat inherent in the context in which placebo treatments are given. Presumably, the degree of threat would contribute to desire for pain relief. Based on comparisons of placebo analgesic effects across studies of different types of pain, both Beecher (1955, 1959) and Jospe (1978) asserted that the magnitudes of analgesic response to an explicit placebo manipulation are, in general, much greater in studies of clinical pain than in experimental trials. Although both authors base their assertion on considerable numbers of studies, a serious limitation of their comparison is that clinical studies rarely take into account the natural history of the subjects' pain. However, among studies of experimental pain that assessed natural history and/or baseline reliability, placebo analgesic effects were greater for forms of experimental pain that lasted longer or were more stressful (Jospe 1978). These types of pain are more likely to simulate the psychological conditions of most acute clinical pains. Thus, placebo treatments produce substantial reductions in experimental pains that continuously increase in intensity over several minutes, such as ischemic limb pain (Grevert et al. 1983). They have smaller effects on brief pains, such as those produced by 5-second heat stimuli applied to the skin (Price et al. 1986b) or 1-second electrical stimuli applied to the tooth pulp (Gracely 1979).

Contrary to their hypothesis, however, Price et al. (1999) could not significantly associate ratings of desire for pain relief with magnitude of placebo analgesia. Although this result casts some doubt on the possible contribution of desire for pain relief on placebo analgesia, there are reasons why the hypothesis should not be completely dismissed at this point. First, nearly all participants of the study had some degree of desire for pain relief, as determined by their ratings of this factor. Second, as discussed above, desire for pain relief may be much more of a critical factor in placebo effects during clinical pain. This factor needs to be assessed in clinical pain studies.

A third reason for not completely rejecting the hypothesis that desire or motivation contributes to placebo analgesia is based on a study by Jensen and Karoly (1991). Although the study was not about pain relief, the authors explicitly assessed the contribution of a desire for symptom change in a study of placebo manipulations consisting of suggestions that the agent had sedative or stimulant effects. Jensen and Karoly (1991) assessed separate contributions of motivation and expectancy to placebo responses. Motivation referred to "the degree to which subjects desire to experience a symptom change," and expectancy was considered the subjects' expectation of symptom change. The authors manipulated both factors by using separate instructions; they later checked (by subject self-ratings) whether either or both factors had been influenced. Thus, the study was a two by two factorial design containing four groups (high motivation plus high expectancy, etc.). They found that motivation accounted for a significant amount of variance in placebo responses that included perceived sedation in the case of placebo tranquilizers or perceived arousal in the case of placebo stimulants.

ALTERNATIVE SPECIFIC MECHANISMS
OF PLACEBO ANALGESIA

Evidence suggests that placebo analgesic effects are largely mediated by expectancy, and in the case of retrospective judgments of pain intensity, memory distortion. In addition, some evidence suggests mediation by a second factor, desire for pain relief. However, questions remain about the exact mechanisms by which psychological factors mediate pain relief. There are several alternative mechanisms by which factors of conditioning, expectancy, and desire for pain relief could mediate placebo analgesia. These alternatives are not necessarily mutually exclusive. One possibility is that desire and expectation are integral components of pain affect and that placebo administration produces a global change in pain-affect by changing one or both of these components. A second possibility is that placebo effects are produced by highly specific response expectancies. A third is that desire for pain relief and/or expectancy simply lead to compliance with the demand characteristics of the experimental or clinical situation (i.e., the perceived need to comply with the responses expected by the investigator or clinician). Finally, desire for pain relief and/or expectancy may be somehow associated with brain mechanisms that trigger descending modulation of the pain-related signal. Except for the third possibility, this last possibility is not inconsistent with any of the other alternatives. The following discussion focuses on these possibilities and some of their implications.

PLACEBO EFFECTS ARE MEDIATED BY GLOBAL
CHANGES IN PAIN AFFECT

Placebo effects mediated by global changes in pain affect could occur if desire for pain reduction and expectancy were integral components of pain affect itself and if placebo administration directly influenced pain affect through changes in these two factors. As discussed in Chapter 3, there is empirical support for the role of these two factors in emotions in general as well as those associated with pain. Remember that the intensities of at least some common types of emotional feelings can be explained on the basis of two major factors: how much we *desire* something to happen or not happen and our level of *expectation* that it will happen or has happened (Price and Barrell 1984; Price et al. 1985a; Price and Fields 1997a,b). These two factors codetermine the valence and magnitude of many ordinary emotions such as anxiety, fear, and disappointment (see Fig. 3).

This desire/expectation model may help to explain not only emotions that occur during pain but also changes in these emotions that result from specific types of placebo manipulations. For example, some types of suggestions could reduce pain unpleasantness by either decreasing desire for pain relief or increasing expectation of obtaining it. These changes would not entail concomitant changes in pain sensation intensity. For example, subjects could simply be told that the therapeutic agent should help them feel better. Under these conditions, placebo effects would involve *only* a reduction in anxiety and consequently a selective reduction in the affective dimension of pain. Anxiety represents a desire to avoid negative consequences coupled with an uncertain expectation of avoiding those consequences (Price et al. 1980, 1985a; Barrell et al. 1985). These two factors comprise the anxiety that is associated with acute clinical pain and some forms of experimental pain. To the extent that patients increase their expectation that a given treatment or agent will reduce general negative consequences associated with pain, their anxiety will decrease when they receive the treatment or when they know they are going to receive a treatment. This reduction in anxiety would be expected to reduce the overall unpleasantness associated with pain (Price 1988). In this way, the direct perception that the placebo agent means a reduction in pain-related unpleasantness, distress, or anxiety is an integral part of the placebo response itself. A selective anti-anxiety effect could occur if the patient were led to expect that the therapeutic agent would make the pain less threatening, bothersome, or distressing but not necessarily less intense (e.g., "I am going to give you something to make it easy to experience the procedure"). An important implication of this global mechanism is that the placebo response would not be localized to one specific region of the body but would be related to the patient's overall sense of well-being or emotional state.

One study has shown a selective effect of a placebo on the affective dimension of pain. As pointed out above, Gracely (1979) found that saline placebo reduced affective, but not sensory ratings of experimental pain. Moreover, this effect was greater toward the low end of the nociceptive stimulus range, a pattern similar to that produced by an anxiety-reducing agent (Gracely et al. 1976) and by cognitive manipulations likely to reduce anxiety (Price et al. 1980). Indeed, the combined factors of desire for relief and uncertainty of relief may at least partly account for the association between the placebo response and anxiety (Bootzin 1985; Evans 1985).

PLACEBO EFFECTS FROM HIGHLY SPECIFIC RESPONSE EXPECTANCIES

When you enter an elevator and push a button for the third floor, there is an implicit but strong response expectancy. If someone were to ask you about the probability that the elevator will now take you to third floor, you would probably respond that you know it will do so or at least that there is a very strong likelihood of getting to the third floor. This is an example of specific response expectancy. You already act *as if* you are going to the third floor. It is possible that placebo responses occur in the same way. You receive an analgesic tablet for pain in the big toe and you "know" that pain relief is just a matter of time. Psychological and neural mechanisms of pain reduction may be a part of the acting *as if* analgesia is happening. This explanation of placebo mechanism contrasts with that of a global change in affect because it proposes (1) a reduction in both sensory and affective dimensions of pain and (2) reduction of pain in a specific part of the body (e.g., the big toe).

Considerable evidence exists for the first proposal. Most studies of placebo analgesia show reductions in sensory-intensive aspects of pain, and placebo studies that measure sensory and affective dimensions show that both are reduced by placebo (e.g., Montgomery and Kirsch 1996b; Price et al. 1999). However, it is still possible that a global change in affect could result in a change in pain sensation intensity, so that this line of evidence alone is not convincing.

Montgomery and Kirsch (1996b) provided critical evidence to support the second proposal. They demonstrated that a placebo applied in the guise of a topical anesthetic produced reduction in pain only at the body site at which it was administered. Controlled mechanical pain stimuli were administered simultaneously to treated and untreated fingers for one group of participants and sequentially for another. For both groups, reduction in pain occurred only on the finger that was treated with the placebo anesthetic, thereby indicating a highly specific mechanism. Therefore, psychological mediation of at least one type of placebo analgesic effect involves much more specific mechanisms than the simple reduction of anxiety or other global effects on emotions. Other global mechanisms, such as the release of hormones, can also be ruled out. The effects were relatively small (about 12–15%) and uniform across intensity and unpleasantness dimensions. The combination of these results indirectly suggests a second general mechanism for placebo analgesia, that of development of a highly specific response expectancy (Kirsch 1990, 1997).

Kirsch (1990) further suggests that response expectancies, defined as the anticipation of nonvolitional responses, are capable of eliciting the expected response in much the same way that intentions elicit voluntary behaviors (cf. Ajzen and Fishbein 1975, 1980; Ohlwein et al. 1996). However, it is not clear whether the results of Montgomery and Kirsch (1996b) distinguish between a specific response expectancy and simple compliance with demand characteristics of the experimental or clinical situation. The latter can be conceptualized as a type of response bias that could mediate apparent placebo analgesic responses. In such cases, patients/participants would reduce their ratings of pain after a placebo treatment in response to both their *desire* to please the person administering the treatment and their *expectation* that reduction of pain ratings would do so. Moreover, they would reduce these ratings for only the body part that was treated with placebo.

DESIRE FOR RELIEF AND EXPECTATION OF PAIN RELIEF IN OPIOID ANTINOCICEPTION

Early studies showed that placebo analgesia is physiologically mediated by endogenous opioid systems. Although somewhat controversial, the first evidence consisted of demonstrations that placebo-induced reductions of experimental and clinical pain could be reversed or antagonized by naloxone, an opioid antagonist (Levine et al. 1978, 1979; Grevert et al. 1983; Grevert and Goldstein 1985). If either desire for or expectation of pain relief is necessary for placebo analgesia and if placebo effects are mediated physiologically by endogenous opioid control systems, then brain states associated with these factors may somehow trigger opioid descending control systems. If so, then we would expect that placebo analgesia would include antinociceptive effects (i.e., reduction of the ascending signal for pain) and not just a response bias or a global change in affective state. Both sensory and affective dimensions of pain would be reduced by this mechanism because opioid pain modulatory systems inhibit nociceptive transmission at the first synapse in pain-related ascending pathways, a site at which sensory and affective dimensions of pain are not differentially represented (see Chapter 6).

Amanzio and Benedetti (1999) investigated the mechanisms underlying the activation of endogenous opioids in placebo analgesia by using a model of human experimental ischemic arm pain. Different types of placebo analgesic responses were evoked by means of cognitive expectation cues, drug conditioning, or a combination of both. Their analysis was elegant because they examined the separate contributions of expectancy cues and conditioning and determined the extent to which each of these factors was associated with endogenous opioid analgesic mechanisms. Their results have bearing on all of the specific mechanisms of placebo analgesia discussed thus far. As shown in Fig. 4, drug conditioning was performed by means of presenting analgesic trials using morphine hydrochloride, either alone or combined with verbal suggestions that a potent painkiller was being given (i.e., expectancy cues). Morphine conditioning trials with no expectancy cues on days 2 and 3 induced a naloxone-reversible placebo effect on day 4 (compare Fig. 4C and D). Morphine conditioning combined with expectancy cues on days 2 and 3 induced a greater placebo effect on day 4 in comparison to the group that received conditioning *without* expectancy cues (compare Fig. 4A and C). This large placebo effect was the combined result of both conditioning and expectancy cues, and it was completely naloxone reversible (Fig. 4A, B). The investigators repeated this analysis using the nonopioid ketorolac. In contrast to morphine conditioning, ketorolac conditioning together with placebo suggestions elicited a placebo effect that was only partially blocked by naloxone. Ketorolac conditioning alone produced a placebo effect that, unlike morphine conditioning, was naloxone insensitive. Finally, expectation cues alone (verbal placebo suggestions) produced a small placebo effect that was completely blocked by naloxone (Fig. 5). This result demonstrates that an expectancy manipulation alone is sufficient to evoke placebo analgesia that utilizes endogenous opioid mechanisms.

Therefore, Amanzio and Benedetti evoked different types of placebo responses that were either completely or partially naloxone reversible or else naloxone insensitive, depending on the procedure used to evoke the placebo effect. They concluded that cognitive factors and conditioning are balanced in different ways in placebo analgesia, and that this balance is crucial for the activation of opioid or nonopioid systems. Verbal placebo suggestions that are likely to induce expectations of analgesia trigger endogenous opioids, whereas conditioning activates specific opioid or nonopioid subsystems. Thus, if conditioning is performed with opioids, placebo analgesia is mediated via opioid receptors, whereas if conditioning is

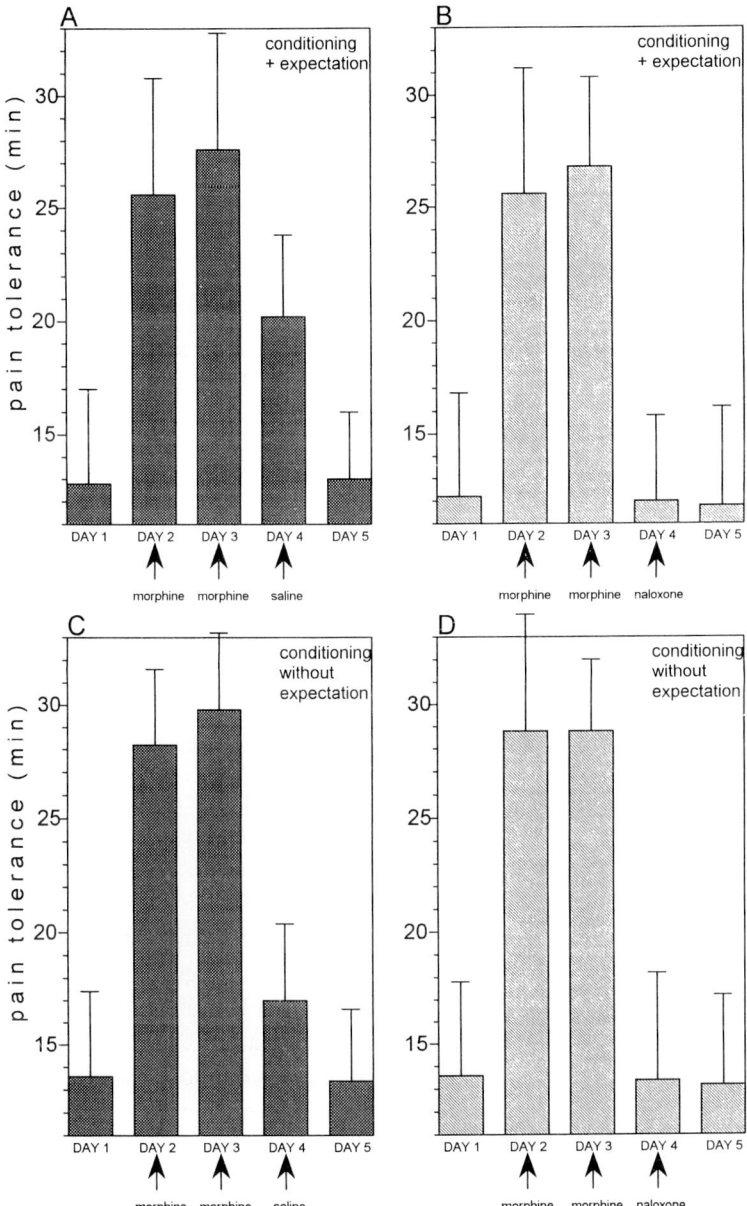

Fig. 4. Results of a study of ischemic arm pain. (A) After morphine conditioning on days 2 and 3, an open injection of saline, which is stated to be morphine, produces an analgesic effect that is over one-half as great as that of morphine itself. (B) If an injection of naloxone is given instead of saline, the placebo analgesic effect is completely abolished. (C) After morphine conditioning on days 2 and 3, an open injection of saline, which is stated to be an antibiotic, produces an analgesic effect that is less than that shown in panel B. (D) An open injection of naloxone, which is stated to be an antibiotic, completely blocks the analgesic effect shown in panel C. Reprinted from Amanzio and Benedetti (1999), with permission.

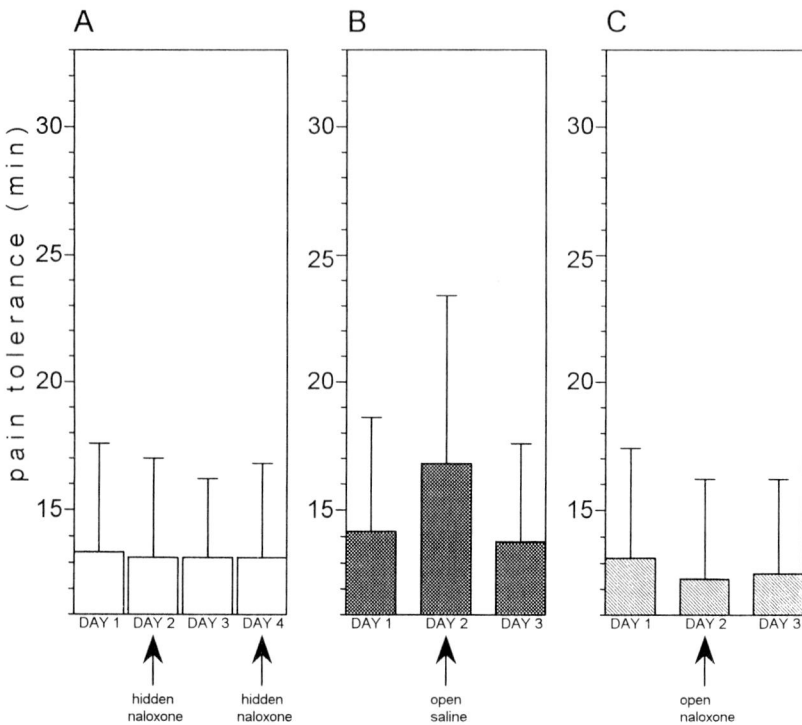

Fig. 5. Expectation-induced placebo analgesia and its blockade by naloxone following morphine conditioning trials. (A) A hidden injection of naloxone on days 2 and 4 produces no change in pain tolerance compared with days 1 and 3, indicating that naloxone per se does not affect this type of experimental pain. (B) Open injection of saline and suggestions that a potent painkiller was being administered resulted in a placebo effect. Days 1 and 3 represent preinjection and postinjection controls. (C) An open injection of naloxone and suggestions that a potent painkiller was being administered did not result in any placebo effect, unlike the results of panel B. Thus, naloxone completely blocked the placebo effect produced by open injection and placebo suggestions. Reprinted from Amanzio and Benedetti (1999), with permission.

performed with nonopioid drugs, other nonopioid mechanisms are activated. It is important to recognize that expectancy could be the proximate cause of analgesia from conditioning, given the evidence cited above that expectancy is a critical mediating factor in conditioning. A limitation of Amanzio and Benedetti's study is that expectations of the participants were not directly assessed but only assumed to result from the manipulations.

Benedetti and colleagues (1999) further clarified the role of expectancy and its relationship to opioid mechanisms in a subsequent study. They examined highly specific expectations of analgesia on four different parts of the body and determined whether the resultant analgesia was mediated by endogenous opioids. In this experiment, both hands and feet were simultaneously stimulated with subcutaneous injection of intradermal capsaicin, producing a moderately intense burning pain at all sites (5–6 on a 10-point scale). Specific expectations of analgesia were induced by applying a placebo cream on only one of these body parts while telling the participants that it was a powerful local anesthetic. Thus, similar to other studies described earlier, they assumed that this procedure produced an expectation directed specifically toward the treated body part. As shown in Fig. 6, a placebo analgesic response occurred on the treated body part but not on the three remaining sites. When the same experiment was repeated after an intravenous infusion of naloxone, this spatially specific placebo effect was completely abolished, indicating that it was mediated by endogenous opioid systems (Fig. 6). These results support both the response expectancy mechanism of placebo analgesia and the role of endogenous opioid mechanisms. Furthermore, since naloxone administration is subjectively undetectable, its reversal of placebo analgesia makes it unlikely that such analgesia is merely a matter of compliance with the demand characteristics of the study.

Reversal of analgesia by naloxone is only one line of evidence implicating endogenous opioid systems in placebo analgesia. Other experiments have demonstrated that blockade of cholecystokinin (CCK) receptors potentiates the placebo analgesic effect, thereby suggesting an inhibitory role of CCK in placebo analgesia (Benedetti 1996). Since CCK is known to inhibit exogenous and endogenous opioid analgesic effects, then the potentiating effects of CCK *antagonists* on placebo analgesia further implicate opioid mechanisms in such analgesia.

These general mechanisms (direct change in affective state, response bias, and activation of descending control mechanisms) all contain the common idea that desire and expectation are proximate psychological mediators of placebo analgesia. However, from the foregoing discussion, it is apparent that desires and expectations may be targeted toward aspects of future experience in the case of concurrent placebo responses, or of past experience for placebo responses based on remembered pain. Furthermore, the desire and expectation may be focused on avoiding general negative consequences associated with the pain condition, on avoiding the pain sensation itself, or even on not disappointing the person who administers the therapeutic agent.

Multiple types of responses to placebo analgesic manipulations may be possible because many types of desires and expectations can be induced in study participants or pain patients by the way in which placebo suggestions are framed. Even the same placebo instructions could lead some individuals to desire and expect reductions in unpleasantness and others to desire and expect reductions in both pain sensation intensity and unpleasantness. Some people may experience only global affective changes as a result of placebo

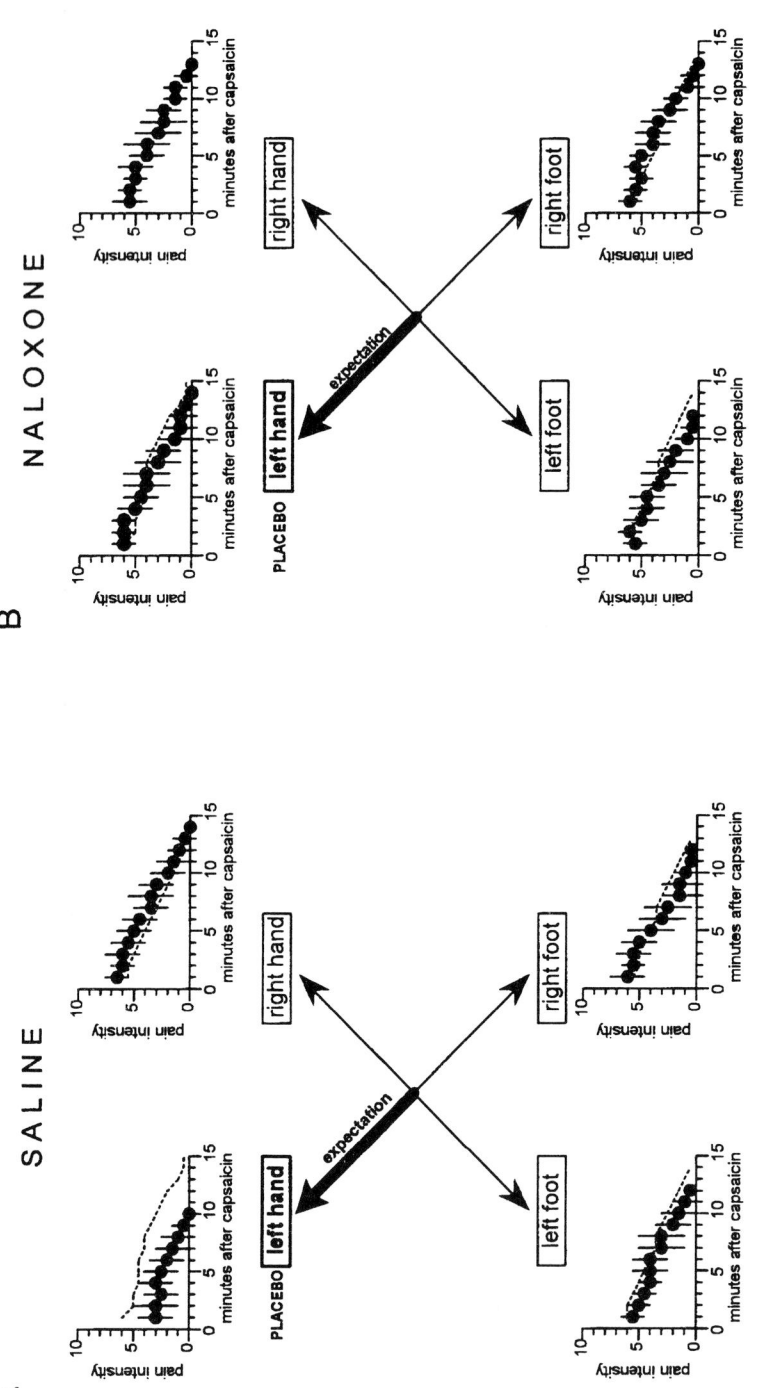

Fig. 6. The effects of a placebo cream. (A) The specific expectation of analgesia on the left hand produced a placebo effect there but not on other parts of the body. (B) This highly specific placebo effect was completely blocked by naloxone. The broken lines show the natural histories of pain from intradermal capsaicin. Reprinted from Benedetti et al. (1999), with permission.

administration, whereas others develop highly specific expectations of pain reduction at single locations or other specific expectations of therapeutic effects. Still others may simply desire and expect to please the person administering the therapeutic agent. This potential diversity in types of placebo responses is indirectly supported by studies of hypnotic analgesia that have proposed the same general possibilities to explain variation in changes in pain reports and behavior after hypnotic analgesic interventions (Barber and Adrian 1982; Price and Barber 1987; Kiernan et al. 1995).

Despite this diversity in specific potential mechanisms of placebo analgesia, some degree of consensus has emerged. Conditioning is a powerful factor in placebo analgesia and is a satisfying model because it provides a potential neurobiology of this phenomenon. However, among human beings, conditioning is powerful only because it leads to specific expectations of analgesic responses. Within clinical contexts, desire for pain relief is likely have at least some additional or interactive influence with expectation. Indeed, the desire/expectation model may provide a more complete account of factors that mediate placebo responses. It may partly account for the diversity of emotional, perceptual, and behavioral responses to placebo manipulations. Indeed, the multiplicative desire/expectation model that has been established for human emotions can be related to expectancy × value theories (Rotter 1954, 1966, 1972; Tolman 1955). To the extent that placebo responses can be conceptualized in terms of changes in emotions, changes in tendency to respond, or learned changes in pain responsiveness, the potential application of a desire/expectancy model to all of these possible variants of placebo analgesic response appears promising and testable.

FUTURE DIRECTIONS AND IMPLICATIONS OF RESEARCH INTO PLACEBO ANALGESIC MECHANISMS

Knowledge about the psychological and neural mechanisms by which placebo treatments reduce pain has far-reaching implications for treatment of medical conditions, including pain. For example, suppose it is true that a specific kind of placebo reduces the magnitudes of the ascending nociceptive signal and pain sensation intensity and not just pain-related emotions or the subject's bias in rating pain. The antinociceptive effects of a placebo administration, exerted at the level of the first synapse in the dorsal horn, implies that the physiological consequences of pain, such as reduced immune response and prolongation of healing, also would be ameliorated (Liebeskind 1991). As a consequence of these general mechanisms, placebo treatments have the potential to influence physiological and pathophysi-

Psychological Mechanisms of Pain and Analgesia, Progress in Pain Research and Management, Vol. 15, by Donald D. Price, IASP Press, Seattle, © 1999.

8

Mechanisms of Hypnotic Analgesia

While cognitive factors such as expectancy, motivation, and memory contribute directly to placebo analgesia, hypnotic analgesia is even more complex and subjective because it may involve subtle changes in consciousness and even in unconscious mechanisms. Studies of hypnotic analgesia have labored under a double burden in that both the independent variables of hypnotic interventions and the multiple components of pain experience, which are the dependent variables, are subjective phenomena. Partly as a consequence, measurement of variables in hypnotic analgesia experiments may lack the precise control that is present in physiological or pharmacological studies. However, in this chapter I present the alternative view that precise analysis and measurement are possible for both the independent and dependent variables associated with hypnotic analgesia. In this context I will present a general explanation of the neural and psychological mechanisms that may underlie this form of analgesia. An understanding of these mechanisms has implications for treating and managing pain by means of psychological approaches.

THE GENERAL NATURE OF HYPNOTIC ANALGESIA

THE RELATIONSHIP OF PAIN RELIEF TO HYPNOTIC STATE

The problem of characterizing the mechanisms of hypnotic analgesia becomes enormously complicated the moment we begin asking questions about the factors that reduce pain as well as about the nature of the pain reduction itself. The factors that evoke pain reduction extend from psychosocial factors, including interactions between hypnotist and subject, to neurophysiological factors that influence the transmission of pain signals within the subject. First I will address the demand characteristics of the hypnotic analgesia situation, second, the role of hypnotic state and the possible interactions between hypnotic state and incorporation of hypnotic suggestions, and third, factors that may be considered potential independent variables of hypnotic analgesia studies. This discussion will be followed by a consideration of how hypnotic interventions influence the multiple dimensions of pain and, at least in a general sense, the neurophysiological processing of pain.

Hypnotic analgesia is not simply the result of demand characteristics of the experiment or clinical situation

One major hypothesis about the nature of hypnotic analgesia is that the phenomenon represents compliance with demand characteristics of the experimental or clinical situation. Thus, after hypnotic induction and suggestions, subjects cognitively re-label their reports of pain as less intense, not because they perceive them to be less intense but simply to act in the role of someone who has less pain (Spanos 1983, 1986). This explanation makes two interrelated claims. The first is that there is nothing special about the hypnotic situation and that a change in conscious state is not required to evoke responses to hypnotic suggestion. The second claim is that there is nothing special about the hypnotic response of reducing one's rating of pain, and that this response does not necessarily involve an actual reduction in pain but rather a willingness to use lowered ratings to describe unaltered pain sensations. According to the "role enactment" theorists, the elaborate ritual of hypnotic induction only serves to strengthen the demand characteristics of the situation and encourage subjects to simply follow instructions and "emit" the desired behavior.

The claim that a change in state of consciousness does not necessarily contribute to hypnotic analgesia is based on studies that compared differences in analgesia between two groups of subjects (Barber and Hahn 1962; Barber and Wilson 1977; Evans and Paul 1985). In both studies, one group was given analgesia suggestions after induction of a hypnotic state and the other received only analgesia suggestions. Both groups of subjects in both studies reduced their pain ratings in response to analgesia suggestions, regardless of whether or not the suggestions were accompanied by hypnotic induction. In fact, no differences were found between effects of the two experimental conditions. On the other hand, there are considerably more studies that demonstrate that greater analgesia occurs when subjects enter a hypnotic state and that hypnotic susceptibility is at least somewhat predictive of hypnotic analgesia (see references in Hilgard and Hilgard 1983). The claim that hypnotically induced reports of reduced pain do not necessarily reflect actual reductions in perceived pain has limited support from observations that physiological responses to pain, such as increased heart rate and blood pressure, often still occur during hypnotically induced reports of greatly reduced pain (Hilgard and Hilgard 1983).

Are hypnotic inductions or states necessary for hypnotic analgesia?

A major question about the nature of hypnotic analgesia has been whether a hypnotic state is required to evoke reductions in pain report. If subjects of hypnotic analgesia experiments are simply enacting an elaborate role, then subjects who are deliberately instructed to simulate analgesia should be able to tolerate intense pain as well as those who undergo the unnecessary ritual of hypnotic induction. Greene and Reyher (1972) tested this hypothesis by assigning highly hypnotizable subjects randomly to hypnotized and simulating groups. They instructed the simulators to remain out of a hypnotic state while deceiving the hypnotist into believing they were hypnotized and to react to the painful stimulus as if they were analgesic. Pain tolerance and pain intensity reports were obtained in response to increasing electric shock intensities. Despite the attempt to behave like hypnotized subjects, the simulators were clearly less tolerant of the pain during each of the several experimental conditions than were the hypnotized subjects. For example, the truly hypnotized and the simulators increased their tolerance of pain by 45% and 16%, respectively, a difference that was highly statistically significant. The shocks were more bearable for the truly hypnotized than for the equally susceptible but unhypnotized role enactors. The results of this experiment cast some doubt on the idea that hypnotized subjects feel pain but report less pain to satisfy the demand characteristics of the hypnotist.

How are responses to suggestions facilitated by a hypnotic state?

Hypnotic states are produced by hypnotic inductions, particularly in subjects who have high scores on standard tests of hypnotic susceptibility (Hilgard and Hilgard 1983). In fact, studies using positron emission tomographic (PET) brain imaging and EEG have recently found hypnotic states to be associated with a pattern of increases in activity in occipital cortical regions and decreases in posterior parietal cortical regions in comparison to nonhypnotic control states (Rainville et al. 1999a). Studies combining brain imaging with analysis of components of hypnotic state have shown that a hypnotic state, without suggestions for analgesia, is not sufficient to produce reduction in pain ratings or reduction in pain-related activity in the cerebral cortex (Hilgard and Hilgard 1983; Rainville et al. 1997, 1998). Conversely, some studies show that subjects with high hypnotic susceptibility scores can develop analgesia in response to analgesic suggestions alone (Tenenbaum et al. 1990; Jacobs et al. 1995). However, it is not altogether clear whether they develop analgesia in the complete absence of a change in consciousness indicative of a hypnotic state.

Considerable evidence points to greater analgesia in response to suggestions in a hypnotic state, particularly when studies combine within-subject and between-subjects comparisons of waking versus hypnotic analgesia (Hilgard and Hilgard 1983; Jacobs et al. 1995). Based on decades of both experimental as well as clinical observations, it is evident that the hypnotic state can at least facilitate the analgesia produced by direct or indirect suggestions (Barber and Adrian 1982; Hilgard and Hilgard 1983; Barber 1996). This brings us to the general question as to *how* a hypnotic state does this. On the basis of experiential and path analysis studies, I proposed the following common elements of a hypnotic state (Price 1996):

1) A feeling of ease or relaxation (manifested as a letting go of "tensions" or becoming at ease and not necessarily physical relaxation).

2) An absorbed and sustained focus of attention on one or few targets.

3) An absence of judging, monitoring, and censoring.

4) A suspension of usual orientation toward time, location, and sense of self.

5) The experiencing of one's own responses as automatic (i.e., without deliberation or effort).

Visual analogue scale (VAS) ratings of these factors have demonstrated strong interrelationships among them, suggesting that some of the common elements are necessary for others (Price and Barrell 1990). Thus, element 1 ("becoming at ease/relaxation") appears to provide a supportive general background for element 2 ("absorbed and sustained focus"), which in turn may result in elements 3 ("absence of judging, monitoring, censoring") and 4 ("suspension of usual orientation toward time and location"). The latter two elements, in turn, appear to maintain element 5 ("automaticity"). Finally, elements 4 and 5 directly contribute to perceived hypnotic depth. The experiential and conceptual basis for this model is generally supported by the work of others who have independently arrived at many of the same common elements (Bowers 1978; Pekula and Kumar 1984). This model also is supported by a neural imaging study in which neural activities in various cerebral cortical regions covaried with some of these dimensions of hypnotic depth (Rainville et al. 1999a).

Returning then to the question as to how a hypnotic state facilitates incorporation of suggestions, such as that for analgesia, this model implicitly provides a basis for *increased responsiveness to suggestion* that is unique and distinguishable from other types of psychologically induced increases in responsiveness to suggestion (e.g., placebo). This basis is directly evident in the phenomenology of the interrelationships between the common elements of this model as follows: A hypnotic state begins with an absorbed and sustained focus on something. At first, it can be effortful, but with time the subject proceeds from an *active* form of concentration to a relaxed *passive* form. There is often (though perhaps not necessarily) an inhibition or reduction in the peripheral range of his or her experience. At the same time, this relaxation and reduction in range of attention support a *lack* of monitoring and censoring of that which is allowed into experience. Hence, inconsistencies are now more tolerable. Contradictory statements, which would normally arrest one's attention and cause confusion or disturbance, no longer do so. The hypnotist's suggestions are accepted without censorship and are not checked against one's own associations. Consequently, the subject no longer chooses or validates the correctness of incoming statements. This allows thinking and "meaning-in-itself" to be disconnected from active reflection. From this way of experiencing, there emerges the sense of *automaticity* wherein thinking does not precede an action; rather, action precedes thought. Thus, if the hypnotist suggests a bodily action, a sensation, or a lack of sensation (e.g., pain), the subject experiences no deliberation of effort but simply and automatically identifies with the suggested action, sensation, or lack of sensation. The possibility of not carrying out the action or not experiencing the suggested changes in sensation is given little or no consideration. In this way, a hypnotic state *facilitates* the incorporation of and responses to suggestions, including that of analgesia.

It may well be that what is unique about hypnotic suggestions is not the end result of the suggestions themselves, such as pain relief, but the way in which the suggestions implicitly or explicitly refer to the source of experiential change as coming automatically from within. This uniqueness perhaps can be illustrated by comparing the nature of hypnotic suggestions with those associated with placebo administration. The "suggestion" provided in the case of placebo analgesia can readily be distinguished from that provided during hypnotic analgesia in that the former refers to an outside authoritative source as the origin of the pain relief. For example, injections or tablets provided by a health care professional indicate that the therapeutic relief comes from a medicine and a person knowledgeable about the efficacy of the treatment. The placebo literature provides some evidence that greater placebo effects are achieved by more believable and technically convincing agents. Thus, placebo injections are more effective than placebo pills, and placebo morphine is more effective than placebo aspirin (Traut and Passarelli 1957). Implicit in the overall suggestion inherent to a placebo analgesic manipulation is the idea that in the absence of this outside authoritative agent, there would be unrelieved pain. The nature of hypnotic suggestions for analgesia, on the other hand, refers to a more innate and *self-directed* capacity to alter one's own experience, often to the effect that one can experience sensations differently and including the possibility that there is no pain to be experienced (Barber and Adrian 1982). All of these types of suggestion are learned, regardless of whether or not they reflect the intentions of the person who administers them.

This experiential distinction between hypnotic and placebo analgesia

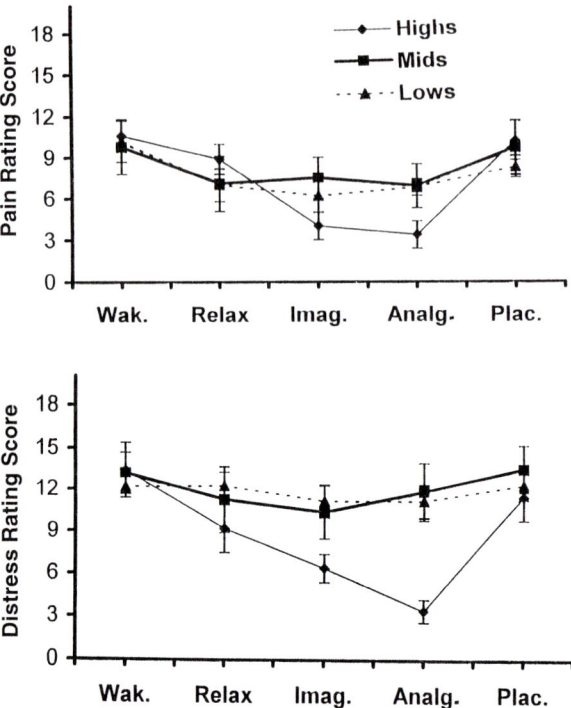

Fig. 1. Mean ratings (± 1 SEM) of pain (top) and distress (bottom) of groups of subjects with high, mid, and low hypnotic susceptibility exposed to five different experimental conditions. Wak. = baseline waking condition; Relax = hypnotic induction followed by suggestions to enter a deeply relaxed condition without pain; Imag. = hypnotic induction followed by suggestions to engage in pleasant visual imagery along with suggestions for dissociating from one's experience of the body; Analg. = hypnotic induction followed by suggestions to experience the hand and arm as if it was in cold water for a long time and was becoming numb and analgesic; Plac. = subjects had their hand dampened with a colored mixture of water and alcohol and it was explained that they were receiving a topical anesthetic that would be effective very quickly in reducing pain perception. Based on data of De Pascalis et al. (2000).

not a simple matter of distraction because the most effective suggestions were for focused analgesia, which requires increased, not decreased, attention to the body region affected. Third, very different types of suggestions for analgesia are effective and are facilitated by hypnotizability.

Each of the types of hypnotic suggestion discussed so far can be given *directly* or *indirectly* (Barber and Adrian 1982; Barber 1996). A direct suggestion for analgesia would be "You will notice that the pain is less intense," whereas an indirect suggestion would be "I wonder if you will notice whether the sensation you once experienced as painful will be experienced as just warmth or pressure or perhaps even numbness." The latter is permis-

sive, ambiguous, and refers to alternative experiences without the implication of a direct instruction. Resistance to hypnotic suggestions may be lower
in the case of *indirect* as compared to *direct* suggestions because the subject
is not directly told what to experience. In contrast, direct suggestions may
be perceived as unnecessarily authoritarian (Barber and Adrian 1982; Barber 1996). Thus we might expect that more people could benefit from a
hypnotic approach that uses indirect suggestions, and there is some evidence that this is so (Barber and Adrian 1982; Fricton and Roth 1985; Barber 1996).

Effects of hypnotic suggestions on sensory and affective dimensions of pain

Just as multiple psychological dimensions contribute to hypnotic analgesia, analgesia itself is likely to have multiple dimensions. The strategy
discussed above for characterizing and measuring the factors in hypnotic
treatments could be interfaced with an assessment of how these factors influence the different dimensions of pain as well as the different general
stages of pain processing (e.g., spinal, cortical). Since pain has sensory-
discriminative, cognitive-evaluative, and affective-motivational dimensions,
a number of questions can be raised about how a hypnotic intervention
influences the various dimensions and stages of pain processing. Does hypnotic analgesia reduce the affective more than the sensory dimension? What
is the relationship of hypnotic susceptibility to hypnotically induced reductions in the intensity and unpleasantness of pain?

Possible differences in the effects of hypnotic suggestion on sensory
and affective dimensions were addressed by Price and Barber (1987). Two
groups of human volunteers made responses on extensively validated visual
analogue scales of pain sensation intensity (sensory VAS) and pain unpleasantness (affective VAS) to noxious skin temperature stimuli (44.5°–51.5°C)
before and after indirect hypnotic suggestions were given for analgesia (Table
I). Group 1 participants were given suggestions for developing a hypnotic
state only once, just before analgesic testing, and did not have significantly
reduced VAS responses to experimental pain after hypnosis (data not shown).
Group 2 participants were continuously given cues for maintaining a hypnotic state during their analgesic testing session and had a mean overall
reduction of 44.5% in pain sensation intensity and 87.4% in pain affect. As
shown in Table I, group 2 subjects had a much larger and more consistent
reduction in pain affect than in pain sensation intensity. A small but statistically reliable correlation was found between hypnotic susceptibility and
overall magnitude of reduction in sensory but not affective VAS ratings

(Table I). Since large reductions in affective ratings occurred in nearly all subjects, the lack of a significant association between hypnotic susceptibility scores and reductions in pain affect ratings is most likely the result of a ceiling effect.

However, it is not immediately apparent why hypnotically induced reductions in affective VAS ratings to experimental pain were greater and more consistent than those in sensory VAS ratings. Affective responses to experimental heat pain were reduced even in participants who had low susceptibility scores and who had very little change in perceived sensation intensities (Table I). The answer may lie in the nature of sensory and affective responses to experimental pain and in the degree of hypnotic involvement required to experience alterations in these pain dimensions. Affective responses associated with pain are more influenced by the perceived context of the experimental situation than are sensory responses (Price 1988). Thus, factors related to a person's psychological context can selectively and often powerfully reduce affective responses to experimental pain (Price et al. 1980; Price 1988). Hypnotic suggestions of this study were directed toward (a) experiencing the testing situation as more pleasant, (b) experienc-

Table I

Hypnotically induced reductions in sensory and affective
VAS ratings of experimental pain according to hypnotic
susceptibility (1 = low; 5 = high)

Subject	Hypnotic Susceptibility	Change in Sensory VAS (%)	Change in Affective VAS (%)
1	1	56.8	74.5
2	1	9.0	90.0
3	1	65.5	100.0
4	1	63.1	100.0
5	1	3.6	100.0
6	2	60.0	100.0
7	2	17.8	91.4
8	2	17.5	78.6
9	3	20.7	51.5
10	3	28.3	78.0
11	3	24.7	74.6
12	3	50.0	100.0
13	3	46.0	100.0
14	4	82.7	99.1
15	5	83.9	62.5
16	5	81.7	98.7
Mean	2.4	44.5	87.4
R_s		0.4	−0.2

Source: Data from Price and Barber (1987).

ing the heat stimuli as more pleasant, and (c) experiencing the heat stimuli as less intense. It is clear that these three alterations in experience would require different degrees of hypnotic involvement (Weitzenhoffer 1953; Shor and Orne 1965). Experiencing the testing situation and test stimuli as less unpleasant would require less hypnotic involvement than would direct reductions in sensations evoked by noxious heat stimuli. In some instances, selective reduction in affect could occur without a hypnotic state. Therefore, one component of a hypnotic intervention may involve responses to suggestions for reduced unpleasantness that do not require a hypnotic state. The reduction in pain-related unpleasantness beyond that associated with a simple reduction in pain sensation intensity, and in some cases without any reduction in pain sensation (e.g., Table I), is not likely to be the result of a reduced pain signal at peripheral or even spinal levels. Rather, it is probably due to alteration in the meanings that normally attend painful experience. As such, the selective reduction in pain affect by cognitive mechanisms is likely to reflect neural events at higher levels of pain processing, including intracerebral mechanisms.

What are the psychological mechanisms of hypnotically induced reductions in pain sensation intensity?

Although it is clear that hypnotic suggestions may exert a more powerful reduction of pain affect than pain sensation, it is also quite apparent that both dimensions are reduced, as has been amply demonstrated in several experimental laboratories (see Hilgard and Hilgard 1983 and Price 1996 for reviews). Moreover, reduction in pain sensation is statistically associated with hypnotic susceptibility, albeit at modest levels. Until very recently, hypnotic analgesia studies have shown that susceptibility to hypnosis is more closely associated with reductions in pain sensation intensity than reductions in pain affect (Hilgard and Hilgard 1983; Price and Barber 1987). Interestingly, the association becomes stronger with increasing levels of pain intensity, as shown in Table II. It makes sense that the reduction in stronger pains requires more hypnotic ability than the reduction in weaker pains. However, the modest association between hypnotic susceptibility and sensory analgesia and the lack of an association between hypnotic ability and reductions in pain affective ratings (Table II) strongly indicate that multiple factors are involved in analgesia that results from a hypnotic intervention. These include some that are unrelated to hypnotic susceptibility and perhaps even to a hypnotic state. Such potential multiple factors are closely related to different proposed mechanisms of hypnotic analgesia. One limitation to most of the studies discussed thus far is that the hypnotic

Table II
Association between hypnotic susceptibility and
reductions in sensory and affective VAS ratings of
increasingly painful experimental heat stimuli

Stimulus Temperature	Spearman Correlation Coefficient, R_s	
	Sensory Analgesia	Affective Analgesia
44.5°C	+0.04	−0.23
47.5°C	+0.21	−0.11
49.5°C	+0.43 ($P < 0.05$)	−0.08
51.5°C	+0.56 ($P < 0.05$)	+0.10

Source: Data from Price and Barber (1987).

suggestions were mixed and included suggestions for altering both sensory and affective dimensions of pain.

A recent study by Rainville et al. (1999b) further clarifies the relationship between different types of hypnotic suggestions for analgesia and the dimensions of pain that are modulated by these suggestions. The authors conducted two experiments, one in which hypnotic suggestions were selectively targeted toward altering the affective dimension of pain and another in which they were targeted toward altering the sensory intensity of pain. In both types of experiments, normal subjects who were trained in receiving hypnosis rated pain intensity and pain unpleasantness produced by a tonic heat pain test (1-minute immersion of the hand in 45.0°–47.5°C water). In the first experiment, pain affect significantly increased or decreased when suggestions were given for these changes; these changes occurred *without* corresponding changes in pain sensation intensity. Moreover, there was a significant correlation between the stimulus-evoked heart rate increase and ratings of pain unpleasantness, but not pain sensation intensity, which suggests a direct functional interaction between pain affect and autonomic activation. In the second experiment, suggestions to modulate pain sensation intensity resulted in significant modulation of pain sensation intensity ratings; pain affect ratings were modulated in parallel. Hypnotic susceptibility (Stanford Hypnotic Susceptibility Scale, Form A) was specifically associated with pain affect modulation in the first type of experiment (directed toward pain affect) and with pain sensation intensity modulation in the second type of experiment (directed toward pain sensation intensity) (Fig. 2).

This study makes three original and critical points. First, unlike previous hypnosis experiments, it showed that hypnotic suggestions can *selectively* and potently modulate the affective dimension of pain. Second, when the sensory dimension is modulated, the affective dimension is modulated in parallel. These results were important in helping to establish the direction of

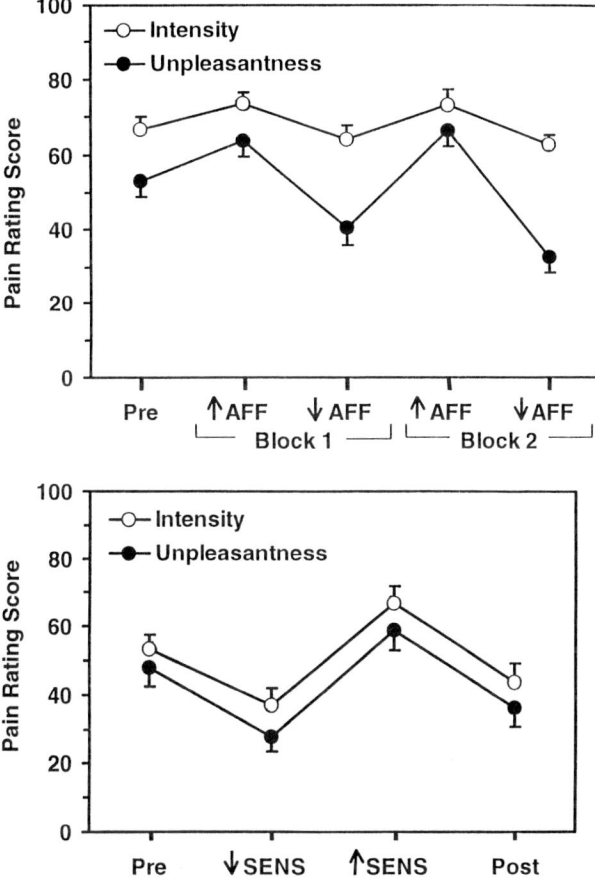

Fig. 2. Top: Mean (± SEM) pain ratings before hypnosis (Pre), and during two successive blocks of trials performed under hypnosis with suggestions to increase (↑AFF) or decrease pain affect (↓AFF). Hypnotic suggestions produced strong modulation of pain unpleasantness with only slight modulation of pain intensity. The order of the suggestion conditions was reversed in half the subjects. Bottom: Mean (± SEM) pain ratings before (Pre), during, and after (Post) suggestions, showing comparable modulation of pain intensity and unpleasantness in response to suggestions to decrease (↓SENS) or increase (↑SENS) pain sensation. The order of the suggestion conditions was reversed in half the subjects. From Rainville et al. (1999b), with permission.

causation between sensory and affective dimensions of pain (discussed in Chapter 3). Third, hypnotic susceptibility is associated with the specific pain dimension toward which the hypnotic suggestions are primarily targeted. Hypnotic susceptibility is required for reductions in pain affect when suggestions are exclusively about affect, but is not required when pain affect is reduced as a passive consequence of reductions in pain sensation. All of these results show important links between the elements of hypnosis and the dimensions of pain toward which suggestions are targeted, providing yet more evidence that hypnotic analgesia is a real and valid phenomenon.

It is useful to consider how results of various hypnotic suggestions help identify the necessary and sufficient psychological factors for hypnotic analgesia. As stated above, hypnotic analgesia cannot work only by means of distraction because suggestions for focused analgesia are among the most effective, particularly among highly hypnotizable participants (Fig. 1). Hypnotic analgesia cannot work only by means of a placebo effect because there is now good evidence that placebo analgesia requires an endogenous opioid pain-inhibitory mechanism and that hypnotic analgesia does not. As discussed in Chapter VII, placebo analgesia is reversible by naloxone in studies of experimental pain, whereas several studies have shown than hypnotic analgesia cannot be reversed by this agent. For example, Barber and Mayer (1977) found that hypnotic suggestions elevated pain thresholds produced by tooth-pulp stimulation and that these elevations were completely unaffected by a dose of naloxone that had previously been reported to reverse acupuncture analgesia (Mayer et al. 1976). Goldstein and Hilgard (1975) also failed to reverse hypnotic analgesia with naloxone. Moreover, placebo analgesia, unlike hypnotic analgesia, is not significantly associated with hypnotic susceptibility. Consideration of the neural mechanisms of hypnotic analgesia provides further insight into psychological mechanisms of hypnotic analgesia.

GENERAL NEURAL MECHANISMS OF HYPNOTIC ANALGESIA

Until very recently, questions about even the most general neural mechanisms of hypnotic analgesia appeared extremely difficult because of intrinsic limitations of techniques that could be used to analyze neural activity during hypnotic analgesia. With the recent advent of neural imaging techniques and improved psychophysiological measures, these limitations have significantly decreased. Several general questions can be asked about the neural mechanisms of hypnotic analgesia. Does hypnotic analgesia utilize an endogenous opioid system? To what extent does it involve descending inhibition of pain transmission at spinal cord levels in contrast to intracortical mechanisms that prevent awareness of pain once nociceptive information has reached the brain? What specific brain structures are affected by hypnotic analgesia? As surprising as it may seem, these questions are at least partly answerable in experiments that use multiple measures of pain experience and, in some cases, physiological indices of pain processing at different levels of the nervous system.

NEODISSOCIATION AND "INTRACEREBRAL" MECHANISMS

Based on current knowledge, there are two general mechanisms by which pain sensations could be reduced in intensity during hypnosis. With regard to the first mechanism, Ernest and Josephine Hilgard (1983) proposed that during hypnotic analgesia awareness of pain diminishes after nociceptive information has reached higher centers. According to this "neodissociation" theory, pain is registered by the body and by covert awareness during hypnotic analgesia. However, an amnesia-like barrier between dissociated streams of consciousness serves to prevent overt experience of pain. This dissociation in awareness has been demonstrated through "automatic writing" and through the phenomenon of the "hidden observer" (Hilgard et al. 1975; Hilgard 1977; Hilgard and Hilgard 1983).

Hilgard and colleagues asked subjects to rate covert levels of cold pressor pain through automatic key pressing, and to estimate the magnitude of overtly experienced pain (Hilgard et al. 1975). *Nonhypnotic* suggestions for analgesia created about a 40% reduction in both overtly and covertly reported pain intensity. Suggestions for analgesia after a hypnotic state was induced further reduced overtly but not covertly reported pain. This additional reduction may reflect amnesia or dissociation mechanisms that are available only during a hypnotic state. A component of the perception of pain may be immediately forgotten or somehow diverted from conscious awareness. This interpretation of hypnotic analgesia as dissociation in consciousness suggests an explanation for the paradox that physiological indices of stress often continue during hypnotic analgesia, even though the subject consciously feels little or no pain. Interestingly, Hilgard and colleagues found that with highly hypnotizable subjects the rise in heart rate caused by cold pressor pain was somewhat less than during waking nonhypnotic control conditions, but that heart rate still increased slightly (Hilgard et al. 1975; Hilgard and Hilgard 1983). This partial reduction is consistent with the Hilgards' observation of two components of pain reduction. The reduction of pain during nonhypnotic conditions may be accompanied by reductions in autonomic and reflex responses to pain, whereas that associated with dissociation mechanisms would not be likely to be accompanied by decreases in autonomic responses.

DESCENDING SPINAL CORD INHIBITORY MECHANISMS

A second general mechanism by which hypnotic suggestions could reduce pain is by activation of an endogenous pain-inhibitory system that descends to the spinal cord, where it prevents the transmission of pain-related information to the brain. There are multiple lines of indirect evidence for and against such a mechanism. The question of whether hypnotic analgesia involves a brain-to-spinal-cord descending control mechanism is indirectly related to another question: Do endogenous opioids mediate hypnotic analgesia? If so, then it would be likely that a descending control system is involved, since it has been well established that opioid analgesic mechanisms rely heavily on a brain-to-spinal-cord descending control system. Several observations indicate that hypnotic analgesia does *not* depend on endogenous opioid mechanisms; for example, different groups of investigators have found that naloxone does not reverse analgesia produced by hypnotic suggestions.

Other characteristic differences also exist between opioid and hypnotic analgesia. Once analgesia is repeatedly established in a highly hypnotizable subject, it can be induced again very quickly (sometimes within seconds) in the same subject and also can be quickly terminated. Endogenous opioid mechanisms, by contrast, typically have a delayed onset to maximum effect (e.g., several minutes) and are slow to dissipate. However, the lack of demonstration of an endogenous opioid mechanism involved in hypnotic analgesia does not exclude the possibility of a descending control system, only that of an opioid descending control mechanism. Nonopioid brain-to-spinal-cord descending control mechanisms are known to exist (Price 1988). Authors of several physiological studies suggest that hypnotic analgesia is associated with a mechanism whereby descending input from the brain inhibits the processing of pain within the spinal cord. However, nearly all of these studies have focused on autonomic (Barber and Hahn 1962), neurochemical (Goldstein and Hilgard 1975; Mayer et al. 1976; Barber and Mayer 1977), or electrocortical changes associated with hypnotic analgesia (Crawford and Gruzelier 1992). A limitation common to all of these studies is that it is difficult to identify the general neuroanatomical sites at which the relevant modulatory mechanisms take place. Evidence that hypnotic analgesia involves a descending inhibition at spinal levels could be simply provided if some measure of spinal nociceptive function and pain perception could be simultaneously provided during hypnotic analgesia. The feasibility of such an approach is indicated by Willer (1977, 1984, 1985), who showed that different types of somatosensory stimulation and attentional manipulations simultaneously reduce pain and the electrically evoked flexion reflex. He also has demonstrated that graded doses of morphine reduce the electrically evoked flexion reflex and pain intensity by about the same percentage, thereby providing a standard of assessing descending pain-inhibitory mechanisms. All of these observations point to the possibility of simultaneous measurement of pain and the flexion reflex during hypnotic analgesia. Indeed, this idea may have originated in Hagbarth and Finer's

(1973) preliminary demonstration of marked suppression of the flexion reflex in a few subjects during hypnotic analgesia. Though this result is pro-
vocative, it was demonstrated in subjects who were aware of the physiological response that was measured. Thus it is possible that their modulation of
the flexion reflex was at least partly deliberate and not dependent on hypnotic factors.

A more recent and extensive investigation of a possible descending
inhibitory mechanism of hypnotic analgesia examined changes in the R-III,
a nociceptive spinal reflex, during hypnotic reduction of pain sensation and
unpleasantness (Kiernan et al. 1995). The R-III was measured in 15 healthy
volunteers who gave sensory and affective VAS ratings of an electrical
stimulus during conditions of resting wakefulness without suggestions and
during hypnosis with suggestions for hypnotic analgesia (Fig. 3). A critically important feature of this study was that subjects were blind to the
physiological index being measured, and when later informed that it was the
R-III flexion reflex, they failed to intentionally reduce the magnitude of this
reflex. As shown in Fig. 4, hypnotic sensory analgesia was partially, yet
reliably related to reduction in the R-III ($R^2 = 0.51$, $P < 0.003$), suggesting
that hypnotic sensory analgesia is at least in part mediated by descending
antinociceptive mechanisms that exert control at spinal levels in response to
hypnotic suggestion. Hypnotic affective analgesia was not quite significantly
related to reduction in R-III ($P = 0.053$) (Fig. 4). Reduction in R-III was 67%

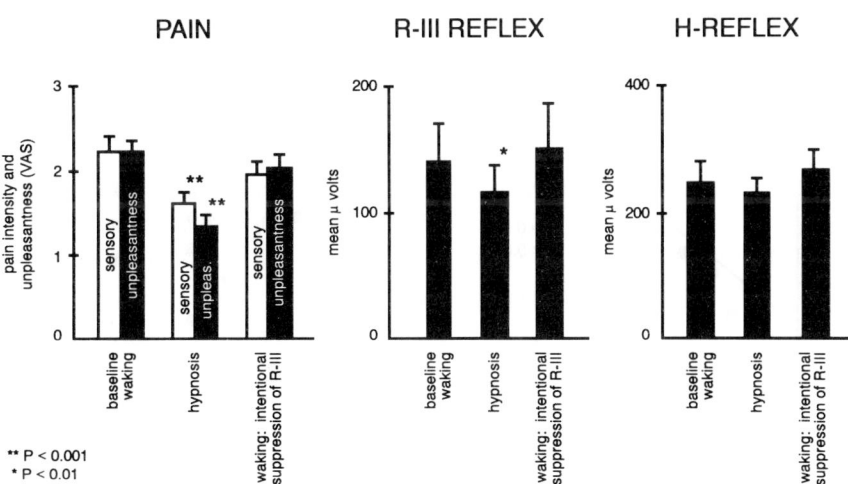

Fig. 3. Pain intensity and unpleasantness VAS ratings and R-III and H-reflex measures
in response to trains of electric shocks delivered under different experimental conditions.
Each bar histogram and vertical line represents the group mean and standard deviation,
respectively, for each response measure. From Kiernan et al. (1995), with permission.

the ascending afferent signal for pain. In the first study, pain unpleasantness ratings and activity in the anterior cingulate cortex (ACC) were modulated in parallel with no change in pain intensity ratings or neural activity levels within somatosensory cortical areas (Rainville et al. 1997). From a psychological perspective, this mechanism is likely to involve changes in the meaning of pain and does not necessarily require much hypnotic ability or involvement, as pointed out above. In the second study, hypnotic suggestions targeted toward pain sensation intensity resulted in parallel changes in ratings of pain sensation intensity and activity within the primary somatosensory cortex (Hofbauer et al. 1998). These results indicate that hypnotic modulation of pain is both psychologically and neurophysiologically multidimensional; that is, different mechanisms target different pain dimensions. Modulation of the affective dimension of pain is at least partly reflected by changes in cortical limbic regional activity (i.e., ACC area 24), independent of modulation of somatosensory processing. Modulation of pain sensation intensity is at least partly reflected by changes in the strength of the incoming signal for pain, as reflected in neural activity levels of the primary somatosensory area (S-1). This result complements that of the flexion reflex study of Kiernan et al. (1995), who provided evidence of inhibition at early levels of nociceptive processing.

THERAPEUTIC IMPLICATIONS OF A REFINED ANALYSIS OF HYPNOTIC ANALGESIA

Taken together, investigations about the psychological and neural mechanisms of hypnotic reduction of pain strongly indicate multiple factors, including those that mediate production of a hypnotic state, those that interrelate hypnotic state with suggestions for analgesia, and those that interrelate hypnotic suggestions with changes in the multiple dimensions of pain experience and behavior. Future studies of hypnotic analgesia should be able to better assess the experiential factors and psychosocial contextual factors that influence the changes in self-reported pain intensity that occur as a result of a hypnotic intervention. New approaches and methods can measure experiential factors such as "perceived automaticity" and "degree of absorption" (Bowers 1978; Pekula and Kumar 1984; Price and Barrell 1990). The factors that optimally influence responses to hypnotic suggestions for analgesia could thus be identified. Moreover, knowledge of these factors could then be more directly and optimally utilized by both patients and health care providers. The concept of "hypnotic therapeutic manipulations" could shift in emphasis from reliance on outside authority to the patients' active participation in developing psychological conditions for therapeutic effects such as analgesia.

More precise analysis of different components of hypnotic analgesic effects also has important therapeutic implications. These different components include selective reduction of pain-related affect (i.e., unpleasantness) by changes in the meaning of sensations and of the contexts in which they occur. It is possible that a hypnotic state is not required for this type of influence, even though it may be an integral part of a hypnotic intervention. Also included are reductions in pain sensation that are related to mechanisms that divert pain from conscious awareness once nociceptive information has reached higher centers. To the extent this component is manifested within an individual, the normal somatomotor reflexes and autonomic, neuroendocrine, and neuroimmunological consequences of pain would *not* be attenuated. Thus, stress-related responses associated with pain would still occur—often to the physiological detriment of the individual. Finally, hypnotic analgesia includes a mechanism wherein pain signals are inhibited at the spinal level of processing; this mechanism would attenuate negative physiological consequences of pain, since inhibition at spinal levels would interrupt the supraspinal activation of brain structures involved in autonomic and neuroendocrine responses to pain. Different individuals may use different proportions of these mechanisms (Kiernan et al. 1995; Price 1988). For example, considerably different proportions of reduction in pain affect and in pain sensation existed among subjects in the Price and Barber (1987) study, as indicated in Table I.

Knowledge about these mechanisms and the factors that influence them has far-reaching implications for treatment of medical conditions, including pain. For example, the discovery that reductions in pain affect are greater and more prevalent than reductions in pain sensation and that the former are unrelated to hypnotic ability indicates that a large percentage of people could benefit by a hypnotic intervention. Furthermore, contrary to standard practice among many clinicians, hypnotic ability may not be a critically limiting factor in deciding who could benefit from a hypnotic intervention. Hypnotic approaches that utilize indirect suggestions for reducing *both* sensory and affective dimensions of pain experience may more effectively optimize the capacities of individuals to alter the overall experience of pain by changing any one of several aspects of their experience. This approach appears to provide more options for changing pain experience than one in which direct suggestions are made for reducing only one dimension of pain experience such as pain intensity. It is important to consider that the efficacy of attempts to induce hypnotic analgesia may differ somewhat depending on susceptibility, the hypnotic approach used, the relationship between the hypnotist and the patient, the pain dimensions assessed, and the level of pain. The observed magnitude of hypnotically induced analgesia, in both clinical and experimental contexts, must be considered in terms of all of these factors (see Barber 1996 for a discussion of clinical applications of hypnosis).

Psychological Mechanisms of Pain and Analgesia, Progress in Pain Research and Management, Vol. 15, by Donald D. Price, IASP Press, Seattle, © 1999.

9

Understanding Pain and Its Mechanisms

Dealing with the presence of pain among our fellow human beings and other animal species is a problem at least as old as human civilization. The problems presented by the existence of pain have been largely conceptualized as mechanistic puzzles to be solved by neuroscientists, psychologists, and clinicians. However, as David Morris (1991) has pointed out, the problem of pain extends well beyond its immediate mechanisms because pain is shaped by individual human minds and by specific human cultures. Yet it is also likely that knowledge of pain mechanisms influences cultural views about pain and can improve the ways in which pain is recognized and managed among human beings. Cultural views of pain and knowledge of pain mechanisms are likely to have reciprocal influences. The purpose of this chapter is to briefly explore some of the implications of new knowledge about pain mechanisms. This exploration is not directly aimed at providing new treatment approaches or new insights about psychological management of pain, but rather at how knowledge of pain mechanisms can shape our relationships to pain and to people who are in pain. I will begin with a summary and interpretation of the general psychological and neural mechanisms of pain, followed by a discussion of how a deeper knowledge of pain mechanisms could be extended by scientific paradigms similar to those proposed for the study of consciousness. Finally, I will explore the relationship between knowledge of pain mechanisms and understanding pain in others.

PAIN MECHANISMS: SOME INTERPRETATIONS

The mechanisms of pain discussed in previous chapters underscore several unique features that distinguish pain as relying on unique sensory mechanisms and at the same time as having multiple and potent affective-motivational characteristics. As discussed in Chapter 2, the psychophysical attributes of pain include (1) reliable stimulus-response relationships that are power functions, (2) refined capacity to discriminate small differences in intensity within the nociceptive range, (3) maintained response to long-duration nociceptive stimulation, (4) slow temporal summation for at least some types of pain, (5) spatial summation across multiple sites and dermatomes, and (6) spatial radiation of painful sensations at nociceptive stimulus intensities above pain threshold. These attributes extend across very different types of pain related to different tissues of cutaneous, muscular, and visceral origin. An attribute of pain that extends across different tissue sources is, of course, referred pain. Many of these attributes, such as temporal summation, spatial summation, and radiation can be exaggerated or abnormally triggered under pathophysiological conditions, as in cases of complex regional pain syndrome, postherpetic neuralgia, or some types of central pain.

The functional significance of these psychophysical attributes can be appreciated further by comparing them with the characteristics of the visual system. The visual system is largely concerned with stimulus features of contrast, edges, and subtleties of spatial dimensions. Intensity is usually important only in the context of these other attributes. The sensory attributes of pain, on the other hand, are largely concerned with intensity, qualities (such as burning, aching, or throbbing), general spatial extent, body location, and duration. The "pain system" is much less concerned with fine details of spatial organization and stimulus contrast, edges, and contours. For example, it probably makes little difference to most cattle whether they are branded with an M or a W. The pain system is designed to support increasing impulse frequencies in nociceptive neurons and recruit large populations of neurons and multiple pathways with increasing levels of pain. This principle has been amply demonstrated for spinal cord dorsal horn neurons, as discussed in Chapter 4 (Figs. 6 and 7) and indirectly for several brain regions, as discussed in Chapter 5 (Figs. 5 and 6).

A fundamental principle of pain encoding is that precise information about nociceptive stimulus intensity is conveyed for as long as or longer than the duration of the stimulus. Nociceptive neurons at all levels of the central nervous system (CNS) have physiological characteristics that support this principle. Yet most spinal cord and brain nociceptive neurons are very likely to participate in *both* nociceptive and non-nociceptive somatosensory functions, including tactile, thermal, and possibly proprioceptive functions. This is biologically adaptive because it conserves the number of neurons and pathways needed to process pain. These mechanisms engage considerable numbers of CNS regions involved in making extensive behavioral responses to potentially injurious stimuli as well as extensive responses *after* injury has occurred. The neural basis for these attributes and mechanisms was discussed in Chapters 4 and 5. This view of pain processing differs radically from that which claims that pain is subserved by neurons and pathways that respond exclusively to nociceptive stimuli and project to discrete centers exclusively involved in pain (Perl 1998).

The psychophysical attributes of pain have several experiential consequences, many of which are manifested during clinical pain. If the physical
stimulus for pain increases or if increasing numbers of nociceptive neurons
are recruited as a function of peripheral or central sensitization, pain fills
the space of our conscious experience, demands our attention, and diverts
attentional and motivational resources away from other agenda. The stimulus-response curves from Coghill et al's (1999) neural imaging study (Chapter 5, Fig. 6) suggest the recruitment of increasing areas of activation with
increasing stimulus intensity. These areas are not exclusively dedicated to
pain processing, so their increased activation by pain probably interferes or
competes with other functions. This possibility is directly supported by
Tommerdahl et al.'s (1998) observation that nociceptive input to primary
somatosensory cortical regions inhibits somatosensory cortical responses to
tactile stimuli (Chapter 5).

Thus, both the neural mechanisms and psychophysical attributes of pain
support a feeling of intrusion. This physically based meaning is tightly linked
with the immediate unpleasantness of pain. At least one component of the
sensory-discriminative dimension is an important constituent of the affective-
motivational dimension of pain. As discussed in Chapters 3 and 5, critical
psychological and neurophysiological evidence supports this assertion. However, just as height is an integral determinant of weight but is not identical
with it, the affective dimension of pain is influenced not only by somatosensory input, but by factors related to perception of other contextual aspects
of the stimulus or conditions in which pain is present. Therefore, an integrated perception of physical and emotional threat represents an additional
component of the immediate unpleasantness of pain. The meanings of intrusion and threat can be conceptualized as cognitive-evaluative factors that
support the immediate affective dimension of pain. However, nociceptive
stimuli also activate neural pathways that have *direct* input to structures
related to production of fear and arousal (e.g., spinoreticular, spinohypothalamic, and spinopontoamygdaloid pathways). Thus, a component of the
affective dimension of pain may be "hard-wired" and may be related to the
immediate fear, sympathetic activation, and arousal that accompanies the
initial phase of pain related to acute injury. The same limbic cortical and
subcortical structures that are activated by these direct inputs are also engaged by cortical structures likely to be involved in cognitive processing of
pain, as shown in the schematic diagram of Chapter 5, Fig. 4. Therefore, the
neural pathways and brain structures related to pain affect may be both in
series and in parallel.

Persistent pain unpleasantness gives rise to reflection, which supports a
secondary stage of pain-related affect. To the extent that these cognitive

factors pertain to the long-term past and long-term future as well as plans for future behavior, frontal cortical areas are likely to be involved in this stage of pain affect. Emotions of depression, anxiety, frustration, despair, and anger arise from reflective meanings that relate to perceptions of life interference and long-term consequences. Pain forces its meaning upon us, and over long periods of time, diminishes other positive aspects of our lives. As Buytendyck (1961) pointed out long ago, pain degrades and impoverishes the human spirit, brings us back to our physicality, and raises the possibility of our annihilation. As pointed out in Chapter 3, psychological factors such as neuroticism and age-related differences in concern for future consequences appear to exert powerful and selective effects on this stage of pain affect. Well-validated instruments for measuring and assessing the various stages and dimensions of pain provide opportunities to determine the effect of various treatments on each of these stages. Thus, if psychological factors exert their greatest influence on the secondary stage of pain affect, psychological therapies could selectively target this stage. This approach also could test possible recursive effects of secondary pain affect on earlier stages of pain processing, analogous to Rainville's hypnosis experiments (Chapters 3, 5, and 8) in which immediate pain unpleasantness was selectively modulated. On the other hand, treatments directed toward reducing pain intensity, the earliest stage of pain processing, would be expected to have successive effects on all subsequent stages of pain processing. However, to the extent that these stages are maintained by factors other than nociception and sensory-discriminative aspects of pain, we have opportunities for refined psychological assessment of persons in pain.

Psychologically mediated modulation of pain also can occur at the earliest levels of pain processing. For example, placebo analgesia can be manifested as a highly specific reduction in pain sensation intensity in a specific area of the body; this analgesia appears to rely on endogenous opioid mechanisms. Such mechanisms are likely to involve circuitry that activates brain-to-spinal-cord pathways and consequent inhibition at the first synapse in the dorsal horn of the spinal gray matter. Hypnotic analgesia also appears to utilize a spinal cord inhibitory mechanism to some extent, although it does not seem to be related to opioid mechanisms. Nevertheless, hypnotic analgesia, like placebo analgesia, can be manifested within a specific region of the body, as in "glove anesthesia." Pain-modulatory mechanisms that use brain-to-spinal-cord circuitry are biologically efficient because all dimensions of pain, physiological responses to pain, and pain-related behavior can be inhibited or facilitated at once.

Psychological modulation of pain sensation intensity may also use neural mechanisms that inhibit pain sensation intensity at higher levels, such as hypnotic dissociative mechanisms that are likely to rely on intracerebral circuitry that diverts the conscious recognition of pain. This type of mechanism may not utilize brain-to-spinal-cord circuitry, as reflected in Danziger et al.'s (1998) hypnotized analgesic subjects whose spinal nociceptive reflexes were not inhibited (see Chapter 8).

Psychological modulation of pain also can be very brief and highly contingent on specific expectations of pain reduction (or enhancement) for a particular area of the body at a specific time. It also can be a widespread bodily phenomenon of long duration, as in some forms of analgesia that result from stress or intense somatosensory stimulation (e.g., acupuncture analgesia). These types of analgesia may be related to release of opioid hormones or other agents. Similar to systemic opioids, they affect the entire body and long outlast their initial onset. Just as there are heterogeneous neural systems that support brief and long term pain, so also there appear to exist "phasic" and "tonic" manifestations of pain modulation. The extent to which these manifestations correspond to different mechanisms and different anatomical systems is not known.

The selective psychological modulation of the immediate and secondary dimensions of pain affect involves modifying the meanings that are common to pain experience, which are highly subjective. If the affective-motivational dimension of pain is based on meanings and if psychological modulation of pain largely consists of modulation of these meanings, then a deeper understanding of pain and pain modulation must take the study of meanings very seriously. The meanings of intrusion and threat that support the immediate affective stage can be reduced or eliminated by substituting alternative positive meanings for potentially unpleasant bodily sensations or by more directly altering negative meanings. Similarly, psychological therapies aimed to reduce the sense of interruption, the difficulty of enduring pain over time, and concern for the future could attenuate the negative emotions of depression, anxiety, frustration, and despair that are associated with persistent pain conditions.

The modulation of pain sensation and pain affect through alteration in meanings and the development of highly specific response expectancies occur even during analgesic responses to conventional treatments. Placebo responses are integral components of opioid analgesia, for example. Meanings and expectations are even likely to modulate opioid analgesic responses of rats, as illustrated by Wiertelak et al.'s (1992) observation that morphine analgesia is potentiated in rats exposed to danger cues and attenuated in rats exposed to safety cues.

AN EXPERIENTIAL APPROACH TO A DEEPER
UNDERSTANDING OF PAIN

That the experience of pain is at least partly the result of physically based as well as more reflective meanings is related to the subjective nature of pain and underlies the claim that pain is a uniquely private and personal experience. A deeper understanding of pain and pain modulation requires that both scientists and health care providers directly address the meanings of pain and how they can be modified. An appropriate starting point may be to reconsider and extend some of the philosophical perspectives that were discussed in Chapter 1. In that chapter, I briefly advanced the thesis that the ontology of pain is subjective and that we know the phenomenon of pain first and foremost through our own direct experience. But if that is true, then our scientific understanding of this phenomenon could be advanced by using a first-person epistemology in the study of pain and interfacing this approach with that of more conventional psychological research. This recommendation requires considerable explanation, and I want to emphasize that it is not a simple matter of armchair reflections on direct experiences of pain. The following discussion considers the feasibility of introducing experiential methods into the study of pain, because such an approach is uniquely suited to the study of meanings that relate to pain. In particular, the phenomenon of pain can be used as a model to study interrelationships between sensation, perception, meaning, emotion, and behavior. Indeed, pain can be used as a model for the study of consciousness itself, as many of the issues concerned with understanding subjective aspects of pain are the same as those involved in understanding consciousness.

THE STUDY OF PAIN AND CONSCIOUSNESS

Pain, like consciousness itself, has long been considered to be at least partially inaccessible to study because of its personal and private nature; there is a subjective quality in an experience of pain, but there are often no external referents for that experience. For example, we can convey our phenomenal sense of the color blue and even define "blue" by pointing to several blue objects. The agreement among independent observers about various blue objects gives us confidence that our phenomenal sense of blue is similar, if not identical, among human beings. Such an agreement is more difficult for pain. Many pains, particularly those arising from pathological events within our bodies, do not have external referents. Yet such pains have phenomenal qualities (qualia), and there is a subjective feel to those pains. If pain is conceptualized as an experience, as indicated by both the IASP definition of pain and the alternative definition provided in Chapter 1, then this lack of accessibility to the referents for pain may limit our understanding of this phenomenon, including our scientific understanding.

However, this problem is not insurmountable, particularly if a method is available for rigorous characterization of different types of human experience. In this chapter I present the view that understanding the nature of pain at least partly depends on recognizing its inherent first-person ontology and on using both a first- and third-person experiential approach to study it. Since pain experience is a state of consciousness, this view is derived from considerations of the "hard" (difficult) problem of consciousness discussed by modern philosophers and from paradigms for the study of human experience.

PHILOSOPHICAL VIEWPOINTS ABOUT CONSCIOUSNESS AND THEIR POTENTIAL RELATIONSHIP TO PAIN

Many of the philosophical issues about understanding the nature of consciousness also apply to the understanding of pain. In fact, many philosophers use the phenomenon of pain to illustrate their points about consciousness. Among contemporary philosophers, some give explicit recognition to the first-person ontological status of consciousness and some of them go further to suggest, albeit sometimes indirectly, that a complete study of consciousness would include a first-person epistemology as well. If so, then their arguments would also be applicable to pain, since pain is a personal and private experience often used to illustrate the phenomenon of consciousness.

John Searle (1995) argues forcefully for a first-person ontological status of consciousness. He proposes that a chief distinction between a system acting *as if* it had experiences, such as a computer, and a system really having experiences (i.e., a mind) is that the latter has an inherent subjective quality. As he points out, beliefs and desires are always *somebody's* beliefs and desires and they are always potentially conscious. He suggests that since the 17th century, the metaphysical presupposition that *reality is objective* has led to framing questions about mental states in terms of the external conditions under which we would *attribute* mental states to some *other* system, as contrasted to framing questions about one's own experiences. Thus, questions such as "What is it like to have a belief?" and "What is it like to have a desire?" are often not regarded as scientifically meaningful. Yet we must explain the phenomenal subjective qualities of experience or consciousness, and this explanation constitutes part of the "hard" problem of consciousness.

David Chalmers (1996) likewise accepts the first-person ontological status of consciousness, but goes further to suggest that in the pursuit of a theory of consciousness we might begin with our own experiences to help formulate theories. He also suggests that we could plausibly rely on indirect information, such as subjects' descriptions of their experiences. It should be pointed out here that such a description would only be "indirect" from the investigator's point of view—not from that of the subject. For Chalmers, the testability of alternative theories of consciousness would include both accurate accounts of first-person experiences as well as the evidence from subjects' reports. An adequate theory would be based on both first- and third-person observations.

All of this implies that pain, like consciousness in general, might be studied from both first- and third-person points of view and that information obtained from these perspectives may be complementary forms of testing hypotheses about the nature of pain. Evidence supports the feasibility of integrating a first-person experiential approach and method into the study of pain and the possibility of combining these paradigms with psychophysical and neural imaging studies.

CLASSIC STUDIES OF PAIN FROM A FIRST-PERSON PERSPECTIVE

One simple line of evidence that first-person studies of pain are feasible is that some classic studies of pain have relied on first-person observation, and the investigators were the subjects of their own experiments. Two studies, one by Henry Head (1920) and the other by Landau and Bishop (1953), have already been discussed in Chapter 4. Landau and Bishop used themselves as investigator-participants to determine the qualities of pain related to stimuli that selectively activated Aδ or C-nociceptive afferents. They found that pains evoked by stimuli that activated only Aδ nociceptive afferents were sharp, well localized, and did not outlast the stimulus, whereas pains evoked by stimuli that activated C-nociceptive afferents had a dull, diffuse quality that was distinctly unpleasant and long outlasted the stimulus. Both Landau and Bishop independently confirmed these results through their own direct observations. Similarly, a study by Lewis and Pochin (1938) on first and second pain demonstrated that the different latencies of the two pains were related to differences in *peripheral* but not *central* conduction velocities of Aδ versus C axons. Both investigators mapped areas of their own bodies wherein the double pain response could be elicited. Each did so without knowing the results of the other investigator. The body maps of both Lewis and Pochin were nearly identical and demonstrated that first and second pain could only be elicited by stimulation of sites in the distal portions of the arm or leg. Double pain could not be evoked by stimulation of sites on the trunk for two reasons. First, the peripheral conduction distance is not sufficient to allow a separation in latencies between the two types of pain. Second, the central conduction of impulses occurs in myelinated axons for *both* first and second pain. Thus, first and second pain can be felt at the elbow but not in the trunk, even though both sites are about the same distance from the brain.

There are three notable points to be made about these studies. First, they arrived at very straightforward observations about the nature of specific types of pain and even made cogent inferences concerning pain mechanisms. Second, the observations have since been incorporated into our body of knowledge of pain and have been replicated in several studies using conventional experimental designs and methods. Finally and most critically, the results were obtained through investigators observing their own experiences of pain and other sensations.

THE POSSIBILITY OF FIRST-PERSON PARADIGMS FOR THE STUDY OF PAIN EXPERIENCE

If straightforward observations can be made of the sensory qualities of pain, then it may be possible for investigators to similarly study other dimensions of pain, including how they perceive the pain in relation to their total experience of themselves, including their emotional feelings. Phenomenological accounts of pain and suffering have made by Buytendyck (1961) and Bakan (1967). Buytendyck describes the ways in which pain calls into question our sense of ourselves and the ways pain generates meanings related to our suffering. Bakan describes the salient meanings of persistent pain and the relationship of pain to our sense of annihilation.

Examples were given in Chapters 1 and 3 of first-person reflections on pain, including accounts made by Buytendyck (1961) and Bakan (1967). In particular, there is general agreement as to the physically based meanings and other experiential dimensions that comprise the immediate unpleasantness of pain. These factors relate in a comprehensible manner to the psychophysical attributes of pain, as discussed above. For example, Bakan used the term "phenomenal distality" to describe the psychological distance between the experienced self and the object of consciousness. Considerations of direct experience provide important hypotheses and insights into the relationships between experienced self, the body, and pain. Overall, these accounts from Buytendyck and Bakan demonstrate how phenomenology, and more importantly, a first-person perspective, can uncover meanings that are at the heart of the affective dimension of human pain and suffering.

Phenomenologists offer reflections on direct experiences that are nearly totally missing in mainstream psychology (Husserl 1952; Buytendyck 1961;

Merleau-Ponty 1962; Sardello 1964; Bakan 1967; Krishnamurti 1967; Lyons 1973). For example, there is relatively little emphasis within mainstream psychology on understanding the experiential structure of emotions, such as frustration, that are intrinsic to chronic pain and suffering. Consequently, there is often no search for underlying causes within the structure of this kind of experience. In fact, emotions such as frustration are considered irreducible and are usually discussed only in relation to their possible external influences. Yet there is no search for the experiential dimensions that underlie these emotions. Phenomenology opens up this search with in-depth reflections of how emotional feelings may be experienced, yet it has stopped short of identifying actual causes imbedded in these experiences, partly because phenomenological analysis has not been interfaced with the methods and practices of natural science (Giorgi 1970). Scientifically and practically, human pain and suffering demands an understanding of these causes.

An experiential paradigm that may fulfill this need has been developed (Barrell and Barrell 1975; Price and Barrell 1980; Price and Barrell 1984; Barrell et al. 1985; Price et al. 1985a). This approach allows for the discovery of common factors or causes within specific types of experiences such as anger, anxiety, and pain as well as for the characterization of the interrelationships among these common factors. The paradigm consists of several stages that include (1) questioning and observing; (2) describing experiences from a first-person perspective; (3) understanding experiences through discovering common factors and their interrelationships (i.e., anxiety, pain); and (4) applying quantitative methods to test generality and functional relationships between common factors. Of these four stages of research, the first three are unique in that the investigators are the subjects of their own research questions (i.e., co-investigators). The last stage utilizes accepted psychometric methods, derived mainly from psychophysics, to test hypotheses in other human subjects. The last stage is no different in principle from conventional psychological research. Hypotheses can be tested with conventional psychometric methods and experiments would be similar in principle to those already used in psychophysical studies. The participants of the experiments would *not* be the investigators and would not have knowledge of the hypotheses of the study. Thus, the last stage of an experiential paradigm would involve a third-person epistemology, but one that is complementary to the first-person exploration stages 1–3 described above. However, it is the combination of these stages that produces direct knowledge about experiential phenomena. This paradigm could be directly applied to the study of consciousness in general and to pain and states of consciousness in particular.

VanKaam (1959), using a similar approach, devised a method of controlled analysis of human experience that consists of describing experiences and reducing the descriptions to their essential elements. The final identification of these common elements was based on the requirements that each element must be: (a) expressed explicitly in some descriptions, (b) expressed explicitly or implicitly in the majority of descriptions, and (c) compatible with descriptions in which the element in question is not expressed, or this element must be shown not to be an expression of the experience under study.

An aim of the experiential methods of both Barrell and Price and VanKaam was to generate qualitative descriptions of given kinds of experience, descriptions that express phenomena as they reveal themselves to the experiencing person. They are to be agreed upon and well understood by all those capable of having the experiences in question. Each final phenomenological-experiential account of a kind of experience (e.g., pain-related frustration) is to contain precise, explicit statements about what is essential for a kind of experience, omitting particulars. These methods also may include a strategy of determining the necessary and sufficient factors for the type of experience in question. Finally, they allow investigators to discover the functional relationships of common factors of given kinds of experience. These factors can be scaled using psychophysical and other psychometric methods, and the scaling of these factors can provide tests of functional hypotheses about the interaction between the various factors.

For example, if we reflect on the experience of simple forms of pain, three interrelated dimensions are apparent—sensations whose qualities are uniquely like those which occur during nociceptive stimulation, meanings of intrusion or threat to the body or self, and unpleasant emotional feelings associated with these meanings. These three dimensions are each necessary and taken together are sufficient for pain. Indeed, pain can be defined in terms of these dimensions and their interrelationships (Chapter 1). Each of these dimensions can be scaled and measured in human observers, including *both* subjects of conventionally designed experiments and the investigators themselves. For example, Landau and Bishop carefully noticed the sensory qualities and unpleasant feelings that were evoked by stimuli that selectively activated $A\delta$ or C nociceptive afferents. They were able to discern *first-hand* what it is like to experience cutaneous pain from C-fiber stimulation. The knowledge obtained from their studies is part of our present knowledge of the physiology of primary nociceptive neurons.

INTEGRATING EXPERIENTIAL AND NATURAL SCIENCE METHODS INTO THE STUDY OF PAIN

Based on the foregoing account of this experiential paradigm, it is evident that investigators who seek to understand the experiential structures of pain and suffering would have to rely on their own experiences of pain or would train groups of pain patients to use the experiential method. Regardless of which alternative is used, a number of obvious questions about the experience of chronic pain and pain-related suffering come to mind. What is it like to experience pain-related feelings of depression, frustration, anxiety, anger, and fear? What is it like to experience one's body, thoughts, and emotional feelings while enduring chronic pain? What are the common meanings that underlie negative emotional feelings during chronic pain? Again, as pointed out above, this approach does not exclude quantitative methods or conventional psychometric methodology, but rather results in more refined analyses of data based on verbal reports and ratings of pain patients. Such an approach has led to the development of a pain questionnaire that assesses several components of the experience of chronic pain (Price 1988; Harkins et al. 1989; Price and Harkins 1992a,b; Wade et al. 1996).

An experiential approach to understanding pain may begin with simple forms of laboratory or acute clinical pain. There is a need for an experiential-phenomenological approach to understand the nature of even simple forms of pain, and this is all the more crucial because pain can provide a model for consciousness. Varela (1996) has provided a "map" of current philosophical positions with respect to the ontology and epistemology of consciousness. He describes his position as an interface between phenomenology and the natural sciences and calls for paradigms and methods that support this interface. The paradigm we briefly describe here and have presented elsewhere (Barrell and Barrell 1975; Price and Barrell 1980; Barrell et al. 1985; Price et al. 1985a) is entirely consistent with Varela's philosophical position. In order to illustrate how an experiential paradigm could be interfaced with conventional neuroscientific methods to study pain, let us imagine an experiment that could interface this paradigm with neural imaging.

The experiment would be an extension of one conducted by Rainville et al. (1997) described in Chapters 5 and 8. Recall that hypnotic suggestions selectively modulated pain unpleasantness and neural activity (measured by regional cerebral blood flow) in area 24 of the anterior cingulate cortex, but not pain sensation intensity and neural activity in the S-1 somatosensory cortex. This experiment represents a strategy designed to identify neural structures differentially involved in two separate dimensions of the experience of pain. It is necessarily overly simplistic because sensory and affective dimensions of pain cover broad and complex experiential territories.

However, this kind of study could be interfaced with the experiential paradigm described above to provide a much more elaborate characterization of neural structures whose activities are associated with the different and subtle subdimensions of pain unpleasantness. Investigator-participants could identify these subdimensions using the first-person experiential approach described above. The subdimensions might include factors such as phenomenal distality, perceived intrusiveness, perceived threat, or simply the extent of desire to remove the source of pain. Once the relevant subdimensions were identified and characterized by investigator-participants, scales could be developed for each dimension, and the usual types of participants of neural imaging experiments could then rate these subdimensions under different experimental conditions. Such conditions would include experimental manipulations designed to selectively modulate a given subdimension or generate variation in its magnitude. Regions of brain activation and patterns of cerebral cortical activity that covary with subdimensions of pain unpleasantness could then be identified and characterized. Questions about *how* patterns of brain activity give rise to subjective experiences such as pain could begin to be answered. This approach represents a synthesis of first- and third-person epistemologies, one grounded in phenomenology and the other in the natural scientific method. Therefore, pain, like consciousness in general, might be studied from both first- and third-person points of view, and information obtained from these viewpoints may provide complementary ways to test hypotheses. This approach may provide important insights about psychological and neural mechanisms of pain.

RECOGNIZING THE HIGHER-ORDER MEANINGS OF PAIN

An experiential method also may be used to investigate the secondary stage of pain affect or pain-related suffering. Morris (1991) discussed the need to recognize pain-related meanings among pain patients and has elaborated on the ways that culture, attitudes, and setting affect these meanings. Patients bring entire constellations of meaning with them when seeking treatments for pain. The author gives a compelling example in a conversation that he had with a chronic pain patient:

> She told me that the high point of her life was playing the organ for her church choir. She lived for the twice-a-week practices and Sunday performances. Now, with pain immobilizing her elbow, she could no longer manage the keyboard. Her days held nothing that she looked forward to. The constant aching had robbed her of any hope. Life seemed empty of everything except pain. When I asked her if she had explained this to the staff of the clinic, she replied that they had not asked. Her medical

history, as one might expect, read exactly like the history of an elbow (Morris 1991, p. 275).

Two points can be made about this narrative. The first is that it illustrates, albeit implicitly, the different stages and dimensions of pain and their interactions. The statement that "the constant aching had robbed her of any hope" illustrates how the qualities and intensity of pain sensation and immediate pain unpleasantness refer directly to a felt sense of interruption and implications for future interruption. Pain had robbed her of life's meaning, and that impoverishment of meaning was in itself a critical meaning of pain. The second is that the patient's medical history contains virtually nothing about the lived meanings that undoubtedly contributed a lot to her suffering. Although the particulars are likely to differ radically across chronic pain patients, it is likely that such individuals experience at least a partial commonality of meanings. If that is true, then it should be possible to assess their presence and perhaps even measure their magnitudes. A scientific analysis of meanings in studies of pain and suffering would be helpful in this regard.

The general meanings of pain-related suffering are not a complete mystery but clearly relate to the dimensions of perceived interruption of one's life, perceived difficulty of enduring pain over time, and concern with future consequences (Chapter 3). These meanings relate in turn to the types of emotional feelings that are an integral part of pain and suffering. Meanings, like dimensions of unpleasantness and sensation intensity, contain the potential for being scaled and measured, as has been amply demonstrated in the history of psychophysics (Shinn 1969; Stevens 1973). It may even be possible to relate the magnitudes of such meanings to neural activity within human brain areas.

KNOWLEDGE OF PAIN MECHANISMS, EMPATHY, AND INFERENCE IN THE COMMUNICATION OF PAIN

The experiential approach wherein first- and third-person observations are interrelated may represent a useful approach for investigating the psychological and neural mechanisms of pain. First- and third-person observations and hypothesis testing represent complementary ways of discovering new knowledge about pain and pain mechanisms. The philosophical foundation of this approach and its rationale also have direct bearing on how we determine the existence of pain and the approximate level of pain in other human beings and in animals. For example, participants of psychophysical pain experiments provide several types of verbal and nonverbal responses that indicate the general level of pain that results from a given stimulus intensity. These behaviors include ratings of pain along multiple dimensions as well as nonverbal behaviors of grimacing and making facial expressions and body movements. Thus, there are multiple ways in which the experimenter can know the approximate levels of pain experienced by the participant. This knowing is partly based on recognition of the general correspondence between pain behavior and pain experience, which includes self-knowledge. For example, I recall that I start to grimace at skin temperatures above 51°C and I know that I rate such stimuli above 6 on a VAS. It is not at all difficult to recognize generally similar levels of pain among participants of studies. Although interpersonal variability may influence pain sensitivity, most pain experimenters know from direct experience that there is a temperature stimulus level that is minimally painful and another stimulus level that is at the point of becoming distinctly aversive—the "squirm" threshold. Regardless of the particular behavioral endpoints that we chose to acknowledge, such as pain threshold, pain tolerance, pain scale ratings, or squirm threshold, all of them have at least general correspondence in our own direct experience. The overall point here is that knowing another's pain in such circumstances can be based on a synthesis of first- and third-person observations.

Contrary to prevailing views that pain and suffering are personal and private and therefore unknowable by persons who do not have pain, an enormous body of literature and scientific evidence points to the feasibility of communicating, measuring, and assessing human pain and suffering (Turk and Melzack 1992). The language of pain experience has been developed to some extent and may continue to be developed. Psychophysical and other psychometric methods to measure pain continue to be developed. Finally, critical new interest is emerging in the study of human experience in general, inspired by recent scientific and philosophical approaches to the study of consciousness. In particular, phenomenological approaches may be interfaced with the methods of natural sciences (Gendlin 1962; Giorgi 1970; Price and Barrell 1980; Varela 1996).

HOW DO WE KNOW ABOUT PAIN AND SUFFERING IN HUMANS AND IN ANIMALS THAT HAVE NO LANGUAGE?

If the fundamental nature of pain is that it is an experience, then *directly* knowing pain can only occur as a result of having it. This leaves us in a very interesting philosophical position with regard to the study of pain and to knowing pain in others. If the ontology of pain is from a first-person, embodied perspective, then both the scientific study of pain and the assessment of pain in patients ultimately need to acknowledge methods or processes by which we know another's pain. Psychologists and neurophysiologists most often carry out research on pain by studying pain-related behaviors. However, this approach implicitly requires the assumption that such behaviors reflect an underlying experience that we understand as pain from our own perspectives. And this is true even when the behavior is the verbal report of pain by someone else. However, even when the behavior is nonverbal, such as grimacing, moans, and protecting an injured body region, we can have a direct sense that these behaviors reflect an experience that contains the common elements of pain. Most of us have learned that when we are exhibiting these same behaviors ourselves, we are perceiving sensations like those that occur when tissue is injured, feeling intrusion and threat associated with these sensations, and experiencing unpleasantness or other negative emotions in relationship to these physically based meanings. That is, we are having an experience of pain. In essence, we translate perceived behaviors of others into a sense of their pain by remembering our experiences of pain when we exhibited the same behaviors.

If this account is accurate, the capacity to know another's pain is not exclusively a matter of inference. An inference of pain would involve obtaining all the relevant objective facts about the person's behavior and circumstances and deducing whether the person was in pain as well as the extent of the pain. The translation of observing another's behavior into a sense of his or her experienced pain may be based on our own memory of the relationship between our direct experience of pain and our experience of our pain behavior. When we see pain behavior, we associate it with the subjective experience of pain. This recognition may be *empathic* in nature. Just as we learn pain throughout life, so also we learn a capacity for recognizing the existence of pain in someone else. For example, part of this capacity is based on the fact that distinctive patterns of facial activity are associated with pain and that these patterns are easily distinguishable from emotions such as fear, anger, and excitement (Craig et al. 1992). Studies have shown that the patterns and magnitudes of these facial expressions are moderately associated with self-reports of pain and pain intensity and that there is often excellent correspondence between separate raters' judgments of the magnitude of another person's expressed pain (Craig et al. 1992). The capacity to recognize pain in each other and to have at least a general recognition of its severity is not restricted to humans; other mammalian species can be seen tending to injured offspring or mates. As Anand et al. (1999) have pointed out, the capacity to recognize the pain of others and respond with compassionate tending behaviors is present in many mammalian species. Such "tending" reactions can be elicited from pet dogs or small infants by exhibiting fake or real pain behaviors. Of course, the relationships between experienced pain and pain-related behaviors are highly imperfect, as reflected in the modest associations between self-reported pain intensity and pain intensity as judged by an outside observer (Van der Does 1989). Constraints of intrapersonal bias and lack of knowledge of behavioral signs of pain may contribute to this modest association. It may be possible to improve these associations by training and educating observers.

Our capacity to know the presence of pain and pain intensity in others represents a combination of empathic understanding and inference, and the latter may be partly based on knowledge of pain mechanisms. For example, I witnessed what I perceived to be pain in my newborn daughter at the time she received a heel lance. When the nurse rubbed her foot vigorously, she did not cry. However, at the exact moment the lance penetrated the skin in her foot, she cried loudly and moved both her arms and legs in an agitated manner. More than that, her crying seemed more emphatic and distressed than when she had cried before. I later realized, after reading some of the papers by Craig et al. (1992), that her face looked distressed because it bore the classic signs of facial pain expression. However, more than empathic recognition was involved in this experience. I knew that rubbing her skin activated tactile and pressure mechanoreceptors and only minimally activated nociceptors. I also knew that penetration of the skin with a heel lance strongly activated several distinct types of nociceptors, including high-threshold mechanical and C-polymodal nociceptors. The physical circumstances of this situation, knowledge of peripheral neural mechanisms of pain, and the exhibited behaviors all indicated to me that the heel lance was painful to her. It is important to recognize from this relatively simple example that knowledge of pain mechanisms, pain behaviors, and empathic sensitivity all help us to know pain in others. This example also supports Cunningham's (1999a,b) contention that verbal communication is not the exclusive means by which another organism's pain can be recognized and assessed.

Rollin (1999) also reminds us that evidence is abundant in our experience that animals perceive pain and that this evidence is not based on inference but can be seen immediately. Yet this powerful, common-sense recognition of pain in animals is strongly buttressed by considerable scientific evidence that physiological mechanisms and neuroanatomical pathways for pain are similar across a wide variety of mammalian species, including rats, monkeys, and humans (see references in Rollin 1999 and Varner 1999). To take just one of many examples, monkeys begin to escape nociceptive heat stimuli at temperature levels (45°–46°C) that are at or just above threshold pain levels in humans (Dubner et al. 1977). Their escape latencies decrease as a monotonic function of heat-induced skin temperatures in the nociceptive range of 45°–51°C (Dubner et al. 1977; Bushnell et al. 1983). Indeed, research on pain mechanisms has helped to determine the presence of pain in organisms that lack verbal capacity. For example, it is now incontrovertible that newborn mammals, including humans, contain the physiological mechanisms that are necessary for pain and that they are more, and not less, sensitive to painful stimuli than adults (Fitzgerald and Jennings 1999). There are countless examples for which the presence or absence of pain in another person or animal could be assisted by knowledge of pain mechanisms, careful attention to the history and circumstances of the other, and empathic sensitivity to the relevant behaviors that are being manifested.

FUTURE CHALLENGES TO UNDERSTANDING PAIN AND ITS MECHANISMS

Pain neuroscience research has shifted its emphasis within the last 10 years from general neuroanatomical and physiological characteristics of pain-related neurons and pathways to detailed neurotransmitter and intracellular mechanisms of normal and abnormal pain processing. During the same time frame, psychological research on pain has shifted its emphasis from behavioral analyses to explorations of the various subjective dimensions of pain experience. This change has been facilitated by increased incorporation of psychophysical methods into pain research and by recent technological advances such as neural imaging. The increasing emphasis of neuroscience research on molecular aspects of pain processing and the tendency of psychological research to focus on subjective aspects of pain need not be at cross-purposes if we continue to recognize the subjective ontological status of pain. Thus, an ultimate goal of pain research is to explain pain mechanisms in relation to how we understand the phenomenon of pain from our own experiential perspective.

The change in emphasis of neuroscience and psychological studies of pain may prove to be beneficial. Molecular and neuropharmacological studies of pain use behavioral indices of pain as their dependent measures, and yet the veracity of these indices depends on their putative relationship to one or more aspects of pain *experience*. For example, measures of paw withdrawal, guarding behavior, and paw-licking in rats are sometimes combined with immunocytochemical analyses of intracellular chemical messengers that are hypothesized to have a role in hyperalgesia and allodynia (Price et al. 1994b). Taken together, these behavioral measures are considered to reflect nociceptive processing and early stages of pain experience itself. More sophisticated paradigms of detection and escape may even be considered to reflect different general dimensions of pain experience in various animal species (Chapter 5). However, the more that is learned about the experiential structure of different kinds of pain, the greater is the possibility for increased interpretability of behavioral indices of pain and for adding new behavioral indices. Furthermore, it is possible that the more we learn about the subjective aspects of pain, the more precise will be our understanding of the relationships between pain behavior and pain experience. As already discussed, knowledge of these relationships has bearing not only on scientific progress in pain research, but also on the potential for improved assessment of pain in our fellow human beings.

References

Adair EE, Stevens JC, Marks LE. Thermally induced pain: the dol scale and the psychophysical power law. *Amer J Psychol* 1968; 81:147–164.

Adams JE. Naloxone reversal of analgesia produced by brain stimulation in the human. *Pain* 1976; 2:161–166.

Ajzen I, Fishbein M. *Belief, Attitude, Intention, and Behavior: an Introduction to Theory and Research.* Reading, MA: Addison-Wesley, 1975, pp 1–221.

Ajzen I, Fishbein M. *Understanding Attitudes and Predicting Social Behavior.* Englewood Cliffs, NJ: Prentice-Hall, 1980.

Akil H, Mayer DJ, Liebeskind J. Comparaison chez le rat entre l'analgesie induite par stimulation de la substance grise periaqueducale et l'analgesie morphinique. *C R Acad Sci* 1972; 274:3603–3605.

Akil H, Mayer DJ, Liebeskind JC. Antagonism of stimulation-produced analgesia by the narcotic antagonist, naloxone. *Science* 1976; 191:961–962.

Albus K, Schott M, Herz A. Interaction between morphine and morphine antagonists after systemic and intraventricular application. *Eur J Pharmacol* 1970; 12:53–64.

Amanzio M, Benedetti F. Neuropharmacological dissection of placebo analgesia: expectation-activated opioid systems versus conditioning-activated specific subsystems. *J Neurosci* 1999; 19:484–494.

Anand KJS, Rovnaghi C, Walden M, Churchill J. Consciousness, behavior, and clinical impact of the definition of pain. *Pain Forum* 1999; 8(2):64–73.

Anderson RA. Inferior parietal lobule function in spatial perception and visuomotor integration. In: Mountcastle VB, Plum F, Geiger SR (Eds). *Higher Functions of the Brain,* Part 2. Handbook of Physiology, Sect. 1, The Nervous System, Vol. V. Bethesda, MD: American Physiology Society, 1987, pp 483–518.

Arendt-Nielsen L. Induction and assessment of experimental pain from human skin, muscle, and viscera. In: Jensen TS, Turner JA, Wiesenfeld-Hallin Z (Eds). *Proceedings of the 8th World Congress on Pain.* Seattle: IASP Press, 1997, pp 393–425.

Arendt-Nielsen L, Graven-Nielsen T, Svennson P, Jensen TS. Temporal summation in muscles and referred pain areas: an experimental human study. *Muscle Nerve* 1997; 10:1311–1313.

Arnold MB. *Feelings and Emotions.* New York: Academic Press, 1970.

Atchison NE, Osgood PF, Carr DB, Szfebein SK. Pain during burn dressing change in children: relationship to burn area, depth, and analgesic regimens. *Pain* 1991; 47:41–45.

Atweh SF, Kuhar MJ. Autoradiographic localization of opiate receptors in the rat brain. II. The brain stem. *Brain Res* 1977; 129:1–12.

Azami J, Llewelyn MB, Roberts MHT. The contribution of nucleus reticularis paragigantocellularis and nucleus raphe magnus to the analgesia produced by systemically administered morphine, investigated with the microinjection technique. *Pain* 1982; 12:229–246.

Bakan D. *On Method.* San Francisco: Jossey-Bass, 1967.

Bakan D. *Disease, Pain, and Sacrifice.* Chicago: University of Chicago Press, 1968.

Baker SL, Kirsch I. Cognitive mediators of pain perception and tolerance. *J Pers Soc Psychol* 1991; 61:504–510.

Barber J (Ed). *Hypnosis and Suggestion in the Treatment of Pain.* New York: W.W. Norton and Company, 1996, pp 117–136.

Barber J, Adrian C. *Psychological Approaches to the Management of Pain.* New York: Brunner/Mazel, 1982.

Barber J, Mayer DJ. Evaluation of the efficacy and neural mechanism of a hypnotic anagesia procedure in experimental and clinical dental pain. *Pain* 1977; 4:41–48.

Barber TX, Hahn KW. Physiological and subjective responses to pain producing stimulation under hypnotically-suggested and waking-imagined "analgesia." *J Soc Psychol* 1962; 65:411–418.

Barber TX, Wilson SC. Hypnosis, suggestions, and altered states of consciousness: experimental evaluation of the new cognitive-behavioral theory and the traditional trance-state theory of "hypnosis." In: Edmonston WE Jr (Ed). *Conceptual and Investigative Approaches to Hypnotic Phenomena,* Annals of the New York Academy of Sciences, Vol. 296. New York: New York Academy of Sciences, 1977, pp 34–47.

Bard P. A diencephalic mechanism for the expression of rage with special reference to the sympathetic nervous system. *Am J Physiol* 1928; 84:490–515.

Baron RM, Kenny DA. The moderator-mediator variable distinction in social psychological research: conceptual, strategic, and statistical considerations. *J Pers Soc Psychol* 1986; 51:1173–1182.

Barrell JJ, Barrell JE. A self-directed approach for a science of human experience. *J Phenomen Psychol;* Fall 1975, 63–73.

Barrell JJ, Jourard S. Being honest with persons we like. *J Individ Psychol* 1976; 32(2):185–193.

Barrell JJ, Neimeyer R. A mathematical formula for the psychological control of suffering. *J Pastoral Counseling* 1975; 10:60–67.

Barrell JJ, Price DD. The perception of first and second pain as a function of psychological set. *Percept Psychophys* 1975; 17:163–166.

Barrell JJ, Madieros D, Barrell JE, et al. Anxiety: an obstacle to performance. *J Humanistic Psychol* 1985; 25:106–122.

Beecher HK. The powerful placebo. *JAMA* 1955; 159:1602–1606.

Beecher HK. Limiting factors in experimental pain. *J Chron Dis* 1956; 4:11–23

Beecher HK. *Measurement of Subjective Responses: Quantitative Effects of Drugs.* New York: Oxford University Press, 1959.

Beitel RE, Dubner R. Response of unmyelinated (C) polymodal nociceptors to thermal stimuli applied to monkey's face. *J Neurophysiol* 1976a; 39:165–175.

Beitel RE, Dubner R. Sensitization and depression of C-polymodal nociceptors by noxious heat applied to the monkey's face. In: Bonica JJ, Albe-Fessard D (Eds). *Advances in Pain Research and Therapy.* New York: Raven Press, 1976b, pp 149–155.

BenDebba M, Torgerson WS, Long DM. Personality traits, pain duration and severity, functional impairment, and psychological distress in patients with persistent low back pain. *Pain* 1997; 72:115–125.

Benedetti F. The opposite effects of the opiate antagonist naloxone and the cholecystokinin antagonist proglumide on placebo analgesia. *Pain* 1996; 64:535–543.

Benedetti F, Arduino C, Amanzio M. Somatotopic activation of opioid systems by target-directed expectations of analgesia. *J Neurosci* 1999; 19(9):3639–3648.

Bennett GJ, Xie YK. A peripheral mononeuropathy in rat that produces disorders of pain sensation like those seen in man. *Pain* 1988; 33:87–107.

Bernard JF, Besson JM. The spino(trigemino) pontoamygdaloid pathway: electrophysiological evidence for an involvement in pain processes. *J Neurophysiol* 1990; 63:473–490.

Bernard JF, Peschanski M, Besson JM. A possible spino (trigemino)-ponto-amygdaloid pathway for pain. *Neurosci Lett* 1989; 100:83–88.

Blitz B, Dinnerstein AJ. Effects of different types of instructions on pain parameters. *J Abnorm Psychol* 1968; 73:276–280.

Bootzin RR. The role of expectancy in behavior change. In: White L, Turskey B, Schwartz GE (Eds). *Placebo: Theory, Research, and Mechanisms.* New York: Guilford Press, 1985.

Boring EG. *A History of Experimental Psychology.* New York: Appleton-Century-Crofts, 1957.

Bowers KS. Hypnotizability, creativity, and the role of effortless experiencing. *Int J Clin Exp Hypn* 1978; 26:184–202.

Buchsbaum MS, Davis GC, Bunney WEJ. Naloxone alters pain perception and somatosensory evoked potentials in normal subjects. *Nature* 1977; 270:620–621.

Burgess PR, Perl ER. Cutaneous mechanoreceptors and nociceptors. In: Iggo A (Ed). *Handbook of Sensory Physiology,* Vol. 2. Heidelberg: Springer, 1973, pp 29–43.

Burstein R, Cliffer KD, Giesler GJ. Direct somatosensory projections from the spinal cord to the hypothalamus and telencephalon. *J Neurosci* 1987; 7:4159–4164.

Bush FM, Harkins SW, Harrington WG, Price DD. Analysis of gender effects on pain perception and symptom presentation in temporomandibular pain. *Pain* 1993; 53:73–80.

Bushnell MC. Thalamic processing of sensory-discriminative and affective-motivational dimensions of pain. In: Besson J-M, Guilbaud G, Ollat H (Eds). *Forebrain Areas Involved in Pain Processing.* Paris: Eurotext, 1995, pp 63–77.

Bushnell MC, Duncan GH. Sensory and affective aspects of pain perception: is medial thalamus restricted to emotional issues? *Exp Brain Res* 1989; 67:415–418.

Bushnell MC, Taylor MB, Duncan GH, Dubner R. Discrimination of innocuous and noxious thermal stimuli applied to the face in human and monkey. *Somatosens Res* 1983; 1:199–219.

Bushnell MC, Duncan GH, Tremblay N. Thalamic VPM nucleus in the behaving monkey. I. Multimodal and discriminative properties of thermosensitive neurons. *J Neurophysiol* 1993; 69:739–752.

Buytendyck FJJ. *Pain.* London: Hutchinson, 1961.

Campbell JN, Raja SN, Meyer RA. Painful sequelae of nerve injury. In: Dubner R, Gebhart GF, Bond MR (Eds). *Pain Research and Clinical Management.* New York: Elsevier, 1988, pp 135–143.

Cannon WB. The James-Lange theory of emotions: a critical examination and an alternative theory. *Am J Psychol* 1927; 39:106–124.

Carmon A, Mor J, Goldberg J. Evoked cerebral responses to noxious thermal stimuli in humans. *Brain Res* 1976; 25:103–107.

Casey KL. Responses of bulboreticular units to somatic stimuli eliciting escape behavior in the cat. *Int J Neurosci* 1971a; 2:15–28.

Casey KL. Escape elicited by bulboreticular stimulation in the cat. *Int J Neurosci* 1971b; 2:29–34.

Casey KL, Keene JJ, Morrow T. Bulboreticular and medial thalamic unit activity in relation to aversive behavior and pain. In: Bonica JJ (Ed). *Advances in Neurology,* Vol. 4 (International Symposium on Pain). New York: Raven Press, 1974, p 197.

Casey KL, Satoshi M, Berger KL, et al. Positron emission tomographic analysis of cerebral structures activated specifically by repetitive noxious heat stimuli. *J Neurophysiol* 1994; 71:802–807.

Casey KL, Minoshima S, Morrow TJ, et al. Comparison of human cerebral activation pattern during cutaneous warmth, heat pain, and deep cold pain. *J Neurophysiol* 1996; 76(1):571–581.

Cesselin F, Bourgoin S, Hamon M, et al. Normal CSF levels of met-enkephalin-like material in a case of naloxone-reversible congenital insensitivity to pain. *Neuropeptides* 1984; 4:217–226.

Chalmers DJ. *The Conscious Mind: in Search of a Fundamental Theory.* New York: Oxford University Press, 1996.

Chapman CR, Casey KL, Dubner R, et al. Pain measurement: an overview. *Pain* 1985; 22:1–31.

Chapman WP, Jones CM. Variations in cutaneous and visceral pain sensitivity in normal subjects. *J Clin Invest* 1944; 23:81–90.

Chatrian GE, Canfield RC, Knauss RA, et al. Cerebral responses to electrical tooth pulp stimulation in man: an objective correlate of acute experimental pain. *Neurology (Minneapolis)* 1975; 25:747–757.

Chung JM, Lee KH, Surmeier DJ, et al. Response characteristics of neurons in the ventral posterior lateral nucleus of the monkey thalamus. *J Neurophysiol* 1986; 56:370–390.

Clarke WC. The psyche in the psychophysics of pain: an introduction to sensory decision theory. In: Boivie J, Hansson P, Lindblom U (Eds). *Touch, Temperature, and Pain in Health and Disease: Mechanisms and Assessments.* Progress in Pain Research and Management, Vol. 3. Seattle: IASP Press, 1994, pp 41–62.

Coghill RC, Mayer DJ, Price DD. Spinal cord coding of pain: the role of spatial recruitment and discharge frequency in nociception. *Pain* 1993a; 53:295–309.

Coghill RC, Mayer DJ, Price DD. Wide dynamic range but not nociceptive specific neurons encode multidimensional features of prolonged repetitive heat stimuli. *J Neurophysiol* 1993b; 69:703–716.

Coghill RC, Price DD, Hayes R, et al. Spatial distribution of nociceptive processing in the rat spinal cord. *J Neurophysiol* 1991; 65:133–140.

Coghill RC, Talbot JD, Evans AC, et al. Distributed processing of pain and vibration by the human brain. *J Neurosci* 1994; 14(7):4095–4108.

Coghill RC, Sang CN, Maisog JM, Iadarola MJ. Pain intensity processing within the human brain: a bilateral distributed mechanism. *J Neurophysiol* 1999; in press.

Cohen RA. *The Neuropsychology of Attention.* New York: Plenum Press, 1993.

Collins WF, Nulsen FE, Randt CT. Relation of peripheral nerve fiber size and sensation in man. *Arch Neurol* 1960; 3:381–385.

Costa PT, McCrae RR. *The NEO Personality Inventory Manual.* Odessa, FL: Psychological Assessment Resources, 1985.

Craig AD. Supraspinal projections of lamina I neurons. In: Besson J-M, Guilbaud G, Ollat H (Eds). *Forebrain Areas Involved in Pain Processing.* Paris: Eurotext, 1995, pp 13–25.

Craig KD, Prkachin KM, Grunau RVE. The facial expression of pain. In: Turk DC, Melzack R (Eds). *Handbook of Pain Assessment.* New York: Guilford Press, 1992, pp 257–274.

Crawford HJ, Gruzelier JH. A midstream view of the neuropsychology of hypnosis: recent research and future directions. In: Fromm E, Nash MR (Eds). *Contemporary Hypnosis Research.* New York: Guilford Press, 1992, pp 227–266.

Cunningham N. Primary requirements for an ethical definition of pain. *Pain Forum* 1999a; 8(2):93–99.

Cunningham N. Inclusion of the non-verbal patient: a matter of moral emergency. *Pain Forum* 1999b; 8(2):110–112.

Dado RJ, Katter JT, Giesler GJ Jr. Spinothalamic and spinohypothalamic tract neurons in the cervical enlargement in rats. II. Responses to innocuous and noxious mechanical thermal stimuli. *J Neurophysiol* 1994; 71:981–1002.

Damasio A. *Descartes Error.* New York: Avon Books, 1994.

Danziger N, Fournier E, Bouhassira D, et al. Different strategies of modulation can be operative during hypnotic analgesia: a neurophysiological study. *Pain* 1998; 75:85–92.

Davis GC, Buchsbaum MS, Bunney WE. Naloxone decreases diurnal variation in pain sensitivity and somatosensory evoked potentials. *Life Sci* 1978; 23:1449–1460.

Defrin R, Urca G. Spatial summation of heat pain: a reassessment. *Pain* 1996; 66(1):23–29.

Dehan H, Willer JC, Boureau F, et al. Congenital insensitivity to pain, and endogenous morphine-like substances. *Lancet* 1977; 2:293–294.

Delfs JM, Kong A, Mestak Y, et al. Expression of mu opioid receptor mRNA in rat brain: an in situ hybridization study at the single cell level. *J Comp Neurol* 1994; 345:46–48.

De Pascalis V, Magurano MR, Bellusci A. Pain perception, somatosensory event-related potentials and skin conductance responses to painful stimuli in high, mid, and low hypnotizable subjects: effects of differential pain reduction strategies. *Pain* 2000; in press.

Dickenson AH, Sullivan AF. Evidence for a role of the NMDA receptor in the frequency dependent potentiation of deep rat dorsal horn nociceptive neurons follwing C fiber stimulation. *Neuropharmacology* 1987; 26:1235–1238.

Dickenson AH, Sullivan AF. Differential effects of excitatory amino acid antagonists on dorsal horn nociceptive neurons in the rat. *Brain Res* 1990; 506:31–39.

Dong WK, Salonen LD, Kawakami Y, et al. Nociceptive responses of trigeminal neurons in SII-7b cortex of awake monkeys. *Brain Res* 1989; 484:314–324.

Dong WK, Chudler EH, Sugiyama K, et al. Somatosensory, multisensory, and task-related neurons in cortical area 7b (PF) of anesthetized monkeys. *J Neurophysiol* 1994; 72:542–564.

Dong WK, Roberts VJ, Hayashi T, et al. Behavioral outcome of posterior parietal cortex injury in the monkey. *Pain* 1996; 64(3):579–587.

Douglass DK, Carstens E, Watkins LR. Spatial summation in human pain perception: comparison within and between dermatomes. *Pain* 1992; 50:197–202.

Dubner R. Neuronal plasticity and pain following peripheral tissue inflammation or nerve injury. In: Bond M, Charlton E, Woolf CJ (Eds). *Proceedings of Vth World Congress on Pain,* Pain Research and Clinical Management. Vol. 5. Amsterdam: Elsevier, 1991, pp 263–276.

Dubner R, Bennett GJ. Spinal and trigeminal mechanisms of nociception. *Annu Rev Neurosci* 1983; 6:381–418.

Dubner R, Bushnell MC, Duncan GH. Sensory-discriminative capacities of nociceptive pathways and their modulation by behavior. In: Yaksh TL (Ed). *Spinal Afferent Processing.* New York: Plenum, 1986, pp 321–331.

Dubreuil D, Kohn P. Reactivity and response to pain. *Pers Individual Differences* 1986; 7:907–909.

Duncan G, Bushnell MC, Levigne G. Comparison of verbal and visual analogue scales for measuring the intensity and unpleasantness of experimental pain. *Pain* 1989; 37:295–303.

Duncan GH, Bushnell MC, Marchand S. Deep brain stimulation: a review of basic research and clinical studies. *Pain* 1991; 45(1):49–59.

Echols DH, Cogclough JA. Abolition of painful phantom limb by resection of the sensory cortex. *JAMA* 1947; 134:1476–1477.

Eide PK, Jorum E, Stubhaug A, et al. Relief of post-herpetic neuralgia with the N-methyl-D-aspartate acid receptor antagonist ketamine: a double blind, crossover comparison with morphine and placebo. *Pain* 1994; 58:347–355.

Ekman G, Sjoberg L. Scaling. *Annu Rev Psych* 1965; 16:451–474.

Ellermeier W, Westphal W. Gender differences in pain ratings and pupil reactions to painful pressure stimuli. *Pain* 1995; 61:435–439.

El-Sobky A, Dostrovsky JO, Wall PD. Lack of effect of naloxone on pain perception in humans. *Nature* 1976; 263:783–784.

Emson PC, Corder SJ, Ratter S, et al. Regional distribution of proopiomelanocortin-derived peptides in the human brain. *Neuroendocrinology* 1984; 38(1):45–50.

Evans FJ. Expectancy, therapeutic instructions, and the placebo response. In: White L, Turskey B, Schwartz GE (Eds). *Placebo: Theory, Research, and Mechanisms.* New York: Guilford Press, 1985.

Evans MB, Paul GL. Effects of hypnotically suggested analgesia on physiological and subjective responses to cold stress. *J Consult Clin Psychol* 1985; 35:362–371.

Eysenck LD. *The Biological Basis of Personality.* Springfield, IL: Thomas, 1967.

Eysenck HJ, Eysenck SBG. *The Manual of Eysenck Personality Questionnaire.* London: Hodder and Stoughton, 1975.

Fanselow MS. Shock-induced analgesia on the formalin test: effects of shock severity, naloxone, hypophysectomy, and associative variables. *Behav Neurosci* 1984; 98(1):79–95.

Fanselow MS. The midbrain periaqueductal gray as a coordinator of action in response to fear and anxiety. In: Depaulis A, Bandler R (Eds). *The Midbrain Periaqueductal Gray Matter.* New York: Plenum Press, 1991, pp 151–173.

Faris P, Komisaruk B, Watkins L, et al. Evidence for the neuropeptide cholecystokinin as an antagonist of opiate analgesia. *Science* 1983; 219:310–312.

Fedele L, Marchinin M, Acaia B, Garagiola U, Tiengo M. Dynamics and significance of placebo response in primary dysmenorrhea. *Pain* 1989; 36:43–47.

Feine JS, Lavigne GJ, Dao TTT, et al. Memories of chronic pain and perceptions of relief. *Pain* 1998; 77:137–141.

Fernandez E, Turk DC. The utility of cognitive coping strategies for altering pain perception: a meta-analysis. *Pain* 1989; 38:123–135.

Fernandez E, Turk DC. Sensory and affective components of pain: separation and synthesis. *Psychol Bull* 1992; 112(2):205–217.

Fields HL. *Pain.* New York: McGraw-Hill, 1987.

Fields HL, Price DD. Toward a neurobiology of placebo analgesia. In: Harrington A (Ed). *Placebo: Probing the Self-Healing Brain.* Boston: Harvard University Press, 1997.

Fields HL, Heinricher MM, Mason P. Neurotransmitters in nociceptive modulatory circuits. *Ann Rev Neurosci* 1991; 14:219–245.

Fillingim RB, Maixner W, Kincaid S, Silva S. Sex differences in temporal summation but not sensory-discriminative processing of thermal pain. *Pain* 1998; 75:121–127.

Fitzgerald M, Jennings E. The postnatal development of spinal sensory processing. *Proc Natl Acad Sci USA* 1999; 96(14):7719–7722.

Foltz EL, White LE. Pain "relief" by frontal cingulumotomy. *J Neurosurg* 1962; 19:89–100.

Foreman RD. Viscerosomatic convergence onto spinal neurons responding to afferent fibers located in the inferior cardiac nerve. *Brain Res* 1977; 137:164–168.

Foreman RD, Schmidt RF, Willis WD. Convergence of muscle and cutaneous input onto primate spinothalamic tract neurons. *Brain Res* 1977; 124:555–560.

Fricton JR, Roth P. The effect of direct and indirect suggestions for analgesia in high and low susceptible subjects. *Am J Clin Hypn* 1985; 27(4):226–231.

Friedman DP, Murray EA, O'Neill JB, et al. Cortical connections of the somatosensory fields of the lateral sulcus of macaques: evidence for a corticolimbic pathway for touch. *J Comp Neurol* 1986; 252(3):323–347.

Gebhart GF (Ed). *Visceral Pain,* Progress in Pain Research and Management, Vol. 5. Seattle: IASP Press, 1995.

Gendlin ET. *Experiencing and the Creation of Meaning: A Philosophical and Psychological Approach to the Subjective*. New York: Free Press, 1962.

Getto CJ, Heaton R. *Psychosocial Pain Inventory*. Odessa, FL: Psychological Assessment Resources, 1985.

Giesler GJ. The spino-hypothalamic tract. In: Besson J-M, Guilbaud G, Ollat H (Eds). *Forebrain Areas Involved in Pain Processing*. Paris: Eurotext, 1995, pp 49–62.

Giesler GJ, Cliffer KD. Postsynaptic dorsal column pathway of the rat. II. Evidence against an important role in nociception. *Brain Res* 1985; 326(2):347–356.

Giorgi A. *Psychology as a Human Science*. New York: Harper and Row, 1970.

Goldstein A, Hilgard ER. Lack of influence of the morphine antagonist naloxone on hypnotic analgesia, *Proc Natl Acad Sci USA* 1975; 72:2041–2043.

Gordon A, Hitchcock ER. Illness behaviour and personality in intractable facial pain syndromes. *Pain* 1983; 17(3):267–276.

Gracely RH. Psychophysical assessment of human pain. In: Bonica JJ, Liebeskind JC, Albe-Fessard DG (Eds). *Advances in Pain Research and Therapy,* Vol. 3. New York: Raven Press, 1979.

Gracely RH. Studies of pain in normal man. In: Wall PD, Melzack R (Eds). *Textbook of Pain,* 3rd ed. London: Churchill-Livingston, 1994, pp 315–336.

Gracely RH, Dubner R. Pain assessment in humans: a reply to Hall. *Pain* 1981; 11:109–120.

Gracely RH, McGrath P, Dubner R. Validity and sensitivity of ratio scales of sensory and affective verbal pain descriptors: manipulation of affect by diazepam. *Pain* 1978; 2:19–29.

Gracely RH, Dubner R, Wolskee PJ, et al. Placebo and naloxone can alter post-surgical pain by separate mechanisms. *Nature* 1983; 306:264.

Gracely RH, Lynch SA, Bennett GJ. Painful neuropathy: altered central processing maintained dynamically by peripheral input. *Pain* 1992; 51:175–194.

Greene LC, Hardy JD. Spatial summation of pain. *J Appl Physiol* 1958; 13:457–464.

Greene RJ, Reyher J. Pain tolerance in hypnotic analgesia and imagination states. *J Abnorm Psychol* 1972; 79:29–38.

Greenspan JD, Joy SE, McGillis SL, et al. A longitudinal study of somesthetic perceptual disorders in an individual with a unilateral thalamic lesion. *Pain* 1997; 72(1-2):13–25.

Grevert P, Goldstein A. Placebo analgesia, naloxone, and the role of endogenous opioids. In: White L, Turskey B, Schwartz GE (Eds). *Placebo: Theory, Research, and Mechanisms*. New York: Guilford Press, 1985.

Grevert P, Baizman ER, Goldstein A. Naloxone effects on a nociceptive response of hypophy-sectomized and adrenalectomized mice. *Life Sci* 1978; 23:723–728.

Grevert P, Albert LH, Goldstein A. Partial antagonism of placebo analgesia by naloxone. *Pain* 1983; 16:129–143.

Groen TV, Wyss JM. Connections of the retrosplenial dysgranular cortex in the rat. *J Comp Neurol* 1992; 315:200–216.

Guilford JP. *Psychometric Methods.* New York: McGraw-Hill, 1954, p 597.

Haddox JD, Kettler RE. Stellate ganglion block: normal saline as placebo. *Anesthesiology* 1987; 67:832–834.

Hagbarth KE, Finer BL. The plasticity of human withdrawal reflexes to noxious skin stimuli in lower limbs. *Prog Brain Res* 1973; 1:65–78.

Haigler HJ, Spring DD. A comparison of the analgesic and behavioral effects of [D-Ala^2] Met-enkephalinamide and morphine in the mesencephalic reticular formation of rats. *Life Sci* 1978; 23:1229–1239.

Halliday AM, Logue V. Painful sensations evoked by electrical stimulation in the thalamus. In: Somjen GG (Ed). *Neurophysiology Studied in Man.* Amsterdam: Excerpta Medica, 1972, pp 221–230.

Hardy JD, Wolff HG, Goodell H. Studies on pain: a new method for measuring pain threshold: observations on spatial summation of pain. *J Clin Invest* 1940; 19:649–657.

Hardy JD, Wolff HG, Goodell H. *Pain Sensations and Reactions.* Baltimore: Williams and Wilkins, 1952.

Harkins SW, Price DD. Assessment of pain in the elderly. In: Turk D, Melzack R (Eds). *Handbook of Pain Measurement and Assessment.* New York: Guilford Press, 1992, pp 315–331.

Harkins SW, Price DD, Martelli M. Effects of age on pain perception: thermonociception. *J Gerontol* 1986; 41:58–63.

Harkins SW, Price DD, Braith J. Effects of extraversion and neuroticism on experimental pain, clinical pain, and illness behavior. *Pain* 1989; 36:209–218.

Harkins SW, Davis MD, Bush FM, Kasberger J. Suppression of first pain and slow temporal summation of second pain in relation to age. *J Gerontol A Biol Sci Med Sci* 1996; 51(5):260–265.

Hassler R. Dichotomy of facial pain conduction in the diencephalon. In: Hassler R, Walker AE (Eds). *Trigeminal Neuralgia.* Philadelphia: Saunders, 1970, pp 123–138.

Hayes RL, Bennett GJ, Newlon PG, et al. Behavioral and physiological studies on non-narcotic analgesia in the rat elicited by certain environmental stimuli. *Brain Res* 1978a; 155:69–90.

Hayes RL, Price DD, Bennett GJ, et al. Differential effects of spinal cord lesions on narcotic and non-narcotic suppression of nociceptive reflexes: further evidence for the physiologic multiplicity of pain modulation. *Brain Res* 1978b; 155:91–101.

Hayes RL, Dubner R, Hoffman DS. Neuronal activity in medullary dorsal horn of awake monkeys trained in a thermal discrimination task II: behavioral modulation of responses to thermal and mechanical stimuli. *J Neurophysiol* 1981; 46:428–443.

Head H. *Studies in Neurology.* London: Oxford University Press, 1920.

Head H, Holmes G. Sensory disturbances from cerebral lesions. *Brain* 1911; 34:102–154.

Heft MW, Parker SR. An experimental basis for revising the graphic rating scale for pain. *Pain* 1984; 19:153–161.

Heft MW, Gracely RH, Dubner R, McGrath PA. A validation model for verbal descriptor scaling of human clinical pain. *Pain* 1980; 9:363–373.

Heilman KM, Watson RT, Valenstein E, et al. Attention: behavior and neural mechanism. In: Mountcastle VB, Plum F, Geiger SR (Eds). *Higher Functions of the Brain,* Part 2. Handbook of Physiology, Sect. 1, The Nervous System, Vol. V. Bethesda, MD: American Physiology Society, 1987, pp 461–481.

Hellon RF, Mitchell D. Convergence in a thermal afferent pathway in the rat. *J Physiol (Lond)* 1975; 248:359–376.

Helmstetter FJ, Tershner SA. Lesions of the periaqueductal gray and rostroventral medulla disrupt antinociceptive but not cardiovascular aversive conditional responses. *J Neurosci* 1994; 14(11):7099–7108.

Hilgard ER. *Divided Consciousness: Multiple Controls in Human Thought and Action.* New York: John Wiley and Sons, 1977, p 300.

Hilgard ER, Hilgard JR. *Hypnosis in the Relief of Pain.* Los Altos, CA: William Kaufmann, 1983, p 294.

Hilgard ER, Morgan AH, Lange AF, et al. Heart rate changes in pain and hypnosis. *Psychophysiology* 1974; 11:692–702.

Hilgard ER, Morgan AH, MacDonald H. Pain and dissociation in the cold pressor test: a study of hypnotic analgesia with "hidden" reports: through automatic key-pressing and automatic talking. *J Abnorm Psychol* 1975; 81:170–174.

Hiller JM, Pearson J, Simon EJ. Distribution of stereospecific binding of the potent narcotic analgesic etorphine in the human brain: predominance in the limbic system. *Res Commun Mol Pathol Pharm* 1973; 6:1052–1062.

Hirshberg RM, Al-Chaer ED, Lawand NB, et al. Is there a pathway in the posterior funiculus that signals visceral pain? *Pain* 1996; 67(2–3):291–305.

Hofbauer RK, Rainville P, Duncan GH, et al. Cognitive modulation of pain sensation alters activity in human cerebral cortex. *Neurosci Abstr* 1998; 24:447.5.

Hoffman DS, Dubner R, Hayes RL, Medlin TP. Neuronal activity in medullary dorsal horn of awake monkeys trained in a thermal discrimination task. I. Responses to innocuous and noxious thermal stimuli. *J Neurophysiol* 1981; 46:409–427.

Hosobuchi Y. Tryptophan reversal of tolerance to analgesia induced by central grey stimulation. *Lancet* 1978; 2:47.

Hosobuchi Y, Adams JE, Linchitz R. Pain relief by electrical stimulation of the central gray matter in humans and its reversal by naloxone. *Science* 1977; 196:183–186.

Hsieh JC, Stahle-Backdahl M, Hagermark O, et al. Traumatic nociceptive pain activates the hypothalamus and the periaqueductal gray: a positron emission tomography study. *Pain* 1996; 64(2):303–314.

Hughes J. Search for the endogenous ligand of the opiate receptor. *Neurosci Res Prog Bull* 1975; 13:55–58.

Husserl E. *Ideas: General Introduction to Pure Phenomenology.* New York: MacMillan, 1952.

Irwin S, Houde RW, Bennett DR, et al. The effects of morphine, methadone and meperidine on some reflex responses of spinal animals to nociceptive stimulation. *J Pharmacol Exp Ther* 1951; 101:132–143.

Ishijima B, Yoshimasu N, Fukushima T, et al. Nociceptive neurons in the human thalamus. *Confin Neurol* 1975; 37:99–106.

Jacobs AL, Kurtz RM, Strube MJ. Hypnotic analgesia, expectancy effects, and choice of design: a reexamination. *Int J Clin Exp Hypn* 1995; 43(1):55–69.

Jacquet YF, Lajtha A. Morphine action at central nervous system sites in rat: analgesia or hyperalgesia depending on site and dose. *Science* 1973; 182:490–491.

Jacquet YF, Lajtha A. Paradoxical effects after microinjection of morphine in the periaqueductal gray matter in the rat. *Science* 1974; 185:1055–1057.

James W. *The Principles of Psychology.* New York: Dover, 1950.

Janal MN, Colt EWD, Clark WC, et al. Pain sensitivity, mood and plasma endocrine levels in man following long-distance running: effects of naloxone. *Pain* 1984; 19:13–26.

Jensen MP, Karoly P. Motivation and expectancy factors in symptom perception: a laboratory study of the placebo effect. *Psychosom Med* 1991; 53:144–152.

Johnson JE. Effects of accurate expectations about sensations on the sensory and distress components of pain. *J Pers Soc Psychol* 1973; 27:261–275.

Jospe M. *The Placebo Effect in Healing.* Lexington, MA: Lexington Books, 1978.

Kelstein DE, Price DD, Hayes RL, et al. Evidence that substance P selectively modulates C-fiber evoked discharges of dorsal horn nociceptive neurons. *Brain Res* 1990; 526:291–298.

Kenshalo DR Jr, Isensee O. Responses of SI cortical neurons to noxious stimuli. *J Neurophysiol* 1983; 50:1479–1496.

Kenshalo DR, Decker T, Hamilton A. Spatial summation on the forehead, forearm, and back produced by radiant and conducted heat. *J Comp Psychol* 1967; 63:510–515.

Kenshalo DR, Giesler GJ, Leonard RB, et al. Responses of neurons in primate ventroposteriolateral nucleus to noxious stimuli. *J Neurophysiol* 1980; 43:1594–1614.

Kevetter GA, Haber LH, Yezierski RP, et al. Cells of origin of the spinoreticular tract in the monkey. *J Comp Neurol* 1982; 207:61–74.

Kiernan BD, Dane JR, Phillips LH, Price DD. Hypnotic analgesia reduces R-III nociceptive reflex: further evidence concerning the multifactorial nature of hypnotic analgesia. *Pain* 1995; 60:39–47.

Kirsch I. *Changing Expectations: a Key to Effective Psychotherapy.* Pacific Grove, CA: Brooks/Cole, 1990.

Kirsch I. Expectancy and conditioning in placebo analgesia: related or independent mechanisms? *Pain Forum* 1997; 6(1):59–61.

Komisaruk BR, Wallman J. Antinociceptive effects of vaginal stimulation in rats: neurophysiological and behavioral studies. *Brain Res* 1977; 137:85–107.

Korcyn AD. Mechanism of placebo analgesia. *Lancet* 1978; 2:1304–1305.

Krishnamurti J. *Talks in Europe.* The Netherlands: Sevire/Wassenaar, 1967.

Kumazawa T, Mizumura K. The polymodal C-fiber receptor in the muscle of the dog. *Brain Res* 1976; 101:489–493.

Kumazawa T, Mizumura K. Thin-fibre receptors responding to mechanical, chemical, and thermal stimulation in the skeletal muscle of the dog. *J Physiol* 1977a; 273:179–194.

Kumazawa T, Mizumura K. The polymodal receptors in the testis of dog. *Brain Res* 1977b; 136:553–558.

La Motte RH, Campbell JN. Comparison of responses of warm and nociceptive C-fiber afferents in monkey with human judgements of thermal pain. *J Neurophysiol* 1978; 41:509–528.

LaMotte RH, Thalhammer JG, Torebjork HE, Robinson CJ. Peripheral neural mechanisms of cutaneous hyperalgesia following mild injury by heat. *J Neurosci* 1982; 2:765–781.

Lamour Y, Willer JC, Guilbaud G. Rat somatosensory (SmI) cortex. I. Characteristics of neuronal responses to noxious stimulation and comparison with responses to non-noxious stimulation. *Exp Brain Res* 1983; 49:35–45.

Landau W, Bishop GH. Pain from dermal, periosteal, and fascial endings and from inflammation. *Arch Neurol Psychiatry* 1953; 69:490–504.

Lander J, Fowler-Kerry S, Hargreaves A. Gender effects in pain perception. *Percept Mot Skills* 1989; 68:1088–1090.

Larson MA, McHaffie JG, Stein BE. Response properties of nociceptive and low threshold mechanoreceptive neurons in the hamster superior colliculus. *J Neurosci* 1987; 7:547–564.

Laska E, Sunshine A. Anticipation of analgesia: a placebo effect. *Headache* 1973; 1:1–11.

Lenz FA, Dostrovsky JO, Tasker RR, et al. Single-unit analysis of the human ventral thalamic nuclear group: somatosensory responses. *J Neurophysiol* 1988; 59:299–316.

Lenz FA, Seike M, Lin YC, et al. Neurons in the area of human thalamic nucleus ventralis caudalis respond to painful heat stimuli. *J Neurophysiol* 1993; 70(1):200–212.

Leon B. Pain perception and extraversion. *Percept Mot Skills* 1974; 38:510–513.

Levine JD, Gordon NC, Fields HL. The mechanism of placebo analgesia. *Lancet* 1978; 654–657.

Levine JD, Gordon NC, Bornstein JC, et al. Role of pain in placebo analgesia. *Proc Natl Acad Sci USA* 1979; 76:3528–3531.

Levine S. *A Gradual Awakening.* New York: Anchor Press, 1979.

Lewin W, Phillips CG. Observations on partial removal of the postcentral gyrus for pain. *J Neurol Neurosurg Psychiatry* 1952; 15:143–147.

Lewis T, Pochin EE. The double response of the human skin to a single stimulus. *Clin Sci* 1938; 67–76.

Li J, Simone DA, Larson AA. Windup leads to characteristics of central sensitization. *Pain* 1999; 79(1):75–82.

Liebeskind JC. Pain can kill. *Pain* 1991; 44:3–4.

Light AR, Perl ER. Spinal termination of functionally identified primary afferent neurons with slowly conducting myelinated fibers. *J Comp Neurol* 1979; 186(2):133–150.

Lu GW. Spinocervical tract-dorsal column postsynaptic neurons: a double-projection neuronal system. *Somatosens Mot Res* 1989; 6(5–6):445–454.

Lyons J. *Experience*. New York: Harper and Row, 1973.

Maixner W, Dubner R, Bushnell MC, et al. Wide-dynamic-range dorsal horn neurons participate in the encoding process by which monkeys perceive the intensity of noxious heat stimuli. *Brain Res* 1986; 374:385–388.

Maixner W, Fillingim R, Sigurdsson A, Kincais S, Silva S. Sensitivity of patients with painful temporomandibular disorders to experimentally evoked pain: evidence for altered temporal summation of pain. *Pain* 1998; 76(1–2):71–81.

Manning BH, Mayer DJ. The central nucleus of the amygdala contributes to the production of morphine antinociception in the formalin test. *Pain* 1995a; 63(2):141–152.

Manning BH, Mayer DJ. The central nucleus of the amygdala contributes to the production of morphine antinociception in the rat tail-flick test. *J Neurosci* 1995b; 15(2):8199–8213.

Mao J, Coghill RC, Price DD, et al. Spatial patterns of spinal cord metabolic activity in a rodent model of peripheral mononeuropathy. *Pain* 1992; 50:89–100.

Mao J, Mayer DJ, Price DD. Patterns of increased brain activity indicative of pain in a rat model of peripheral mononeuropathy. *J Neurosci* 1993; 13(6):2689–2702.

Mark VH, Ervin FR, Hackett TP. Clinical aspects of stereotactic thalamotomy in the human. I. The treatment of severe pain. *Arch Neurol* 1960; 3:351–367.

Marks LW. *Sensory Processes: The New Psychophysics*. New York: Academic Press, 1974.

Mathias BJ, Dillingham TR, Zeiger DN, et al. Topical capsaicin for neck pain, a pilot study. *Am J Phys Med Rehabil* 1995; 74:39–44.

Mayer DJ, Hayes R. Stimulation-produced analgesia: development of tolerance and cross tolerance to morphine. *Science* 1975; 188:941–943.

Mayer DJ, Manning BH. The role of opioid peptides in environmentally-induced analgesia. In: Tseng LF (Ed). *The Pharmacology of Opioid Peptides*. Chur, Switzerland: Harwood, 1995, pp 345–395.

Mayer DJ, Price DD. Central nervous system mechanisms of analgesia. *Pain* 1976; 2:379–404.

Mayer DJ, Price DD. The neurobiology of pain. In: Snyder-Mackler L, Robinson AJ (Eds). *Clinical Electrophysiology*. Baltimore: Williams and Wilkins, 1994, pp 35–68.

Mayer DJ, Wolfle TL, Akil H, et al. Analgesia from electrical stimulation in the brainstem of the rat. *Science* 1971; 174:1351–1354.

Mayer DJ, Price DD, Becker DP. Neurophysiological characterization of the anterolateral spinal cord neurons contributing to pain perception in man. *Pain* 1975; 1:51–58.

Mayer DJ, Price DD, Barber J, Rafii A. Acupuncture analgesia: evidence for activation of a pain inhibitory system as a mechanism of action. In: Bonica JJ, Albe-Fessard D (Eds). *Advances of Pain Research and Therapy*, Vol. 1. New York: Raven Press, 1976, pp 751–754.

McHaffie JG, Larson MM, Stein BE. Response properties of nociceptive and low-threshold neurons of rat trigeminal pars caudalis. *J Comp Neurol* 1994; 347(3):409–425.

McMillan SC. The relationship between age and intensity of cancer-related symptoms. *Oncol Nurs Forum* 1989; 16(2):237–241.

Melzack R, Casey KL. Sensory, motivational, and central control of determinants of pain. In: Kenshalo DR (Ed). *The Skin Senses*. Springfield, IL: Charles C. Thomas, 1968, pp 423–439.

Melzack R, Torgerson WS. On the language of pain. *Anesthesiology* 1971; 34:50–59.

Melzack R, Wall PD. Pain mechanisms: a new theory. *Science* 1965; 150:971–979.

Melzack R, Wall PD. *The Challenge of Pain*. New York: Basic Books, 1983.

Melzack R, Rose G, McGinty D. Skin sensitivity to thermal stimuli. *Exp Neurol* 1962; 6:300–314.

Mendell LM. Physiological properties of unmyelinated fiber projections to the spinal cord. *Exp Neurol* 1966; 16:971–979.

Mense S, Schmidt RF. Muscle pain: which receptors are responsible for the transmission of noxious stimuli? In: Rose JE (Ed). *Physiological Aspects of Clinical Neurology.* Oxford: Blackwell, 1977, pp 265–276.

Mense S, Stahnke M. Responses in muscle afferent fibres of slow conduction velocity to contractions and ischaemia in the cat. *J Physiol* 1983; 342:383–397.

Merleau-Ponty M. *The Phenomenology of Perception.* New York: Humanities Press, 1962.

Merskey H, Bogduk N. *Classification of Chronic Pain,* 2nd ed. Seattle: IASP Press, 1994.

Mesulam MM. Spatial attention and neglect: parietal, frontal, and cingulate contributions to the mental representations and attentional targeting of salient extrapersonal events. *Philos Trans R Soc Lond B Biol Sci* 1999: 354(1387):1325–1346.

Meyer RA, Campbell JN. Myelinated nociceptive afferents account for the hyperalgesia that follows a burn to the hand. *Science* 1981; 213:1527–1529.

Milne RJ, Foreman RD, Giesler GJ, Willis WD. Convergence of cutaneous and pelvic visceral nociceptive inputs onto primate spinothalamic tract neurons. *Pain* 1981; 11:163–183.

Miron D, Duncan GH, Bushnell MC. Effects of attention on the intensity and unpleasantness of thermal pain. *Pain* 1989; 39:345–352.

Montgomery GH, Kirsch I. Classical conditioning and the placebo effect. *Pain* 1996a; 72:103–113.

Montgomery GH, Kirsch I. Mechanisms of placebo pain reduction: an empirical investigation. *Psychol Sci* 1996b; 7:174–176.

Montgomery GH, Tomoyasu N, Bovbjerg DH, et al. Patients' pretreatment expectations of chemotherapy-related nausea are an independent predictor of anticipatory nausea. *Ann Behav Med* 1998; 20:104–109.

Morris DB. *The Culture of Pain.* Berkeley: University of California Press, 1991, pp 1–342.

Morrow TJ, Paulson PE, Danneman PJ, et al. Regional changes in forebrain activation during the early and late phase of formalin nociception: analysis using cerebral blood flow in the rat. *Pain* 1998; 75(2–3):355–365.

Mountcastle VB. Pain and temperature sensibilities. In: Mountcastle VB (Ed). *Medical Physiology,* Vol. 1, 13th ed. Saint Louis: Mosby, 1974, pp 348–381.

Mowrer OH. *Learning Theory and Behavior.* New York: Wiley, 1960.

Mumford JM. Pain perception threshold and adaptation of normal human teeth. *Arch Oral Biol* 1965; 10:957.

Mundinger F, Becker P. Long-term results of central stereotactic interventions for pain. In: Sweet WH, Obrador S, Martin-Rodriguez JG (Eds). *Neurosurgical Treatment in Psychiatry, Pain and Epilepsy.* Baltimore: University Park Press, 1977, p 685.

Murgatroyd D. *Spatial Summation of Pain for Large Body Areas,* Defense Atomic Support Agency Report, October, 1964.

Nashold BS, Wilson WP, Slaughter DG. Stereotactic midbrain lesions for central dysesthesia and phantom pain: preliminary report. *J Neurosurg* 1969; 30:116–126.

Nashold BS Jr, Wilson WP, Slaughter G. The midbrain and pain. In: Bonica JJ (Ed). *Advances in Neurology,* Vol. 4 (International Symposium on Pain). New York: Raven Press, 1974, p 191.

Neal JW, Pearson RC, Powell TP. The ipsilateral cortico-cortico connections of area 7 with the frontal lobe in the monkey. *Brain Res* 1990; 509(1):31–40.

Nielsen J, Arendt-Nielsen L. Spatial summation of heat induced pain within and between dermatomes. *Somatosens Mot Res* 1997; 14(2):119–125.

Noordenbos W. *Pain.* Amsterdam: Elsevier, 1959, pp 1–182.

Ohlwein AL, Stevens MJ, Catanzarao SJ. Self-efficacy, response expectancy, and temporal context: moderators of pain tolerance and intensity. *Imagination, Cognition, and Personality* 1996; 16:3–23.

Oley N, Cordova C, Kelly ML, et al. Morphine administration to the region of the solitary tract nucleus produces analgesia in rats. *Brain Res* 1982; 236:511–515.

Palecek J, Paleckova V, Dougherty PM, et al. Responses of spinothalamic tract cells to mechanical and thermal stimulation of skin in rats with experimental peripheral neuropathy. *J Neurophysiol* 1992; 67:1562–1573.

Paxinos G, Watson C. The rat brain in stereotaxic coordinates. New York: Academic Press, 1986.

Pekula RJ, Kumar VK. Predicting hypnotic susceptibility by a self-report phenomenological instrument. *Am J Clin Hypn* 1984; 27:114–121.

Penfield W, Boldrey E. Somatic motor and sensory representation in the cerebral cortex of man. *Brain* 1937; 60:116–126.

Perl ER. Myelinated afferent fibres innervating the primate skin and their response to noxious stimuli. *J Physiol (Lond)* 1968; 197:593–615.

Perl ER. Afferent basis of nociception and pain: evidence from the characteristics of sensory receptors and their projections to the spinal dorsal horn. In: Bonica JJ (Ed). *Pain*. New York: Raven Press, 1980, pp 471–482.

Perl ER. Getting a line on pain: is it mediated by dedicated pathways? *Nat Neurosci* 1998; Jul 1(3):177–178.

Pert A, Yaksh T. Sites of morphine induced analgesia in the primate brain: relation to pain pathways. *Brain Res* 1974; 80:135–140.

Pert CB, Snyder SH. Opiate receptor: demonstration in nervous tissue. *Science* 1973; 179:1011–1013.

Pert CB, Snowman AM, Snyder SH. Localization of opiate receptor binding in synaptic membranes of rat brain. *Brain Res* 1974; 70:184–188.

Pert CB, Kuhar MJ, Snyder SH. Autoradiographic localization of the opiate receptor in rat brain. *Life Sci* 1975; 16:1849–1854.

Pittius CW, Seizenger BR, Pasi A, et al. Distribution and characterization of opioid peptides derived from proenkephalin A in human and rat central nervous system. *Brain Res* 1984; 304(1):127–136.

Pons TP, Garraghty PE, Friedman DP, et al. Physiological evidence for serial processing in somatosensory cortex. *Science* 1987; 237(4813):417 420.

Porro CA, Cavazzuti M, Galetti A, et al. Functional activity mapping of the rat brainstem during formalin-induced noxious stimulation. *Neuroscience* 1991; 41:667–680.

Porro CA, Cettolo V, Francescato MP, et al. Temporal and intensity coding of pain in human cortex. *J Neurophysiol* 1998; 80(6):3312–3320.

Pretel S, Piekut DT. ACTH and enkephalin axonal input to paraventricular neurons containing C-fos-like immunoreactivity. *Synapse* 1991; 8(2):100–106.

Price DD. *Psychological and Neural Mechanisms of Pain*. New York: Raven Press, 1988.

Price DD. Selective activation of A-delta and C nociceptive afferents by different parameters of nociceptive heat stimulation: a tool for analysis of central pain mechanisms. *Pain* 1996a; 68:1–4.

Price DD. The neurological mechanisms of hypnotic analgesia. In: Barber J (Ed). *Hypnosis and Suggestion in the Treatment of Pain*. New York: W.W. Norton, 1996b, pp 117–136.

Price DD, Barber JJ. An analysis of factors that contribute to the efficacy of hypnotic analgesia. *J Abnorm Psychol* 1987; 96:46–51.

Price DD, Barrell JJ. An experiential approach with quantitative methods: a research paradigm. *J Human Psychol* 1980; 20(3):75–95.

Price DD, Barrell JJ. Some general laws of human emotion: interrelationships between intensities of desire, expectation, and emotional feeling. *J Pers* 1984; 52(4):389–409.

Price DD, Barrell JJ. The structure of the hypnotic state: a self-directed experiential study. In: Barrell JJ (Ed). *The Experiential Method: Exploring the Human Experience*. Acton, MA: Copely, 1990, pp 85–97.

Price DD, Browe AC. Responses of spinal cord neurons to graded noxious and non-noxious stimuli. *Exp Neurol* 1975; 48:201–221.

Price DD, Dubner R. Neurons that subserve the sensory discriminative aspects of pain. *Pain* 1977; 3:307–388.

Price DD, Fields HL. The contribution of desire and expectation to placebo analgesia: implications for new research strategies. In: Harrington A (Ed). *Placebo: Probing the Self-Healing Brain*. Boston: Harvard University Press, 1997a.

Price DD, Fields HL. Where are the causes of placebo analgesia? An experiential behavioral analysis. *Pain Forum* 1997b; 6(1):44–52.

Price DD, Harkins SW. The combined use of experimental pain and visual analogue scales in providing standardized measurement of clinical pain. *Clin J Pain* 1987; 3:1–8.

Price DD, Harkins SW. Psychological approaches to pain measurement and assessment. In: Turk DC, Melzack R (Eds). *Handbook of Pain Assessment*. New York: Guilford Press, 1992a, pp 111–134.

Price DD, Harkins SW. The affective-motivational dimension of pain: a two stage model. *APS J* 1992b; 1(4):229–239.

Price DD, Mayer DJ. Evidence for endogenous opiate analgesic mechanisms triggered by somatosensory stimulation (including acupuncture) in humans. *Pain Forum* 1995; 4(1):40–43.

Price DD, Dubner R, Hu JW. Trigeminothalamic neurons in nucleus caudalis responsive to tactile, thermal, and nociceptive stimulation of monkey's face. *J Neurophysiol* 1976; 39:936–953.

Price DD, Hu JW, Dubner R, et al. Peripheral suppression of first pain and central summation of second pain evoked by noxious heat pulses. *Pain* 1977; 3:57–68.

Price DD, Hayes RL, Ruda MA, Dubner R. Spatial and temporal transformations of input to spinothalamic tract neurons and their relation to somatic sensation. *J Neurophysiol* 1978; 41:933–947.

Price DD, Barrell JJ, Gracely RH. A psychophysical analysis of experiential factors that selectively influence the affective dimension of pain. *Pain* 1980; 8:137–149.

Price DD, McGrath PA, Rafii A, Buckingham B. The validation of visual analogue scales as ratio scale measures for chronic and experimental pain. *Pain* 1983; 17:45–56.

Price DD, Barrell JE, Barrell JJ. A quantitative-experiential analysis of human emotions. *Motivation and Emotions* 1985a; 9:19–38.

Price DD, von der Gruen A, Miller J, Rafii A, Price C. A psychophysical analysis of morphine analgesia. *Pain* 1985b; 22:320–330.

Price DD, Harkins SW, Baker C. Sensory-affective relationships among different types of clinical and experimental pain. *Pain* 1986a; 28:291–299.

Price DD, Harkins SW, Rafii A, Price C. A simultaneous comparison of fentanyl's analgesic effects on experimental and clinical pain. *Pain* 1986b; 24:197–203.

Price DD, McHaffie JG, Larson MA. Spatial summation of heat induced pain: influence of stimulus area and spatial separation of stimuli on perceived pain sensation intensity and unpleasantness. *J Neurophysiol* 1989a; 62:1270–1279.

Price DD, Bennett GJ, Rafii A. Psychophysical observations on patients with neuropathic pain relieved by a sympathetic block. *Pain* 1989b; 36:209–218.

Price DD, Long S, Huitt C. Sensory testing of pathophysiological mechanisms of pain in patients with reflex sympathetic dystrophy. *Pain* 1992a; 49:163–173.

Price DD, McHaffie JG, Stein BE. The psychophysical attributes of heat-induced pain and their relationships to neural mechanisms. *J Cogn Neurosci* 1992b; 4:1–13.

Price DD, Mao J, Frenk H, et al. The N-methyl-D-aspartate receptor antagonist dextromethorphan selectively reduces temporal summation of second pain in man. *Pain* 1994a; 59:165–174.

Price DD, Mao J, Mayer DJ. Central neural mechanisms of normal and abnormal pain states. In: Fields HL, Liebeskind JC (Eds). *Pharmacological Approaches to the Treatment of Chronic Pain: New Concepts and Critical Issues,* Progress in Pain Research and Management, Vol. 1. Seattle: IASP Press, 1994b, pp 61–84.

Price, DD, Bush FM, Long S, Harkins SW. A comparison of pain measurement characteristics of mechanical visual analogue and simple numerical rating scales. *Pain* 1994c; 56:217–226.

Price DD, Long S, Wilsey B, et al. Analysis of peak magnitude and duration of analgesia produced by local anesthetics injected into sympathetic ganglia of complex regional pain syndrome patients. *Clin J Pain* 1998; 14(3):216–226.

Price DD, Milling LS, Kirsch I, et al. An analysis of factors that contribute to the magnitude of placebo analgesia in an experimental paradigm. *Pain* 1999; 84(1):110–113.

Procacci P, Bozza G, Buzzelli G, et al. The cutaneous pricking pain threshold in old age. *Gerontology Clinics* 1970; 12:213–214.

Rainville P, Feine JS, Bushnell, MC, et al. A psychophysical comparison of sensory and affective responses to four modalities of experimental pain. *Somatosens Motor Res* 1992; 9(4):265–277.

Rainville P, Duncan GH, Price DD, Carrier B, Bushnell MC. Pain affect encoded in human anterior cingulate but not somatosensory cortex. *Science* 1997; 277:968–971.

Rainville P, Hofbauer RK, Paus T, et al. Cerebral mechanisms of hypnotic induction and analgesia. *J Cogn Neurosci* 1999a; 11(1):110–125.

Rainville P, Carrier B, Hofbauer RK, et al. Dissociation of sensory and affective dimensions of pain using hypnotic modulation. *Pain* 1999b; 82(2):159–171.

Reiss S. Pavlovian conditioning and human fear: an expectancy model. *Behav Ther* 1980; 11:380–396.

Rescorla RA. Pavlovian conditioning: it's not what you think it is. *Am Psychol* 1988; 43:151–160.

Reynolds DV. Surgery in the rat during electrical analgesia induced by focal brain stimulation. *Science* 1969; 164:444–445.

Richardson DE, Akil H. Pain reduction by electrical brain stimulation in man. Part I: Acute administration in periaqueductal and periventricular sites. *J Neurosurg* 1973; 47:178–183.

Riley J, Robinson ME, Wise EA, et al. Sex differences in perception of noxious experimental stimuli: a meta-analysis. *Pain* 1998; 74(2–3):181–187.

Robinson CJ, Burton H. Somatic submodality distribution within the second somatosensory (SII), 7b, retroinsular, postauditory, and granular insular cortical areas of *M. fascicularis. J Comp Neurol* 1980; 192:93–108.

Robinson CJ, Torebjork HE, La Motte RH. Psychophysical detection and pain ratings of incremental stimuli: a comparison with nociceptor responses in humans. *Brain Res* 1983; 274:87–106.

Rodgers RJ. Elevation of aversive threshold in rats by intra-amygdaloid injection of morphine sulphate. *Pharmacol Biochem Behav* 1977; 6:385–390.

Rodgers RJ. Influence of intra-amygdaloid opiate injections on shock thresholds, tail-flick latencies and open field behaviour in rats. *Brain Res* 1978; 153:211–216.

Rollin BE. Some conceptual and ethical concerns about current views of pain. *Pain Forum* 1999; 8(2):78–83.

Rollin BE. Reply to Varner and Kopelman. *Pain Forum* 1999; 8(2):91–92.

Rotter JB. *Social Learning: Clinical Psychology*. Englewood Cliffs, New Jersey: Prentice-Hall, 1954.

Rotter JB. Generalized expectancies for internal versus external control of reinforcement. *Psychological Monographs,* 80(1, Whole No. 609), 1966.

Rotter JB. *Applications of Social Learning Theory of Personality.* New York: Holt, Rinehart, and Winston, 1972.

Rubins JL, Friedman ED. Asymbolia for pain. *Arch Neurol Psychiatr* 1948; 60:554–560.

Samanin R, Valzelli L. Increase of morphine-induced analgesia by stimulation of the nucleus raphe dorsalis: comment. *Eur J Pharmacol* 1971; 16:298–302.

Sardello RJ. The role of direct experience in contemporary psychology. *Phenom Psychol* 1964; 43:1:30–49.

Satoh M, Takagi H. Effect of morphine on the pre- and postsynaptic inhibitions in the spinal cord. *Eur J Pharmacol* 1971; 14:150–154.

Schacter S, Singer J. Cognitive, social, and physiological determinants of the emotional state. *Psychol Rev* 1962; 36:379–399.

Scott J, Huskisson EC. Graphic representation of pain. *Pain* 1976; 2:175–184.

Searle JR. *The Rediscovery of the Mind.* Cambridge, MA: MIT Press, 1995.

Seymour RA, Simpson JM, Charlton JE, Phillips ME. An evaluation of length and end-phrase of visual analogue scales in dental pain. *Pain* 1985; 21:177–186.

Sherman ED, Robillard E. Sensitivity to pain in relationship to age. *J Am Geriatr Soc* 1964; 12:1037.

Sherrington DS. *The Integrative Action of the Nervous System.* New York: Scribner's, 1906.

Shinn AM. An application of psychophysical scaling techniques to the measurement of national power. *J Politicus* 1969; 31:932–951.

Shor RE, Orne MT. *The Nature of Hypnosis: Selected Basic Readings.* New York: Holt, Rhinehart, and Winston, 1965, p 345.

Sikes RW, Vogt BA. Nociceptive neurons in area 24 of rabbit cingulate cortex. *J Neurophysiol* 1992; 68:1720–1732.

Simone DA, Sorkin LS, Oh U, et al. Neurogenic hyperalgesia: central neural correlates in responses of spinothalamic tract neurons. *J Neurophysiol* 1991; 66:228–246.

Sorkin BA, Rudy TE, Hanlon RB, et al. Chronic pain in old and young patients: differences appear less important than similarities. *J Gerontol* 1990; 45(2):64–68.

Spanos NP. The hidden observer as an experimental creation. *J Pers Soc Psychol* 1983; 44:170–176.

Spanos NP. Hypnotic behavior: a social-psychological interpretation of amnesia, analgesia, and "trance logic." *Behav Brain Sci* 1986; 9:440–467.

Stein BE, Meredith MA. *The Merging of the Senses.* Cambridge, MA: MIT Press, 1993.

Stein BE, Price DD, Gazzaniga M. Pain perception in a man with total corpus callosum transection. *Pain* 1989; 38:51–55.

Stein JF. Representation of egocentric space in the posterior parietal cortex. *Q J Exp Physiol* 1989; 74:583–606.

Sternbach RA, Tursky B. Ethnic differences among housewives in psychophysical and skin potential responses to electric shock. *Psychophysiology* 1965; 1:241–246.

Stevens JC, Marks LE. Spatial summation and the dynamics of warmth sensation. *Perception Psychophysics* 1971; 9:291–298.

Stevens SS. *Psychophysics. Introduction to its Perceptual, Neural, and Social Prospects.* New York: John Wiley & Sons, 1975.

Stohler CS, Kowalski CJ. Spatial and temporal summation of sensory and affective dimensions of deep somatic pain. *Pain* 1999; 79:165–173.

Takagi H. The nucleus reticularis paragigantocellularis as a site of analgesic action of morphine and enkephalin. *Trends Pharmacol Sci* 1980; 1:182–184.

Takagi H, Doi T, Akaike A. Microinjection of morphine into the medial part of the bulbar reticular formation in rabbit and rat: inhibitory effects on lamina V cells of spinal dorsal horn and behavioral analgesia. In: Kosterlitz HW (Ed). *Opiates and Endogenous Opioid Peptides.* Amsterdam: North-Holland, 1976, pp 191–200.

Talbot JD, Marrett S, Evans AC, et al. Multiple representations of pain in human cerebral cortex. *Science* 1991; 251:1355–1358.

Tenenbaum SJ, Kurtz RM, Bienias JL. Hypnotic susceptibility and experimental pain reduction. *Am J Clin Hypn* 1990; 33(1):40–49.

Terenius L. Stereospecific interaction between narcotic analgesics and a synaptic plasma membrane fraction of rat cerebral cortex. *Acta Pharmacol Toxicol* 1973; 32:317–320.

Thompson S, Robertson RT. Organization of subcortical pathways for sensory projections to the limbic cortex. I. Subcortical projections to the medial limbic cortex in the rat. *J Comp Neurol* 1987; 265:175–188.

Thompson SWN, Woolf CJ. Primary afferent-evoked prolonged potentials in the spinal cord and their central summation: role of the NMDA receptor. In: Bond MR, Carlton J, Woolf CJ (Eds). *Proceedings of the VIth World Congress on Pain.* Amsterdam: Elsevier, 1990.

Tolle TR, Kaufmann T, Seissmeier T, et al. Region-specific encoding of sensory and affective components of pain in the human brain: a positron emission tomography correlation analysis. *Ann Neurol* 1999; 45(1):40–47.

Tolman EC. Principles of performance. *Psych Rev* 1955; 62:315–326.

Tommerdahl M, Delemos KA, Vierck CJ, et al. Anterior parietal cortical response to tactile and skin heating stimulation. *J Neurophysiol* 1996; 75(6):2662–2670.

Tommerdahl M, Delemos KA, Favorov OV, et al. Response of anterior parietal cortex to different modes of same-site skin stimulation. *J Neurophysiol* 1998; 80(6):3272–3283.

Torebjork HE, Hallin RG. Identification of afferent C units in intact human skin nerves. *Brain Res* 1974; 67:387–403.

Traut EF, Passarelli EW. Placebos in the treatment of rheumatoid arthritis and other rheumatic conditions. *Ann Rheumatic Diseases* 1957; 16:18–22.

Travell JG, Simmons DG. *Myofascial Pain and Dysfunction: The Trigger Point Manual.* Baltimore, MD: Williams & Wilkins, 1983.

Treede RD, Meyer RA, Campbell JN. Myelinated mechanically insensitive afferents from monkey hairy skin: heat-response properties. *Neurophysiology* 1998; Sept 80(3):1082–1093.

Tsou K. Antagonism of morphine analgesia by the intracerebral microinjection of nalorphine. *Acta Physiol Sinica* 1963; 26:332–337.

Tsou K, Jang CS. Studies on the site of analgesic action of morphine by intracerebral micro-injection. *Sci Sinica* 1964; 13:1099–1109.

Turk DC, Melzack R (Eds). *Handbook of Pain Assessment.* New York: Guilford Press, 1992, pp 1–491.

Turner JA, Deyo RA, Loeser JD, et al. The importance of placebo effects in pain treatment and research. *JAMA* 1994; 271(20):1609–1614.

Van der Does AJ. Patients' and nurses' ratings of pain and anxiety during burn wound care. *Pain* 1989; 39(1):95–101.

VanKaam AL. Phenomenal analysis exemplified by a study of the experience of really feeling understood. *J Individ Psychol* 1959; 15:66–72.

VanRee JM. Multiple brain sites involved in morphine antinociception. *J Pharm Pharmacol* 1977; 29:765–766.

Varela F. Neurophenomenology: a methodological remedy for the hard problem. *J Consciousness Studies* 1996; June.

Varner G. How facts matter: on the language condition and the scope of pain in the animal kingdom. *Pain Forum* 1999; 8(2):84–86.

Vierck CJ, Cannon RL, Fry G, Maixner W, Whitsel BL. Characteristics of temporal summation of second pain sensations elicited by brief contact of glabrous skin by a pre-heated thermode. *J Neurophysiol* 1997; 78(2):992–1002.

Vogt BA, Rosene DL, Pandya DN. Thalamic and cortical afferents differentiate anterior from posterior cingulate cortex in the monkey. *Science* 1979; 204(4389):205–207.

Vogt BA, Sikes RW, Vogt LJ. Anterior cingulate cortex and the medial pain system. In: Vogt BA, Gabriel M (Eds). *Neurobiology of Cingulate Cortex and Limbic Thalamus: a Comprehensive Handbook.* Boston: Birkhauser, 1993.

Voudouris NJ, Peck CL, Coleman G. The role of conditioning and expectancy in the placebo response. *Pain* 1990; 43:121–128.

Wade JB, Price DD. Non-pathologic factors in chronic pain: implications for assessment and treatment. In: Gatchel RJ, Weisberg JN (Eds). *Personality Characteristics of Pain Patients.* New York: American Psychological Press, 1999, in press.

Wade JB, Dougherty LM, Archer CR, Price DD. Assessing the stages of pain processing: a multivariate approach, *Pain* 1986; 68:157–168.

Wade JB, Price DD, Hamer RM, Schwartz SM, Hart RP. An emotional component analysis of chronic pain. *Pain* 1990; 40:303–310.

Wade JB, Dougherty LM, Hart RP, et al. A canonical correlation analysis of the influence of neuroticism and extroversion on chronic pain, suffering, and pain behavior. *Pain* 1992; 51:67–74.

Wade JB, Dougherty LM, Archer CR, et al. Assessing the stages of pain processing: a multivariate analytical approach. *Pain* 1996; 62:1–8.

Wall PD. On the relation of injury to pain (The First John J. Bonica Lecture). *Pain* 1979; 6:253–264.

Wall PD. Mechanisms of acute and chronic pain. In: Kruger L, Liebeskind JC (Eds). *Advances in Pain Research and Therapy,* Vol. 6. New York: Raven Press, 1984, pp 95–104.

Wall PD. The placebo and the placebo response. In: Wall PD, Melzack R (Eds). *Textbook of Pain.* New York: Churchill Livingstone, 1994.

Watkins LR, Mayer DJ. Involvement of spinal opioid systems in footshock-induced analgesia: antagonism by naloxone is possible only before induction of analgesia. *Brain Res* 1982a; 242:309–316.

Watkins LR, Mayer DJ. Organization of endogenous opiate and nonopiate pain control systems. *Science* 1982b; 216:1185–1192.

Watkins LR, Cobelli DA, Mayer DJ. Classical conditioning of front paw and hind paw footshock induced analgesia (FSIA): naloxone reversibility and descending pathways. *Brain Res* 1982a; 243:119–132.

Watkins LR, Cobelli DA, Mayer DJ. Opiate vs non-opiate footshock induced analgesia (FSIA): descending and intraspinal components. *Brain Res* 1982b; 245:97–106.

Watkins LR, Young EG, Kinscheck IB, et al. The neural basis of footshock analgesia: the role of specific ventral medullary nuclei. *Brain Res* 1983; 276:305–315.

Watkins LR, Kinscheck IB, Mayer DJ. Potentiation of opiate analgesia and apparent reversal of morphine tolerance by proglumide. *Science* 1984; 224:395–396.

Weinstein EA, Kahn RL, Slate WH. Withdrawal, inattention, and pain asymbolia. *Arch Neurol Psychiatr* 1995; 74:235.

Weitzenhoffer AM. *General Techniques of Hypnotism.* New York: Grune and Stratton, 1953.

Whipple B, Komisaruk B. Elevation of pain thresholds by vaginal stimulation in women. *Pain* 1985; 21(4):357–367.

Whipple B, Ogden G, Komisaruk BR. Physiological correlates of imagery-induced orgasm in women. *Arch Sex Behav* 1992; 21(2):121–133.

White JC, Sweet WH. *Pain and the Neurosurgeon.* Springfield, IL: Thomas, 1969.

White L, Turskey B, Schwartz GE (Eds). *Placebo: Theory, Research, and Mechanisms.* New York: Guilford Press, 1985.

Wickramasekera I. A conditioned response model of the placebo effect: predictions from the model. In: White L, Turskey B, Schwartz GE (Eds). *Placebo: Theory, Research, and Mechanisms.* New York: Guilford Press, 1985.

Wiertelak EP, Maier SF, Watkins LR. Cholecystokinin antianalgesia: safety cues abolish morphine analgesia. *Science* 1992; 256(5058):830–833.

Willer JC. Comparative study of perceived pain and nociceptive flexion reflex in man. *Pain* 1977; 3:69–80.

Willer JC. Studies on pain. Effects of morphine on a spinal nociceptive flexion reflex and related pain sensation in man. *Brain Res* 1985; 331:105–114.

Willis WD Jr. *The Pain System.* New York: Karger, 1985.

Woodrow KM, Friedman GD, Siegelaub AB, et al. Pain tolerance: differences according to age, sex and race. *Psychosom Med* 1972; 34(6):548–556.

Woolf CJ, Thompson SWN. The induction and maintenance of central sensitization is dependent on N-methyl-D-aspartic acid receptor activation; implications for the treatment of post-injury pain hypersensitivity states. *Pain* 1991; 44:293–299.

Yaksh TL, Rudy TA. Chronic catheterization of the spinal subarachnoid space. *Physiol Behav* 1976; 17:1031–1036.

Yaksh TL, Rudy TA. Studies on the direct spinal actin of narcotics in the production of analgesia in the rat. *J Pharmacol Exp Ther* 1977; 202:411–428.

Yaksh TL, Yeung JC, Rudy TA. Systematic examination in the rat of brain sites sensitive to the direct application of morphine: observation of differential effects within the periaqueductal gray. *Brain Res* 1976; 114:83–104.

Yeung JC, Rudy TA. Sites of antinociceptive action of systemically injected morphine-involvement of supraspinal loci as revealed by intracerebroventricular injection of naloxone. *J Pharmacol Exp Ther* 1980a; 215:626–632.

Yeung JC, Rudy TA. Multiplicative interaction between narcotic agonisms expressed at spinal and supraspinal sites of antinociceptive action as revealed by concurrent intrathecal and intracerebroventricular injections of morphine. *J Pharmacol Exp Ther* 1980b; 215:633–642.

Young RF, Feldman RA, Kroening R, et al. Electrical stimulation of the brain in the treatment of chronic pain in man. In: Liebeskind JC, Kruger L (Eds). *Advances in Pain Research and Therapy: Neural Mechanisms of Pain.* New York: Raven Press, 1984, p 289.

Zatzick DF, Dimsdale JE. Cultural variations in response to painful stimuli. *Psychosom Med* 1990; 52(5):544–557.

Zorman G, Belcher G, Adams JE, et al. Lumbar intrathecal naloxone blocks analgesia produced by microstimulation of the ventromedial medulla in the rat. *Brain Res* 1982; 236:77–89.

Zotterman Y. Studies in the peripheral nervous mechanism of pain. *Acta Med Scand* 1933; 80:185–242.

Index